“*The Pharmagellan Guide to Analyzing Bi*
research tool. This excellent book belongs on the desk of anyone involved—directly or tangentially—in the biopharma industry. With exhaustive research and clear language, this is the best explainer of biotech clinical trials I've ever seen. It spills all the secrets to clinical trial analysis! Now everyone will know how to do it well, and my job will be in jeopardy. Buy this book; you'll be smarter for it.”

—Adam Feuerstein, Senior Writer, STAT

“This is a hugely helpful book highlighting the ins and outs of drug development, trial design, and data interpretation. I wish I'd had a book like this earlier in my career.”

—Sir Mene Pangalos, Executive VP, Biopharmaceuticals R&D, AstraZeneca

“*The Pharmagellan Guide to Analyzing Biotech Clinical Trials* is a terrific primer for those looking to better evaluate new therapies. Readers get the tools they need to make informed decisions about the data and identify potential red flags. This is a must-read for non-experts to level up your understanding of drug development.”

—Daphne Zohar, Founder and CEO, PureTech Health

“The biotech sector is booming, and during the pandemic we've witnessed its impact on health globally. Never before have so many people learned so quickly about the importance of clinical trials and been confronted with learning the process for demonstrating the safety and efficacy of drugs and vaccines. *The Pharmagellan Guide to Analyzing Biotech Clinical Trials* is a special resource for interpreting the results of clinical trials. It can be used to learn about the field all in one place, or as a refresher, or as a reference for looking up specific topics. This book is a crisp and clear explainer of key concepts in clinical trials, without a flood of detail on statistical methods (those are available through an extensive reference list). And the reader will find wise advice on when to rely on clinical data and when to be skeptical. I enthusiastically endorse this guide for biotech management, investors, bench scientists, journalists, or anyone interfacing with the world of biopharma clinical trials.”

—Michael Rosenblatt, Senior Partner, Flagship Pioneering

“If you have struggled, like me, to make sense of the disconnect between the celebratory tone of a press release and the concomitant negative stock market reaction, *The Pharmagellan Guide to Analyzing Biotech Clinical Trials* is a source of much-needed illumination.”

—Dan Lepanto, Senior Managing Director, M&A, SVB Leerink

THE PHARMAGELLAN GUIDE TO ANALYZING BIOTECH CLINICAL TRIALS

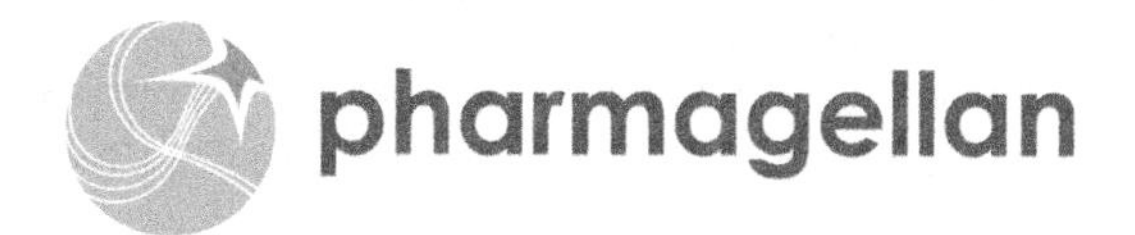

Frank S. David

This book may be purchased for educational, business, or sales promotional use. For information, please visit www.pharmagellan.com.

First edition

Edited by Robert Simison

Designed by Denise Clifton. Cover illustration by Sutton Long.

ISBN-13: 978-0-9984075-2-4

10 9 8 7 6 5 4 3 2 1

Printed in the United States of America

CONTENTS

INTRODUCTION

In God we trust. All others bring data. —W. Edwards Deming*

WHEN A BIOTECH OR PHARMA COMPANY discloses new information about a clinical trial of an experimental drug, it sets off a flurry of activity among folks who want to understand the results. The greenest readers use the first few lines of a press release or the abstract of a published paper to adjust their view of the drug's odds of clinical, regulatory, or commercial success. Others may be more experienced in biopharma but don't feel confident methodically assessing the information on their own, so they wait for experienced journalists, financial analysts, physicians, and R&D experts to tell them what to think. And others wade bravely into the weeds of tables, figures, and methods and try to dissect what the findings tell them about the drug's efficacy and safety.

The underlying premise of this book is that you can—and should—form your own opinions about trial results, even if you're not an expert in clinical medicine, study design, and biostatistics. But this isn't easy! Key details are often lacking, especially in press releases and media reports, and even articles in peer-reviewed journals vary widely in how clearly and completely they disclose how the study was designed, executed, and analyzed. To compound matters, investigators and companies are under enormous pressure to highlight positive aspects

---

* Deming was an American scholar and teacher best known for his work on evidence-based quality management within organizations. Although this quote is commonly attributed to him, there are no objective data to confirm that he ever uttered it. We recognize the irony.

of candidate drugs and minimize negative ones, which can sometimes cross the line from "glass half-full" optimism to outright misconduct.

On top of all these challenges, until now there hasn't been a good roadmap to help non-experts evaluate clinical trial results of new therapies. We've read hundreds of books and journal articles about interpreting clinical studies—and found them all lacking for this audience. Many try to do too much, covering not just interventional trials of new therapies but also retrospective analyses, meta-analyses, and other studies that are important for clinical care but are less critical for drug development. Others focus on how to design trials and are intended for biostatisticians at the front end of the process, not readers at the back end.

This book is written primarily to help educated non-experts—professional consumers of drug trial data who lack formal training in biostatistics—interpret clinical trial results of new therapies in development and make informed decisions based on them, even when they are incomplete and imperfect.

How this book is organized

This book is divided into two sections:

Part 1: How to systematically assess biotech clinical trials provides guidance on interpreting each major aspect of a study report. This section starts with a roadmap that will help you evaluate each key component and make sure you don't miss anything in a press release, meeting presentation, investor deck, or journal article. Within each subsequent chapter, you'll find general information about why and how the topic is important, frequently encountered terms and concepts, and potential sins of both omission and commission.

Part 2: Special topics covers specific technical points in more detail. This is where you'll find key statistical and methodological concepts discussed in slightly more detail but still at an appropriate level for non-statisticians with basic algebra skills.

Who should read this book?

If you are in one of these categories, you fall squarely into our bull's-eye of educated non-experts who will probably benefit the most from this guide:

Investors, financial analysts, consultants, and journalists who are trying to draw informed conclusions about the prospects of development-stage drugs and companies based on results of clinical studies.

Biotech and pharma industry professionals who engage with clinical trial results regularly as part of their jobs but are not experts in trial design and analysis, including folks in senior management, preclinical and translational research, regulatory affairs, business development, marketing, and finance.

Students and academic professionals in medicine, science, economics, business management, and related fields who want to gain a biopharma industry perspective on how to interpret clinical trial results of new drugs.

Folks in government, public policy, advocacy, and related areas who want to expand their understanding of key aspects of drug development.

There are three sets of individuals for whom this book may not be suitable. First, we've written this for *readers* of trial results, not the people who *generate* the results. If you are an expert in pharma clinical development or biostatistics who designs studies or analyzes raw data for a living, you probably need a highly technical reference, and this ain't it. Second, most of our examples and references come from the U.S., and in particular, regulatory discussions relate to the U.S. Food and Drug Administration (FDA) except as explicitly noted otherwise. (In the same vein, throughout this book we refer to drugs by their U.S. brand names.) Readers with specific interest in other geographies should do additional diligence in this regard. And finally, this book is not intended to help doctors or patients make decisions about clinical care.

PRIMER ON BIOTECH DRUG DEVELOPMENT

THIS GUIDE ASSUMES that readers have at least an "advanced beginner" understanding of how new drugs are developed, approved, and commercialized. For those who may be earlier in their careers or desire a brush-up on basic concepts, this chapter provides a basic introduction to aspects of trial phases, regulatory considerations, and market access issues that are referred to throughout the rest of the book.

Trial phases

A new drug typically goes through three sequential phases of clinical study before entering the market.[1] Each trial's specific phase is typically defined by the sponsor, and this provides some insights into why the study is being conducted and what role it is intended to play in the drug's journey from lab to clinic.

Phase 1: The first phase of clinical study for a new drug is intended to determine a range of safe and potentially effective doses for subsequent trials. In most therapeutic areas, these "first-in-human" trials are run in healthy volunteers, although in oncology and some non-cancer diseases they are typically carried out in people with the specific disease or condition of interest.

Most Phase 1 studies involve testing the drug at increasing dose levels to understand its pharmacologic properties and monitor for unwanted side effects.[2]

The starting dose typically has strong evidence from preclinical studies in animals that it will be safe for patients. Outside of oncology, these are referred to as single ascending dose (SAD) studies, which administer a single dose of the drug to each participant, and multiple ascending dose (MAD) studies, which administer repeat doses to reach steady-state levels of the drug. These studies typically measure the concentration of the drug in the blood and other tissues at various time points. They often also assess some aspect of its pharmacologic effect, such as the ability to modulate the activity of the drug's target or some other downstream readout that indicates the therapy is having an intended effect. Collectively, the outputs of these studies are referred to as pharmacokinetics (PK) and pharmacodynamics (PD).

In oncology Phase 1 studies are typically designed to determine the maximum tolerated dose (MTD) of the experimental therapy, above which the side-effect profile is deemed intolerable due to dose-limiting toxicities (DLTs).[3] This information then informs the choice of the recommended Phase 2 dose (RP2D). Many oncology Phase 1 studies use a so-called 3+3 design, in which investigators determine the MTD by treating three patients at a time at steadily increasing doses until DLTs appear, although alternate approaches are increasingly used to reduce the required time and number of patients.[4]

Each Phase 1 study typically includes a few dozen patients or more, and depending on the therapeutic area, a company may run several of them to assess various aspects of the drug's effects. Depending on complexity and size, a Phase 1 study in healthy volunteers may last a few weeks to a few months. These trials are often run at single centers, and healthy volunteer studies are typically executed at sites that specialize in Phase 1 studies.

Phase 1 studies in oncology have several important distinguishing characteristics compared with those in other therapeutic areas. First, Phase 1 trials in cancer are virtually always conducted in individuals with cancer rather than in healthy volunteers. Second, because patients with terminal cancer are generally believed to be more accepting of the adverse effects of a therapy than those with benign conditions, Phase 1 oncology studies typically increase the dose of the therapy until the MTD is reached, based on a pre-specified and relatively permissive definition of "tolerability." Finally, almost all contemporary first-in-human studies in oncology are designed as seamless Phase 1/2 trials, in which the same patients advance into the Phase 2 portion (see below) once the RP2D is identified.

Phase 1 studies typically provide three pieces of information. First, they define a range of safe and well-tolerated drug dosages suitable for subsequent Phase 2 studies. Second, they begin to describe the specific side effects that arise as a result of taking the drug. And finally, they usually provide some supporting evidence that the drug can reach a potentially effective concentration in the blood or tissues of interest and have an expected and desired effect.

Overall, about 60% of Phase 1 studies of new drugs typically advance into Phase 2.[5] The main reasons why programs are terminated after this phase are poor safety, strategic reasons ("portfolio rationalization"), and poor pharmacokinetics or bioavailability.[6]

Phase 2: The middle phase of clinical development is typically intended to provide initial evidence that the drug is having its intended biochemical, physiological, or clinical effect. Many companies refer to different types of Phase 2 trials as "proof of mechanism" (POM) or "proof of concept" (POC) studies. Outside of oncology, many early Phase 2 "dose-finding" studies are designed to define the most appropriate dose to take into subsequent efficacy trials.[7] In contrast with the healthy volunteer studies that are common in Phase 1, Phase 2 studies test the drug in patients with the indication of interest who could plausibly derive a clinical benefit.

There is extremely wide variability in the design, size, and execution of Phase 2 studies. The simplest ones might be small, single-arm trials run at a single site, whereas others may be large, complex, international studies that are virtually indistinguishable from those in Phase 3 (see below). Some companies refer to trials as "Phase 2a" or "Phase 2b" to indicate on which end of the spectrum they lie, but these terms do not have precise or generally accepted definitions. A sponsor may run a variable number of Phase 2 studies for a given new-drug candidate, depending on the therapeutic area and the data obtained from each trial.

Most Phase 2 programs are intended to help sponsors either reduce the risk of subsequent investment in large and expensive Phase 3 studies or decide to abandon the program because additional development is not likely to be fruitful. These trials usually aim to identify one or two target doses for later trials where there is some evidence of efficacy with acceptable tolerability. They also typically help define the patient population and likely effect size for follow-up studies. Phase 2 trials often use endpoints that are likely to correlate with bona fide clinical benefits but are not necessarily sufficient for approval by regulators, although there are scenarios in which drugs can be approved on the basis of Phase 2 results, as discussed later in this primer.

The success rate for new drugs in Phase 2 is about 36%.[8] Over half the drugs that fail to advance to Phase 3 are abandoned due to poor efficacy or clinical safety.[9]

Phase 3: The final phase of development is typically intended to demonstrate sufficient efficacy and an appropriate efficacy/safety balance to support a submission to regulators for approval. In most scenarios outside of oncology and rare diseases with limited treatment options, regulators require sponsors to demonstrate efficacy in at least two independent Phase 3 studies.

Phase 3 studies, often referred to as "pivotal" trials, are designed primarily to measure an efficacy outcome that will be relevant to approval agencies and also satisfy payers, physicians, and patients. Depending on the clinical indication, they can last as long as several years and include hundreds or even thousands of patients, although they may be shorter or smaller depending on the specific disease and the outcome being measured. The criteria for selecting study subjects generally define the population that will be reflected in the drug's label if it is approved. These trials are almost always conducted at multiple sites and frequently include patients from different countries.

Besides generating efficacy data on key outcome measures, Phase 3 studies yield additional safety and tolerability data on a much larger number of patients, which are important to both regulators and prospective prescribers and patients.

About 63% of Phase 3 programs are successful, but this statistic hides a great deal of variability.[10] Several large analyses have found ~20-percentage-point spreads in Phase 3 success rates across different therapeutic areas.[11,12,13]

Phase 4: Sponsors often run Phase 4, or post-marketing surveillance, studies on drugs after initial approval. This designation refers to a study in an indication and patient subset in which the drug has already been approved. A study in a different indication or population would typically be denoted as either Phase 2 or Phase 3, depending on its intention and design.

Some Phase 4 studies are required by regulators as a condition for approval and are intended to generate additional safety or efficacy data over a longer period and in more patients. The initial application may have been deemed incomplete on such metrics but not so deficient as to pose a barrier to market authorization. In other cases, a sponsor might choose to run a Phase 4 study for strategic reasons to differentiate the drug from competitors with additional long-term efficacy and safety data or evidence of positive effects on ancillary measures that were not measured in the original trials. Other Phase 4 studies are intended to provide evidence of improved quality of life or cost-effectiveness that can help justify the drug's price to payers. Although Phase 4 studies generally resemble Phase 3 trials in terms of overall size and scope, they are extremely heterogeneous due to the variety of underlying goals.

Exceptions: Although the Phase 1–Phase 2–Phase 3 paradigm is classic for most new drugs, some development programs skip one of the last two steps. Regulators may clear a drug without Phase 3 data under a special pathway like accelerated approval (see below) if a Phase 2 trial demonstrates efficacy on an endpoint that plausibly predicts clinical impact. Less commonly, a sponsor may move directly from Phase 1 to Phase 3. Due to the high cost of Phase 3 trials, most companies opt to reduce the risks of the program with a Phase 2 study, but there is no formal requirement for this intermediate step.

In other cases, sponsors combine trial phases into "Phase 1/2" or "Phase 2/3" instead of running the two phases as discrete trials in sequence. These so-called seamless studies use a single trial protocol to cover both phases, and patients from the first portion roll over directly into the next. For example, a Phase 1/2 study might include a dose escalation phase followed immediately by an expansion of the trial at the selected dose. Similarly, a Phase 2/3 study might evaluate a short-term endpoint intended to demonstrate proof of concept but then continue to allow for a longer-term endpoint suitable for assessment of a regulatory filing. Seamless studies are discussed in more detail in Chapter 15 on adaptive trials.

Regulatory considerations

Sponsors interact with regulatory agencies at various points along the way from initiating clinical trials to gaining approval to commercialize a new drug. These interactions are an integral part of drug development and provide important context for understanding the goals and implications of many clinical studies of new therapies. In this section, we summarize the main policies and processes relevant to first approvals of new drugs in the U.S.

Although much of modern drug development is conducted globally, this chapter focuses on policies and processes of the FDA. There is broad conceptual overlap with the policies, programs, and processes of other regulatory bodies, like the European Medicines Agency (EMA), the National Medical Products Administration (NMPA) in China, and the Pharmaceuticals and Medical Devices Agency (PMDA) in Japan. The details differ in each country or region and should be individually researched as needed.

As a final caveat, this discussion does not cover other aspects of drug regulation like label expansions for already-approved therapies; first approvals for generic medicines, devices, or diagnostics; or special situations that are specific to particular therapeutic classes or disease areas.

Required regulatory interactions

For a new drug to reach the market in the U.S., two regulatory interactions are required. At the outset, to initiate first-in-human clinical studies, a sponsor needs to obtain the FDA's approval of an **investigational new drug (IND) application.**[14] The IND application includes results of preclinical animal tests, information about the consistency and quality of manufacturing, and detailed protocols for first-in-human studies. Based on this information, the FDA determines whether the product is likely to expose humans in early-stage clinical trials to unnecessary risks. Information related to specific IND applications is not released by the agency, but sponsors often disclose that an IND application has been approved in press releases or investor presentations.

Once the pivotal trials are complete, the sponsor asks for permission to market the new therapy by submitting a **new drug application (NDA)**[15] for small molecule drugs or a **biologics license application (BLA)**[16] for biologic agents, including proteins, therapeutic antibodies, cell-based products, and vaccines. Although these two pathways cover different classes of therapeutics and are administered by different branches of the FDA, the processes are largely similar. In both cases, the sponsor submits all its clinical data to support its claim that the new therapy has an appropriate efficacy-safety balance to merit approval for commercialization, as well as information on the proposed labeling. Based on the NDA or BLA, the agency can either approve the drug or issue a **complete response (CR) letter**, which is essentially a rejection. CRs may be issued because the FDA finds that the efficacy-safety balance of the drug is inadequate, but they can also be due to issues unrelated to the clinical trial data, such as defects in manufacturing. In response to a CR letter, a sponsor can request a meeting with the agency and then either fix any deficiencies or withdraw the application. The agency does not disclose the content of CR letters or even that one was issued; any public information comes from the company. The FDA maintains databases for approved drugs, and the NDA and BLA numbers can be used to search for labels, FDA reviews, approval letters, and other key documents.[17,18]

Other common regulatory interactions

Besides filing the IND application and NDA or BLA, sponsors are permitted to ask for formal meetings with the FDA at any time during the drug development process to get feedback on key aspects of the clinical development plan for a new therapy.[19] Sponsors commonly request these meetings at the end of Phase 2 to get sign-off on key design elements of an "approvable" pivotal trial, or before submitting an IND application, NDA, or BLA. Companies sometimes publicly disclose that these meetings have taken place in press releases or financial filings, but the FDA does not proactively report their occurrence, content, or outcomes.

Sponsors also commonly ask the FDA for a **special protocol assessment (SPA)**, in which the agency and sponsor reach formal agreement on the design and size of a planned clinical trial that would support approval.[20] The agency reserves the right to rescind an SPA if a "substantial scientific issue" arises after the study is initiated, but historically less than 1% of SPAs have suffered this fate. As with other formal regulatory interactions, details of discussions related to SPAs may be disclosed by sponsors, but they are not publicized by the FDA.

Before NDA approval, the FDA sometimes convenes a **scientific advisory committee ("AdComm")** made up of outside experts in the field.[21] These public meetings are typically called when the FDA believes the issues raised by the NDA are controversial, have significant public interest, or require extremely specialized input that is not available within the agency. AdComm meetings typically include presentations by FDA staff, the sponsor, and other interested parties, and they usually include one or more votes by committee members on focused questions related to the risk-benefit profile of the drug. All background materials, presentations, discussions, and voting outcomes are publicly available. The FDA is not bound to follow the AdComm's recommendations, although it does so about 80% of the time.[22]

Sometimes the FDA issues a **clinical hold** on an IND application[23] or an ongoing trial.[24] In the IND scenario, this is typically because the agency has found deficiencies in the application and has delayed approving the application until key issues are resolved. During clinical studies, the most common reason for a clinical hold is if a new safety signal emerges that makes the agency believe that study subjects would be exposed to "an unreasonable and significant risk of illness or injury." Although the FDA does not comment on clinical holds, companies typically disclose them promptly via press releases.

Special regulatory pathways and programs

During the drug development process, sponsors have the option of applying to the FDA for various special programs that accelerate or otherwise enable the path to approval, although in some cases their effects on clinical trial design and evaluation are indirect:

- **Accelerated approval:** This program allows drugs that target certain high-need indications to be approved based on a demonstrated effect on a surrogate or intermediate clinical endpoint that is "reasonably likely" to predict a bona fide clinical benefit, but the actual benefit has not yet been demonstrated. Sponsors of drugs that are approved under this pathway are typically required to perform confirmatory Phase 4 studies (see above) to validate the clinical benefit of the new therapy.[25]
- **Breakthrough therapy:** A drug candidate can receive this designation if it has shown preliminary clinical evidence of efficacy on at least one of several possible measures. Such evidence can include improvement in irreversible morbidity or mortality; a surrogate or intermediate endpoint that is at least "reasonably likely" to confer a true clinical benefit; or a pharmacodynamics biomarker that "strongly suggests the potential" for a meaningful clinical effect. Breakthrough therapy can also be granted for treatments with evidence of significantly improved safety and comparable efficacy. Recipients of this designation receive the benefits of fast-track designation (see below), plus increased FDA commitment and intensive guidance on clinical development starting as early as Phase 1. As with fast track, a breakthrough designation does not have any direct effect on study design or execution or the criteria for eventual approval.[26]
- **Emergency use authorization:** The FDA can grant emergency use authorization (EUA) for unapproved products that address situations of high military or public health priority. The secretary of Health and Hu-

man Services defines which indications are eligible and updates the list as the nation's needs evolve. At the time of writing, EUAs were in effect for COVID-19 therapies, vaccines, diagnostics, and related medical devices; treatments for several other infectious agents, including the Ebola, H7N9 influenza, and Zika viruses; freeze-dried plasma; and nerve agent antidotes. For a product to receive an EUA, there must be "no adequate, approved, and available alternative," and there must be evidence that the product "may be effective," a lower, ill-defined regulatory standard that evaluators apply on a case-by-case basis.[27,28]

- **Fast track:** Programs can receive this designation if they are in a clinical area with no available therapies or have evidence of clear advantages over current treatments, such as superior efficacy or fewer side effects. It does not have any direct effects on the design, execution, or efficacy bar for clinical trials, although companies do gain access to more frequent interactions with the FDA to discuss the development plan. Fast track also speeds up the approval process by allowing the sponsor to submit an NDA or BLA for rolling review instead of waiting for the entire application to be complete.[29]
- **Priority review:** For drugs that have shown "significant improvement" in efficacy or safety in clinical studies, the sponsor can apply for expedited review, which shortens the review time for the NDA or BLA. This program has no effect on the criteria for FDA approval or any other factors related to clinical development.[30]

Pricing and market access issues

In most countries, once regulators authorize a drug it still needs to be found cost-effective by a governmental health technology assessment (HTA) body before it can be sold. The U.S. is a notable exception, where a manufacturer can set a price and enter the market immediately after drug approval without an official HTA. However, U.S. politicians and private payers are beginning to use independent HTAs by the Boston-based Institute for Clinical and Economic Review (ICER) to assess whether a drug's price is appropriate. Consequently, manufacturers are increasingly considering the prospect of HTAs in their U.S. development and commercialization plans.[31]

HTA bodies conduct cost-benefit analyses to assess whether the proposed price of a new therapy is justified by its purported health economic value. Examples of HTA reports that demonstrate the analytical approach are available online from ICER and the National Institute for Health and Care Excellence in the United Kingdom. These analyses integrate information from clinical trials with data from published literature and analyses of real-world sources like electronic medical records and patient registries.

For sponsors developing new medicines, the need to satisfy HTA authorities can influence several aspects of clinical trial design, most notably the choice of comparator and endpoints.[32] Most HTA bodies seek to assess a new therapy's efficacy relative to the current standard of care. Thus, although regulators may approve a drug based on a clinical trial that lacks a control arm or uses a placebo or other comparator that is not representative of current practice, these designs can sometimes make it difficult for sponsors to demonstrate a magnitude of benefit over available therapies that will justify their proposed price. Similarly, some studies that measure surrogate or short-term endpoints may not be viewed as relevant by HTA bodies, which typically assess the value of a drug based on its effect on clinical endpoints related to increasing patients' duration or quality of life.[33]

---

[1] Step 3: Clinical research. U.S. Food and Drug Administration. https://www.fda.gov/patients/drug-development-process/step-3-clinical-research. Updated January 4, 2018. Accessed October 15, 2021. Permalink: https://perma.cc/QQN3-JYFD.

[2] Gieser GS. Clinical pharmacology 1: Phase 1 studies and early drug development. FDA Clinical Investigator Course, November 13–15, 2012. https://www.fda.gov/media/84920/download. Permalink: https://perma.cc/39CJ-SWSL.

[3] Le Tourneau C, Lee JJ, Siu LL. Dose escalation methods in phase I cancer clinical trials. J Natl Cancer Inst. 2009 May 20;101(10):708–720. doi: 10.1093/jnci/djp079. Epub 2009 May 12. PMID: 19436029; PMCID: PMC2684552.

[4] Kurzrock R, Lin CC, Wu TC, Hobbs BP, Pestana RC, Hong DS. Moving beyond 3+3: The future of clinical trial design. Am Soc Clin Oncol Educ Book. 2021 Jun;41:e133–e144. doi: 10.1200/EDBK_319783. PMID: 34061563.

[5] David FS, Robey S, Matthews A. *The Pharmagellan Guide to Biotech Forecasting and Valuation.* 1st ed. Pharmagellan; 2016.

[6] Waring M, Arrowsmith J, Leach AR, Leeson PD, Mandrell S, Owen RM, Pairaudeau G, Pennie WD, Pickett SD, Wang J, Wallace O, Weir A. An analysis of the attrition of drug candidates from four major pharmaceutical companies. Nat Rev Drug Discov. 2015 Jul;14(7):475–486. doi: 10.1038/nrd4609. Epub 2015 Jun 19. PMID: 26091267.

[7] Viele K, Connor JT. Dose-finding trials: Optimizing Phase 2 data in the drug development process. JAMA. 2015 Dec 1;314(21):2294–2295. doi: 10.1001/jama.2015.16702. PMID: 26624828.

[8] David FS, Robey S, Matthews A. *The Pharmagellan Guide to Biotech Forecasting and Valuation.* 1st ed. Pharmagellan; 2016.

[9] Waring M, Arrowsmith J, Leach AR, Leeson PD, Mandrell S, Owen RM, Pairaudeau G, Pennie WD, Pickett SD, Wang J, Wallace O, Weir A. An analysis of the attrition of drug candidates from four major pharmaceutical companies. Nat Rev Drug Discov. 2015 Jul;14(7):475–486. doi: 10.1038/nrd4609. Epub 2015 Jun 19. PMID: 26091267.

[10] David FS, Robey S, Matthews A. *The Pharmagellan Guide to Biotech Forecasting and Valuation.* 1st ed. Pharmagellan; 2016.

[11] DiMasi JA, Feldman L, Seckler A, Wilson A. Trends in risks associated with new drug development: Success rates for investigational drugs. Clin Pharmacol Ther. 2010 Mar;87(3):272–277. doi: 10.1038/clpt.2009.295. Epub 2010 Feb 3. PMID: 20130567.

[12] Hay M, Thomas DW, Craighead JL, Economides C, Rosenthal J. Clinical development success rates for investigational drugs. Nat Biotechnol. 2014 Jan;32(1):40–51. doi: 10.1038/nbt.2786. PMID: 24406927.

[13] Biotechnology Innovation Organization, Informa Pharma Intelligence, and QLS Advisors. Clinical development success rates and contributing factors, 2011–2020. February 2021. https://pharmaintelligence.informa.com/~/media/informa-shop-window/pharma/2021/files/reports/2021-clinical-development-success-rates-2011-2020-v17.pdf.

[14] Investigational new drug (IND) application. U.S. Food and Drug Administration. https://www.fda.gov/drugs/types-applications/investigational-new-drug-ind-application. Updated February 24, 2021. Accessed October 15, 2021. Permalink: https://perma.cc/UYQ4-WFLA.

[15] New drug application (NDA). U.S. Food and Drug Administration. https://www.fda.gov/drugs/types-applications/new-drug-application-nda. Updated June 10, 2019. Accessed October 15, 2021. Permalink: https://perma.cc/7TMK-Q6LK.

[16] Biologics license applications (BLA) process (CBER). U.S. Food and Drug Administration. https://www.fda.gov/vaccines-blood-biologics/development-approval-process-cber/biologics-license-applications-bla-process-cber. Updated January 27, 2021. Accessed October 15, 2021. Permalink: https://perma.cc/X38D-Q84G.

[17] Drugs@FDA: FDA-approved drugs. U.S. Food and Drug Administration. https://www.accessdata.fda.gov/scripts/cder/daf/index.cfm. Accessed October 15, 2021.

[18] Purple Book database of licensed biological products. U.S. Food and Drug Administration. https://purplebooksearch.fda.gov/. Updated October 8, 2021. Accessed October 15, 2021.

[19] Formal meetings between the FDA and sponsors or applicants of PDUFA products: Guidance for industry (draft guidance). U.S. Food and Drug Administration. December 2017.

[20] Special protocol assessment: Guidance for industry (Revision 1). U.S. Food and Drug Administration. April 2018.

[21] Guidance for industry: Advisory committees: Implementing Section 120 of the Food and Drug Administration Modernization Act of 1997. U.S. Food and Drug Administration. October 1998.

[22] Zhang AD, Schwartz JL, Ross JS. Association between Food and Drug Administration advisory committee recommendations and agency actions, 2008–2015. Milbank Q. 2019 Sep;97(3):796–819. doi: 10.1111/1468-0009.12403. Epub 2019 Jul 14. PMID: 31304643; PMCID: PMC6739629.

[23] IND application procedures: Clinical hold. U.S. Food and Drug Administration. https://www.fda.gov/drugs/investigational-new-drug-ind-application/ind-application-procedures-clinical-hold. Updated October 9, 2015. Accessed October 15, 2021. Permalink: https://perma.cc/MRE2-J6QD.

[24] 21 C.F.R. § 312.42.

[25] Accelerated approval. U.S. Food and Drug Administration. https://www.fda.gov/patients/fast-track-breakthrough-therapy-accelerated-approval-priority-review/accelerated-approval. Updated January 4, 2018. Accessed October 15, 2021. Permalink: https://perma.cc/3JUR-9D6X.

[26] Breakthrough therapy. U.S. Food and Drug Administration. https://www.fda.gov/patients/fast-track-breakthrough-therapy-accelerated-approval-priority-review/breakthrough-therapy. Updated January 4, 2018. Accessed October 15, 2021. Permalink: https://perma.cc/RHW7-BJA8.

1.

OVERVIEW: ROADMAP TO EVALUATING A BIOTECH CLINICAL TRIAL

NEWS ABOUT BIOTECH CLINICAL TRIALS comes in waves. When a sponsor kicks off a study, you might get some insights into the planned trial from a press release, an abstract at a medical meeting outlining the main design elements, or a record in a clinical trials registry like clinicaltrials.gov. Sometime later, press releases, investor presentations, or scientific meeting presentations often provide key, top-line findings, but usually without a lot of supporting details. Finally—sometimes much later—you may get to read a full article in a medical journal containing detailed methods and much more complete results, although even then, certain aspects may remain vague or poorly described.

At each stage, it's important to learn as much as possible about the study to assess the new information, highlight gaps that still need to be filled, and identify red flags that raise concerns about how to interpret the results. Importantly, this process doesn't end when a paper is published in a major medical journal. Even with the full results of a trial in hand, there will almost always be unanswered questions and unaddressed concerns about the drug's efficacy and safety, its relevance to clinical care, and its prospects for regulatory approval, market authorization, and commercial success.

This section provides an overview of how to systematically evaluate planned, in-progress, and completed studies of new drugs. In this chapter, we take a bird's-eye view of the various trial components and summarize four overarching questions you should ask to determine the intent of a clinical trial, whether it was designed and executed to meet its goals, and the meaning and impact of the results. In the subsequent chapters we do a deep dive on each of the components.

1. What is the intent of the study?

Relevant chapter: 2, Goals and Rationale

Every clinical trial of a new drug has defined goals. Understanding them is critical to evaluating the study's design and results. Many early-stage studies are intended for the sponsor to understand basic pharmacologic parameters of the drug, inform "go/no-go" decisions about further development, and help optimize the design of future trials. Later studies often aim to optimize how regulators, market access authorities, physicians, and patients will view the agent versus already-available therapies.

It's important to be as specific as possible about how the intent of the study affects the bar for success and how that bar might vary depending on one's perspective. For example, a company may design a study to detect a certain amount of efficacy that it thinks is meaningful and achievable, but this level may not be sufficient for regulators to grant approval or for physicians to prescribe and patients to use the new medicine. Setting precise, quantitative thresholds for how one thinks various parties will assess the results of a trial is critical to understanding its significance once results are in hand, as discussed later.

Key sub-questions:

- **Rationale:** What was the sponsor's rationale for running the study?
- **Bar for success:** What was the sponsor's likely bar for success at the outset of the trial?

2. Is the study designed to achieve its goals?

Relevant chapters: 3, Patient Population; 4, Study Design; 5, Endpoints

The next key question is whether the study is capable of achieving its goals. Is the research plan designed to answer the intended question about the new therapy? Or is there a mismatch between the study's goals and its setup?

Finding these mismatches requires digging into the details of the trial's methods. The choices of which patients to include and exclude, what therapy to use as a comparator, and what endpoints to measure have huge implications for what type of results one might plausibly expect to emerge and how one might interpret them. For example, if a pivotal study is designed to test a drug's effect on endpoint A, but regulators mainly care about endpoint B, then even the most statistically convincing positive result probably won't achieve the study's goal of enabling the drug to reach the market.

More commonly, these decisions are shades of gray, and evaluating a study's design requires understanding the sponsor's approach to balancing various types of risks and opportunities. A drug might be most likely to work in an extremely small subset of patients with particular characteristics, but the trial might be designed to also include additional subjects where the odds of success are lower to broaden the therapy's potential market opportunity. One might ideally want to know how a drug performs head-to-head against an available, widely used, and highly active alternative, but a trial versus placebo or a weaker agent might be cheaper, faster, and more likely to succeed. The sponsor might decide not to study a drug's effect on extending or improving life if regulators are likely to accept some other surrogate endpoint as good enough to grant approval. A large trial might increase the odds of detecting a small effect, but this strategy could increase the risk that prescribers, regulators, or payers consider the amount of improvement insufficient. A major part of assessing how a study's design fits with its goals is understanding how sponsors handle these trade-offs.

Key sub-questions:

- **Patient selection criteria:** How were patients identified, included, and excluded, and why?
- **Validation of tests:** How well validated are the tests or biomarkers that were used to define the patient population?
- **Study design:** What was the study design? Were the comparator and length of treatment appropriate? Did the study use any specialized design features such as a run-in period, crossover, or interim analysis, and if so, why?
- **Endpoints:** What were the endpoints, and which was the primary one? How were they selected and measured? What is their relevance?

- **Effect size:** What effect size in the primary endpoint was the trial designed to detect, and why was it chosen?
- **Design implications:** How might the study's design affect its ability to inform further development or support regulatory approval, pricing, and market access, or commercial success?

3. Was the study executed and analyzed properly?

Relevant chapters: 6, Execution; 7, Analysis

Even the best-designed drug study can fall flat if there are issues with how it was run or how the data were analyzed. Once a trial is completed, it's important to assess the mechanics of execution and analysis to ensure that there are no lingering doubts about how to interpret the findings.

These issues are hard for outsiders to evaluate because we never get access to the level of detail seen by trial investigators, sponsors, and regulators. Nonetheless, careful readers of biotech clinical trials can answer important questions about which patients finished the study, dropped out, and were included in the final analysis, as well as the likely trustworthiness of results in specific patient subsets.

Key sub-questions:

- **Enrollment and dropouts:** How many enrolled patients completed the study? How many dropouts occurred, at what points, and why?
- **Subject characteristics:** What were the characteristics of participating patients? Were the control and experimental arms balanced for key characteristics?
- **Analysis:** Did the analysis include all enrolled patients? If not, which patients were excluded and why?
- **Sub-groups:** How and why were sub-groups chosen for analysis? Were they pre-specified or defined after the fact?

4. What is the significance of the study's results?

Relevant chapters: 8, Results—Efficacy; 9, Results—Safety

Many newbie readers of biotech clinical trial news jump immediately to the results, but that's a big mistake. Just because the *P* value on the primary endpoint looks good and a company rep, academic expert, journalist, or equity analyst says the study "succeeded" or "failed" doesn't necessarily tell the whole story.

Instead of reflexively accepting top-line findings, it's important to consider whether the study's design, execution, or analytic approach might make one more skeptical of apparently positive findings or more hopeful about negative ones. And even if the results seem kosher, it's crucial to return to the first question about the study's goals and view the findings in light of the trial's intent. There are many consumers of clinical data—the sponsors themselves, regulators, market access authorities, prescribers, patients, investors, and so forth—and they may have extremely different views of the study's significance and implications.

Key sub-questions:

- **Significance:** Were the drug's effects statistically and clinically significant? What might be the caveats to nominally "positive" or "negative" results?
- **Safety:** What was the safety and tolerability profile of the intervention?
- **Consistency and plausibility:** Were the results consistent and plausible across key subgroups?
- **Perception of findings:** Did the study meet the sponsor's goals? How are the results likely to be perceived by various consumers of the trial results?

2.

GOALS AND RATIONALE

EVERY CLINICAL TRIAL OF A POTENTIAL NEW THERAPY has a defined purpose, and understanding it is critical to assessing the study's design, results, and impact. Of course, from a drugmaker's perspective, the goal is to develop blockbuster treatments that will generate billions of dollars of profits. But it can take many years and hundreds of millions of dollars of at-risk investment to bring a new drug to the market, and the duration, cost, and odds of success of clinical development can vary widely depending on how the studies are designed and executed. As managers consider whether and how to develop a new therapy, decisions about clinical trials have a significant impact on the potential return on investment and ultimate business case around every potential new product.

Another consideration for readers is that the "success" bar for a study is different if it is a first-in-human trial, the first clinical test of whether the new drug could plausibly work in an indication, or a pivotal experiment intended to support regulatory approval, market access, and commercial uptake. Thus, when evaluating clinical study results it is crucial to consider the sponsor's intent and how the trial fits into the overall strategy for the drug and the company.

In this chapter, we first discuss the possible strategic rationales a sponsor might have for running a clinical study. We then highlight key questions one should answer about the scientific, clinical, and business context for a new drug before evaluating the design or results of a clinical trial.

Reasons to run a clinical study

Given the cost of clinical trials, drug companies need to have good business and scientific reasons for running them. These reasons have a direct impact on how the sponsor designs, executes, and interprets the study—and how you, as the reader, should evaluate it as well. Before diving into a press release, abstract, journal article, or investor presentation, it's worth considering the sponsor's likely goals and how they might affect different aspects of the trial. Based on how the study fits into the overall development plan, what is the trial's intent, and what decisions by the sponsor, regulators, market access authorities, physicians, or patients are likely to be triggered as a result of it?

In general, there are three main reasons that companies run clinical studies, which are not mutually exclusive:

- **Provide evidence to justify or enable further R&D:** Drug development is a costly and risky endeavor, and most non-pivotal trials are intended to generate additional information to justify continued investment.[1,2] At the earliest stage of drug development, many trials are designed to answer two critical "go/no-go" questions about whether it is feasible and potentially profitable enough to develop the drug. First, can the treatment be dosed so that it reaches an appropriate level, for the right length of time, in the right anatomical location without excess safety or tolerability concerns? And second, is there some early evidence for "proof of mechanism," that the drug is having its intended biochemical, cellular, or physiologic effect? A major focus for readers of these early clinical studies is determining exactly what type and level of evidence sponsors expect to surmount these hurdles and continue investing in development, and whether their thresholds are set appropriately. A Phase 1 study of Ribon Therapeutics' PARP7 inhibitor RBN-2397 showed that the drug led to an increase in CXCL10 mRNA in treated tumors over pre-treatment levels, as predicted based on its mechanism of action,[3,4] but readers would need to do additional diligence and background research to decide whether they think the observed 1.5- to 8-fold increase validates the mechanistic hypothesis enough to justify further studies.

  Once proof of mechanism has been established, sponsors typically design follow-up studies to define one or two doses that provide "clinical proof of concept" by showing enough efficacy to justify investing in a larger, registration-enabling trial. This can sometimes be accomplished via a small-scale clinical study that is intended to provide a glimmer of evidence that the drug is effective using the intended Phase 3 endpoint, without the enormous expense of a large-scale trial designed to generate a statistically significant result. Alternatively, a proof-of-concept study might use an endpoint that is not of high relevance to regulators, patients, or physicians but may enable the company to more quickly and cheaply determine whether there is any reason to believe that the drug has an effect on the disease of interest. The impact of the study's results on the company's decision to move forward is not typically clear-cut and depends on the predictive power of the endpoint and the magnitude of the effect. These issues are discussed in more detail in Chapter 5 on endpoints.

Finally, another frequent goal of both early- and mid-stage clinical trials is to test the drug in a broad range of opportunities to see which ones seem most promising for further pursuit. This "signal-seeking" strategy is particularly common in areas like cancer and rheumatology, where a drug's mechanism of action may not point to a specific tumor type or indication. It also applies to scenarios in which a sponsor plans to see whether particular patient subsets yield results that could inform the population selection strategy for a follow-up trial. The study of RBN-2397, for example, was designed to include patients with a broad range of tumor types, and the observation of a partial response in a patient with squamous lung cancer most likely informed Ribon's plan to expand the study to explicitly test the drug's activity in a larger cohort of patients with this cancer type. As discussed further in Chapter 8 on efficacy results, these types of studies are intended to generate hypotheses, not validate them, and as such, they often lack strong statistical guardrails against false positive results.

- **Gain regulatory approval:** Most Phase 3 studies are designed to surmount regulatory hurdles. Almost all companies seeking U.S. approval request an "end of Phase 2 meeting" with the U.S. Food and Drug Administration (FDA) to discuss the path forward. If that meeting is productive and the agency's advice is heeded, one can usually have a reasonable level of certainty that the number of planned Phase 3 studies and their design, endpoints, control arms, populations, sizes, and other parameters would support registration if the results are positive. Importantly, a trial that satisfies regulatory requirements may not necessarily fully support the sponsor's commercial ambitions, so in practice, pivotal trials incorporate additional factors beyond those that are strictly required by regulators.

Notably, in the modern era many earlier-stage trials are also intended to leave the door open for the drug to qualify for a special regulatory pathway that could enable accelerated approval, particularly in cancer and rare diseases.[5]

- **Support successful commercialization:** Many aspects of a trial's design and execution may be mainly intended to bolster the drug's commercial prospects. In highly competitive markets, for example, the choice of comparator and target effect size might be driven largely by the need to convince prescribers, patients, and payers of a drug's value. This is particularly an issue in regions where HTA agencies regulate a drug's price and market access, because these bodies' standards for a trial's comparator and endpoints often differ from those of regulators.[6,7]

  Some aspects of a study may be intended to produce data for inclusion in the drug's label that can then be used in sales and marketing. This is a particular issue with quality-of-life endpoints and patient-reported outcomes, where regulators in different regions have different standards for what level of evidence suffices for label inclusion.[8]

  For marketed drugs, there can be commercial benefits to studies in new indications that never lead to formal regulatory approval. Under certain circumstances, sponsors are allowed to disseminate journal article reprints on studies exploring "off-label" uses.[9] A study designed for this purpose might have very different patients, endpoints, and statistical power than one intended to inform R&D decision-making or support full marketing authorization.

Assessing the scientific, clinical, and business context of a trial

Before executing a trial of a new drug, virtually all companies conduct a comprehensive assessment of the relevant scientific, clinical, and business landscape. This provides important information that feeds directly into the sponsor's choices in all aspects of study design. For external readers it can be helpful to put oneself in the company's shoes to understand managers' perspective on the strength of evidence linking the drug's mechanism to the disease it purports to treat, where the opportunities lie for a new therapy, and the key design factors and efficacy hurdles for a clinical trial to satisfy the needs of patients, physicians, regulators, payers, and R&D funders and decision makers.

A full discussion of how to assess the relevant landscape for a drug in clinical development is beyond our scope. Most trial sponsors conduct a comprehensive review of secondary research, including journal articles, clinical references like UpToDate, regulatory documents, and "gray" literature, and supplement it with primary interviews and surveys of experts, practicing physicians, patients, and other key stakeholders. Instead of focusing on the mechanics, we summarize here some of the most important questions to address in interpreting a planned, in-progress, or completed study:

1. **What is known about the pathophysiology of the disease?** What is the rationale for thinking that this specific drug could affect particular subsets of patients at particular stages of illness? What mechanistic and clinical endpoints are likely to be modulated by the drug? What precedents and comparators might be relevant to this drug in terms of common target molecules or pathways? Based on the underlying science, what is the overall strength of the scientific and clinical hypothesis for this drug, and what is the pretest likelihood that the drug will work?
2. **How are patients identified and diagnosed?** How are patients segmented based on stage of progression, severity, prognosis, underlying pathophysiology, line of therapy, or other factors? What are the defining clinical characteristics of patients in each subset? How well defined are the criteria for making the diagnosis and for defining different subsets of patients, and how homogeneous or heterogeneous are these subsets?

How is the landscape evolving in terms of the disease's epidemiology, diagnosis, and segmentation?

3. **How are patients treated?** For each patient group, what treatment options are available? How do they differ from one another, and what are the key factors that drive the choices of physicians, patients, and payers? Which options are viewed as standard of care? How is the treatment landscape likely to evolve based on other development-stage programs?
4. **What are the current unmet needs?** How do the main treatments perform on various metrics that are important to physicians, patients, and payers? In which domains and specific sub-populations is there room for improvement? What level of performance would be seen as "better" by physicians, patients, regulators, and payers? How are these needs likely to evolve as additional therapeutic options in development are validated and become available?
5. **What is known about clinical development, market access, and regulatory approval in this area?** What are the most widely cited and accepted clinical trials for proof of mechanism, proof of concept, regulatory approval, and market authorization? What endpoints, comparators, and levels of improvement are likely to be required at each stage based on historical precedents? How might the threshold for success change as the therapeutic landscape advances?

These questions are directly relevant to evaluating key components of the design and results of a clinical trial. For example, the choice of patient population for a study is affected by how one thinks various sub-groups fit with one's knowledge of the disease pathophysiology and drug mechanism, how they are currently diagnosed and classified, how they perform with current and evolving clinical options, and how they fit with historical and evolving standards for regulatory approval and market access. Performing this foundational research on the scientific, clinical, and business context of a drug and a specific trial is critical to being able to assess the sponsor's likely goals, whether the study was designed to address them, and whether the results indicate success or failure.

[1] Cook D, Brown D, Alexander R, March R, Morgan P, Satterthwaite G, Pangalos MN. Lessons learned from the fate of AstraZeneca's drug pipeline: A five-dimensional framework. Nat Rev Drug Discov. 2014 Jun;13(6):419–431. doi: 10.1038/nrd4309. Epub 2014 May 16. PMID: 24833294.

[2] Morgan P, Brown DG, Lennard S, Anderton MJ, Barrett JC, Eriksson U, Fidock M, Hamrén B, Johnson A, March RE, Matcham J, Mettetal J, Nicholls DJ, Platz S, Rees S, Snowden MA, Pangalos MN. Impact of a five-dimensional framework on R&D productivity at AstraZeneca. Nat Rev Drug Discov. 2018 Mar;17(3):167–181. doi: 10.1038/nrd.2017.244. Epub 2018 Jan 19. PMID: 29348681.

[3] RBN-2397, an oral PARP7 inhibitor, in patients with solid tumors, FIH, MAD study. ClinicalTrials.gov identifier: NCT04053673. Updated August 26, 2021. Accessed October 15, 2021.

[4] Falchook GS, Patel MR, Yap TA, McEachern K, Kuplast-Barr K, Utley L, Cleary L, Manyak E, Bozon V, Parasuraman S, Johnson ML. A first-in-human Phase 1 study of a novel PARP7 inhibitor RBN-2397 in patients with advanced solid tumors. J Clin Oncol. 2021 May 20;39(15 suppl):3000. doi: 10.1200/JCO.2021.39.15_suppl.3000.

[5] Accelerated approval. U.S. Food and Drug Administration. https://www.fda.gov/patients/fast-track-breakthrough-therapy-accelerated-approval-priority-review/accelerated-approval. Updated January 4, 2018. Accessed October 15, 2021. Permalink: https://perma.cc/3JUR-9D6X.

[6] Wang Y, Qiu T, Zhou J, Francois C, Toumi M. Which criteria are considered and how are they evaluated in health technology assessments? A review of methodological guidelines used in Western and Asian countries. Appl Health Econ Health Policy. 2021;19:281–304. doi: 10.1007/s40258-020-00634-0. Epub 2021 Jan 11.

[7] Comparators and comparisons: Direct and indirect comparisons (adapted version). European Network for Health Technology Assessment. November 2015. Available at https://www.eunethta.eu/comparators-comparisons-direct-and-indirect-comparisons-amended-ja1-guideline-final-nov-2015/. Permalink: https://perma.cc/TD4J-BSM7.

[8] Gnanasakthy A, Barrett A, Evans E, D'Alessio D, Romano CD. A review of patient-reported outcomes labeling for oncology drugs approved by the FDA and the EMA (2012–2016). Value Health. 2019 Feb;22(2):203–209. doi: 10.1016/j.jval.2018.09.2842. PMID: 30711065.

[9] Guidance for industry: Distributing scientific and medical publications on unapproved new uses—recommended practices (revised draft guidance). U.S. Food and Drug Administration. February 2014.

3.

PATIENT POPULATION

PRESS REPORTS commonly refer to clinical studies in "lung cancer," "depression," or "asthma," but most trials restrict enrollment to more specific subsets of patients. For example, a lung cancer trial might specifically include or exclude patients with brain metastases or a particular oncogenic mutation. A new depression therapy might be studied in "first-line" patients, or those who have already failed to respond to selective serotonin reuptake inhibitors (SSRIs). And an asthma trial might focus on high-severity patients as defined by oral steroid usage and the number of hospitalizations per year.

These choices and others like them about the patient population are attempts to manage the balance between risk and reward in drug development. In each case, more-restrictive criteria for patient inclusion change the study's odds of clinical, regulatory, and commercial success. Almost every specific detail of the patient population affects one or more of these factors, and each sponsor makes different decisions about how to define the trial population to manage the tradeoffs and optimize what it thinks is most important.

Most readers of clinical trials are not privy to the full study protocol and instead learn details about the patient population from lists of inclusion and exclusion criteria in clinicaltrials.gov or the methods section of a published report. These lists do not necessarily include every factor that influences the study population, but they typically include the most critical ones. This permits a reader to put the study in context with the target indication, prior trials, and the regulatory and commercial landscape.

In this chapter, we first highlight some key issues to consider when placing the patient population of a trial into its broader context. We then consider the main factors related to R&D success and execution, regulatory approval, and commercial success that play a role in how sponsors define the patient population for a particular trial. We also discuss the difference between prognostic and predictive biomarkers and the impact of this distinction on the evaluation of study protocols and results.

How to put the patient population in context

In examining the target patient population for a planned or completed study, it is first important to do background research to understand the clinical, regulatory, and commercial context. Some key issues that should be investigated are summarized below:

- **Scientific rationale:** In many situations, there are reasons to think a drug will work better in certain subgroups of patients based on its mechanism of action, clinical or pathophysiological characteristics of various patient subsets, supporting preclinical data, or other factors. Particularly common scenarios involve drugs that are likely to work in patients with high expression of the drug's target or a particular genetic background that is relevant to the therapy's activity. Similarly, drugs that are intended to reverse or slow the progression of chronic organ damage are often more likely to work in patients at earlier disease stages before the damage becomes irreversible.
- **Current clinical management:** The context for understanding the study population for a clinical trial is often grounded in an understanding of how physicians identify, diagnose, and categorize patients, and then use this information to pick among the appropriate and available treatment options. This helps the reader of a trial figure out how the patients who are included and excluded overlap with existing standards and approaches. In areas that lack clear clinical guidelines, there may be substantial challenges with predicting the homogeneity of participating patients, as well as putting the study's design and results in context with

available knowledge. And even if current clinical approaches to diagnosing and segmenting patients are relatively well established, if a study incorporates a new diagnostic modality, then the drug's success may hinge on the technical performance of the novel test and physicians' and payers' acceptance of it.

A study's choice of patients also defines what agents prescribers are likely to view as an appropriate comparator to the new drug. This affects the drug's commercial opportunity by defining not just the level of improvement prescribers will expect over available alternatives but also how HTA bodies will use the trial's design and results to decide whether to grant market access and set an appropriate price for the new drug.

- **Comparator and competitor studies:** Looking at the study population of prior successful and failed trials in the same indication, particularly for drugs that are closely related, can help one determine which patient selection criteria are more generally used in a disease area versus customized for a particular trial. Less-standardized approaches typically warrant additional attention to understand the rationale and implications of the unusual requirements. Even in areas with long histories of pivotal trials, like major depression, there are often differences in the tests used to classify patients and the specific cutoffs used to include and exclude patients.
- **Regulatory landscape:** Approved and draft guidance documents often provide extremely specific insights into regulators' recommendations on which patients to include and exclude in pivotal trials. For example, the U.S. Food and Drug Administration (FDA) recommends that studies of therapies for "routine" dry eye base inclusion on both objective signs and subjective symptoms and exclude patients with eyelid inflammation or dry eye due to scarring or vitamin A deficiency.[1]
- **Fit with earlier studies of the drug:** A common contributor to the failure of Phase 3 studies is a change in the patient population compared with a prior Phase 2 study that adds heterogeneity or uncertainty into the pivotal trial.[2] Differences in inclusion and exclusion criteria can sometimes increase the risk that the earlier success may not translate into a positive result in the later trial.

R&D, regulatory, and commercial impact of the patient population

The choice of patient population is at the heart of every new-drug clinical trial. When assessing the different components of the trial's inclusion and exclusion criteria, it is often helpful to systematically ask how each parameter might affect aspects of the study's design, execution, interpretation, and impact along various dimensions as discussed below.

Odds of success

Trials of new drugs often limit the study population to patients with particular clinical or molecular characteristics to focus on individuals who are more likely to respond to the investigational agent. An obvious example would be a trial of an agent that specifically inhibits activated forms of oncogenic proteins. In the early 2000s—before the relationship between molecular genetics and clinical response for targeted therapies was fully understood—the original Phase 3 trials of the first-generation epidermal growth factor receptor (EGFR) inhibitors erlotinib (Tarceva; Roche/Astellas) and gefitinib (Iressa; AstraZeneca) were run in unselected lung cancer patients regardless of EGFR mutational status.[3] Although erlotinib managed to achieve a positive result in the broad population (unlike gefitinib), this was a high-risk strategy based on what we now know about the biology of EGFR-driven lung cancer.

In the modern era, it is increasingly common for drug developers to focus first on the subset of patients most likely to respond and only later test the treatment in a broader population where the odds and magnitude of response are likely to be lower. But this is far from a universal axiom in the industry. When Merck tested its PD-1 inhibitor pembrolizumab (Keytruda) in first-line lung cancer, the company chose to restrict study entry to patients whose tumors were at least 50% positive for expression of PD-1's binding partner, PD-L1. Bristol Myers Squibb opted instead to test its PD-1 inhibitor nivolumab (Opdivo) in the entire unselected population, irrespective of PD-L1 expression. Pembrolizumab's success and nivolumab's failure set the stage in 2016 for Merck to capture significant share of the checkpoint inhibitor market overall, despite having launched after Bristol Myers Squibb.[4]

A less common but sometimes-employed strategy for choosing the population to maximize the odds of success is a so-called multi-population trial, in which a single study tests a drug in both a broader population and one or more predefined subsets. With the appropriate design, such a study can provide additional "shots on goal" without compromising overall statistical integrity. (The challenges of multiple hypothesis testing are discussed more fully in Chapter 7.) The Phase 3 SATURN study of erlotinib in second-line lung cancer, published in 2010, measured two co-primary endpoints, either of which would have qualified as a positive result: progression-free survival (PFS) in the "all-comers" population, and PFS in the EGFR-overexpressing subset.[5] The APEX study of whether the anticoagulant betrixaban (Bevyxxa; Portola) prevented venous clots in acutely ill patients used a different approach to achieve the same result of studying multiple populations within the same trial.[6] That Phase 3 trial, published in 2016, recruited patients age 40 or older with various combinations of pro-clotting risk factors. The statistical plan stipulated that the analysis would serially consider populations of increasing breadth, provided the preceding result was positive: first those with elevated D-dimer, a protein fragment that indicates clots are being actively made and dissolved; then those with either elevated D-dimer or age over 75; and finally, the entire study population.

Besides restricting the population to a particular biomarker-defined group, another common strategy to boost the odds of success in chronic indications is to restrict the study population to patients at a particular disease stage. Phase 3 studies of drugs intended to prevent or delay progression in diseases like chronic renal insufficiency, fibrotic diseases in the lungs and liver, and Alzheimer's disease often seek to exclude later-stage patients in whom end-organ damage may be irreversible and the clinical course may be less likely to be modifiable.

Finally, it is important to note that although such scenarios seek to boost efficacy by restricting the patient population, in some cases it may be desirable to cast a broad net. In some cancer and rheumatology indications, early-phase "signal-seeking" trials intentionally recruit a diverse set of patients to explore a wide range of hypotheses that could be confirmed in later studies. In 2019, Sierra Oncology reported top-line results from two Phase 1/2 trials in "advanced cancer" of its Chk1 inhibitor, SRA737, which together included 265 patients with various tumor types.[7] The studies found that SRA737 plus low-dose gemcitabine yielded response rates of 30% (3/10) in anogenital cancer and 25% (4/16) in patients with FA/BRCA gene network mutations across multiple histologies.[8] In this situation, the relatively loose inclusion criteria allowed the sponsor to identify potentially promising signs of efficacy in specific cancers that it intended to explore with partners in focused Phase 2 follow-up trials.[9]

Risk of adverse events

Many studies seek to avoid treating patients who are more likely to experience adverse safety events. If the experimental drug is metabolized by the cytochrome P450 system in the liver, many studies exclude patients taking certain other medicines that inhibit these enzymes to prevent patients from accumulating excess levels of the experimental therapy.[10] Other trials exclude patients with poor function or prior events related to specific organs if there is already evidence of organ-specific toxicity or other worrisome pharmacologic properties from preclinical studies or prior trials. The most common scenarios involve kidney, liver, and heart toxicity. In the last category, many cancer drugs and other therapies increase the risk of arrhythmias by prolonging the QT interval, which is the time it takes for the heart to fire an electrical impulse through the ventricles and then recover.[11,12] Preclinical evidence showed that the tyrosine kinase inhibitor vandetanib (Caprelsa; Sanofi) induced QT prolongation in dogs, and some subsequent clinical trials attempted to mitigate the risk of sudden cardiac death by excluding patients on "current therapy with any medication known to be associated with Torsades de pointes," the most severe clinical manifestation of QT interval prolongation.[13,14]

Other exclusions based on laboratory values, multiple co-morbid medical conditions, or other clinical criteria are also nominally intended to reduce the risk of safety events, although the rationale may be weaker. Restrictions based on laboratory evidence of liver dysfunction (based on liver aspartate aminotransferase [AST] or alanine aminotransferase [ALT] levels) or kidney dysfunction (based on estimated glomerular filtration rate [eGFR] or creatinine clearance [CrCl]) are extremely common in drug trials. These patients may be at higher risk of toxicity from the study drug, even if the dose is adjusted to compensate for their kidney or liver function. However, there is often little evidence behind the cutoffs, and the real-world trade-off of these exclusions is missing the opportunity to learn about the drug's safety and efficacy in these prevalent patient subsets.

for 16- and 17-year-olds because the Comirnaty trials included that age group and others did not.[25,26]

A more complex and common scenario is when a sponsor is forced to choose a study population that either maximizes the drug's commercial opportunity or its odds of success, but not both. That was the situation with pembrolizumab in lung cancer, as discussed earlier, where Merck limited its study to a smaller population enriched for likely responders instead of running a higher-risk trial in a larger population. It successfully leapfrogged Bristol Myers Squibb, which reached the market earlier but lagged commercially after making the opposite strategic choice.[27] A similar example was the Phase 2 RELIEF study of the P2X3 antagonist BLU-5937 (Bellus Health) in chronic cough, initiated in 2019. This trial enrolled patients with a broad range of disease severity, even though an earlier study of another drug in the same class, gefapixant (AF-219/MK-7264; Merck), reported in 2014 that patients with the highest baseline cough frequency drove the vast majority of the response.[28] RELIEF failed to meet its primary endpoint, and a post hoc subset analysis found that, as one might have expected, the most meaningful effect was indeed observed in the most symptomatic patients.[29] The company's follow-up Phase 2b SOOTHE trial initiated in December 2020 focuses exclusively on these higher-severity patients.[30]

Beyond affecting the size of the future addressable market, a trial's patient population also affects how easy or challenging it will be for a company to capture share within that market. The simplest situation is when the drug's label fits seamlessly with established clinical practice guidelines for diagnosis and classification, but the situation can be challenging if the criteria to categorize patients in clinical care are emerging or evolving. In 2007, Ception initiated a Phase 2/3 study of its anti-interleukin-5 treatment, reslizumab (Cinqair), for severe asthma. The trial required that enrolled patients have a biopsy showing a high level of allergic inflammation, defined as at least 24 eosinophils per high-powered microscopic field.[31] But that same year, an expert consensus group formally defined the disease based on a lower threshold of only 15 eosinophils per high-powered field.[32] The reslizumab study failed,[33] but if it had been successful, it most likely would have led to disagreements in the field about which cutoff to use for subsequent studies and difficulties comparing across trials using different inclusion criteria.

A similar situation arose with immune checkpoint inhibitors in non-small cell lung cancer, where different companies' studies used different assays and cutoffs for PD-L1 expression as part of their inclusion criteria. As a result, there was confusion among clinicians and laboratory personnel about how to determine which patients were potentially eligible for which therapies. Although some progress has been made in benchmarking these assays against one another,[34] the situation is still evolving and may continue to affect the uptake of some of these drugs in certain regions.

Importantly, although Phase 1 and 2 trials may use various unapproved and experimental tests to define the study population, any test that will be used in a pivotal study needs to be approved and available at the same time as the new therapy. A full discussion of the regulatory and commercial issues related to companion diagnostics is beyond our scope here, but is covered in FDA guidance documents[35,36,37] and other sources.[38]

Predictive and prognostic biomarkers

Many clinical trials use some sort of diagnostic test to select whom to include or exclude or to define patient segments within the studied population. We can refer to all these objective tests as "patient selection biomarkers," regardless of whether the assessment is based on laboratory, imaging, clinical, or other techniques. Importantly, these are different from biomarkers that are assayed as surrogate endpoints to assess a drug's efficacy. The differences between patient selection and efficacy biomarkers, as well as technical aspects of how they are validated, are covered in depth in several review articles.[39,40]

There are two types of patient selection biomarkers that are important to appreciate—predictive and prognostic:

- **Predictive biomarkers:** Most trials of so-called targeted therapies or personalized medicines use predictive biomarkers to identify patients who are more likely to benefit from the experimental therapy. Going back to an earlier example, an inhibitor of the EGFR receptor tyrosine kinase is expected to act mainly or exclusively against tumors that depend on EGFR signaling for growth or progression. So if one wants to enrich a trial for likely responders, it would make logical sense to select patients only if their cancers express high levels of EGFR or hyperactivated forms of it while excluding patients whose tumors do not express this biomarker.

- **Prognostic biomarkers:** In contrast, prognostic biomarkers can be used to identify patients with a particular course of disease progression, independent of the experimental therapy. For example, in a chronic, progressive disease, it might be advantageous to know which patients are "slow progressors" and which are "fast progressors." Testing a new drug in fast progressors might make it feasible to detect a clinical effect more quickly. Importantly, prognostic biomarkers in clinical trials are often unrelated to a specific drug's mechanism of action.

A common challenge in clinical trials is when a biomarker has or might have both predictive and prognostic implications. Selpercatinib (Retevmo; Lilly) was approved in 2020 for RET fusion-positive lung and thyroid cancer based on results from single-arm studies in patients selected for expression of RET.[41] But RET positivity in lung cancer may also identify a subgroup of patients with longer survival than those without it.[42] In the absence of knowing how these patients perform with standard of care, it's impossible to conclusively interpret results from single-arm trials, although in this particular case, the ambiguity didn't stop regulators from approving the drug or oncologists from prescribing it. It also complicates the design of future controlled trials because power and sample size calculations depend on accurate predictions of the likely control arm performance and therapeutic effect size.

---

[1] Dry eye: Developing drugs for treatment: Guidance for industry (draft guidance). U.S. Food and Drug Administration. December 2020.

[2] 22 case studies where Phase 2 and Phase 3 trials had divergent results. U.S. Food and Drug Administration. January 2017.

[3] Martinez-Marti A, Navarro A, Felip E. Epidermal growth factor receptor first generation tyrosine-kinase inhibitors. Transl Lung Cancer Res. 2019 Nov;8(Suppl 3):S235–S246. doi: 10.21037/tlcr.2019.04.20. PMID: 31857948; PMCID: PMC6894987.

[4] Palmer E. BMS loses its lung cancer lead to Merck as Opdivo data come up short. FiercePharma. August 5, 2016. https://www.fiercepharma.com/pharma/bms-sees-reversal-fortunes-merck-as-opdivo-comes-up-short-trial. Accessed November 23, 2021.

[5] Cappuzzo F, Ciuleanu T, Stelmakh L, Cicenas S, Szczésna A, Juhász E, Esteban E, Molinier O, Brugger W, Melezínek I, Klingelschmitt G, Klughammer B, Giaccone G; SATURN investigators. Erlotinib as maintenance treatment in advanced non-small-cell lung cancer: a multicentre, randomised, placebo-controlled phase 3 study. Lancet Oncol. 2010 Jun;11(6):521–529. doi: 10.1016/S1470-2045(10)70112-1. Epub 2010 May 20. PMID: 20493771.

[6] Cohen AT, Harrington RA, Goldhaber SZ, Hull RD, Wiens BL, Gold A, Hernandez AF, Gibson CM; APEX Investigators. Extended thromboprophylaxis with betrixaban in acutely ill medical patients. N Engl J Med. 2016 Aug 11;375(6):534–544. doi: 10.1056/NEJMoa1601747. Epub 2016 May 27. PMID: 27232649.

[7] Sierra announces promising preliminary efficacy in SRA737 clinical program and outlines potential path to registration. Sierra Oncology press release. June 1, 2019. https://investor.sierraoncology.com/news-releases/news-details/2019/Sierra-Announces-Promising-Preliminary-Efficacy-in-SRA737-Clinical-Program--Outlines-Potential-Path-to-Registration/default.aspx. Accessed October 15, 2021. Permalink: https://perma.cc/35KS-WZ4K.

[8] Sierra Oncology (SRRA). Form 10-Q for quarterly period ending June 30, 2019. https://www.sec.gov/Archives/edgar/data/0001290149/000119312519216008/d765310d10q.htm.

[9] Sierra Oncology launches campaign exploring non-dilutive strategic options to support development of its DDR assets. Sierra Oncology press release. June 27, 2019. https://investor.sierraoncology.com/news-releases/news-details/2019/Sierra-Oncology-Launches-Campaign-Exploring-Non-Dilutive-Strategic-Options-to-Support-Development-of-its-DDR-Assets/default.aspx. Accessed October 15, 2021. Permalink: https://perma.cc/84BU-84Y3.

[10] Lynch T, Price A. The effect of cytochrome P450 metabolism on drug response, interactions, and adverse effects. Am Fam Physician. 2007 Aug 1;76(3):391–396. PMID: 17708140.

[11] Lester RM, Paglialunga S, Johnson IA. QT Assessment in early drug development: The long and the short of it. Int J Mol Sci. 2019 Mar 15;20(6):1324. doi: 10.3390/ijms20061324. PMID: 30884748; PMCID: PMC6471571.

[12] Moslehi JJ. Cardiovascular toxic effects of targeted cancer therapies. N Engl J Med. 2016 Oct 13;375(15):1457–1467. doi: 10.1056/NEJMra1100265. PMID: 27732808.

[13] Thornton K, Kim G, Maher VE, Chattopadhyay S, Tang S, Moon YJ, Song P, Marathe A, Balakrishnan S, Zhu H, Garnett C, Liu Q, Booth B, Gehrke B, Dorsam R, Verbois L, Ghosh D, Wilson W, Duan J, Sarker H, Miksinski SP, Skarupa L, Ibrahim A, Justice R, Murgo A, Pazdur R. Vandetanib for the treatment of symptomatic or progressive medullary thyroid cancer in patients with unresectable locally advanced or metastatic disease: U.S. Food and Drug Administration drug approval summary. Clin Cancer Res. 2012 Jul 15;18(14):3722–3730. doi: 10.1158/1078-0432.CCR-12-0411. Epub 2012 Jun 4. PMID: 22665903.

[14] Evaluation of efficacy, safety of vandetanib in patients with differentiated thyroid cancer (VERIFY). ClinicalTrials.gov identifier: NCT01876784. Updated April 9, 2021. Accessed October 15, 2021.

[15] Enrichment strategies for clinical trials to support determination of effectiveness of human drugs and biological products: Guidance for industry. U.S. Food and Drug Administration. March 2019.

[16] Kirby S, Burke J, Chuang-Stein C, Sin C. Discounting Phase 2 results when planning Phase 3 clinical trials. Pharm Stat. 2012 Sep–Oct;11(5):373–385. doi: 10.1002/pst.1521. Epub 2012 May 29. PMID: 22641524.

[17] Indications and usage section of labeling for human prescription drug and biological products—content and format: Guidance for industry (draft guidance). U.S. Food and Drug Administration. July 2018.

[18] Canevelli M, Rossi PD, Astrone P, Consorti E, Vanacore N, Cesari M. "Real world" eligibility for aducanumab. J Am Geriatr Soc. 2021 Oct;69(10):2995–2998. doi: 10.1111/jgs.17390. Epub 2021 Jul 31. PMID: 34331706.

[19] Evaluating inclusion and exclusion criteria in clinical trials. Duke-Margolis Center for Health Policy. National Press Club, April 16, 2018. https://healthpolicy.duke.edu/sites/default/files/2020-03/master_slide_deck_presenter_slides2.pdf. Accessed October 15, 2021. Permalink: https://perma.cc/R2CA-ARUR.

[20] Sequist LV, Yang JC, Yamamoto N, O'Byrne K, Hirsh V, Mok T, Geater SL, Orlov S, Tsai CM, Boyer M, Su WC, Bennouna J, Kato T, Gorbunova V, Lee KH, Shah R, Massey D, Zazulina V, Shahidi M, Schuler M. Phase III study of afatinib or cisplatin plus pemetrexed in patients with metastatic lung adenocarcinoma with EGFR mutations. J Clin Oncol. 2013 Sep 20;31(27):3327–3334. doi: 10.1200/JCO.2012.44.2806. Epub 2013 Jul 1. PMID: 23816960.

[21] Sumi E, Asada R, Lu Y, Ito-Ihara T, Grimes KV. A qualitative study on the differences between trial populations and the approved therapeutic indications of antineoplastic agents by 3 regulatory agencies from 2010 to 2018. Clin Ther. 2020 Feb;42(2):305–320.e0. doi: 10.1016/j.clinthera.2020.01.002. Epub 2020 Jan 31. PMID: 32008723.

[22] Xigris [package insert]. Eli Lilly. November 2001. https://s3-us-west-2.amazonaws.com/drugbank/fda_labels/DB00055.pdf. Accessed October 15, 2021. Permalink: https://perma.cc/X6AH-PFBL.

[23] A Phase 1/2 open-label dose-escalation study to evaluate safety, tolerability, pharmacokinetics, and efficacy of intracerebroventricular BMN 190 in patients with late-infantile neuronal ceroid lipofuscinosis (CLN2) disease. ClinicalTrials.gov identifier: NCT01907087. Updated March 8, 2019. Accessed October 15, 2021.

[24] Brineura [package insert]. BioMarin Pharmaceutical. April 2017. https://www.accessdata.fda.gov/drugsatfda_docs/label/2017/761052lbl.pdf. Accessed October 15, 2021. Permalink: https://perma.cc/4K46-6M5X.

[25] Weiland N, LaFraniere S, Mandavilli A. The F.D.A. is set to authorize the Pfizer-BioNTech vaccine for those 12–15 years old by early next week. New York Times. May 3, 2021. https://www.nytimes.com/live/2021/05/03/world/covid-vaccine-coronavirus-cases/pfizer-covid-vaccine-teens. Accessed October 15, 2021.

[26] Comirnaty [package insert]. Pfizer/BioNTech. August 2021. https://www.fda.gov/media/151707/download. Accessed October 15, 2021. Permalink: https://perma.cc/7Q3D-3Z6K.

[27] LaMotta L. How biomarkers cost Bristol-Myers the lung cancer market. BioPharma Dive. February 13, 2017. https://www.biopharmadive.com/news/biomarkers-bristol-myers-opdivo-lost-lung-cancer/435891/. Accessed November 23, 2021.

[28] Abdulqawi R, Dockry R, Holt K, Layton G, McCarthy BG, Ford AP, Smith JA. P2X3 receptor antagonist (AF-219) in refractory chronic cough: A randomised, double-blind, placebo-controlled phase 2 study. Lancet. 2015 Mar 28;385(9974):1198–1205. doi: 10.1016/S0140-6736(14)61255-1. Epub 2014 Nov 25. PMID: 25467586.

[29] Bellus Health. BLU-5937: RELIEF Phase 2 topline data (investor presentation). July 6, 2020. https://ir.bellushealth.com/static-files/bbafa076-4bba-42aa-b905-db56f7ee036d. Accessed October 15, 2021. Permalink: https://perma.cc/W4BV-WB3M.

[30] Bellus Health announces first patient dosed in its Phase 2b SOOTHE trial of BLU-5937 for the treatment of refractory chronic cough. Bellus Health press prelease. December 8, 2020. https://ir.bellushealth.com/news-releases/news-release-details/bellus-health-announces-first-patient-dosed-its-phase-2b-soothe. Accessed October 15, 2021. Permalink: https://perma.cc/GY24-8PCL.

[31] Efficacy and safety study of reslizumab to treat eosinophilic esophagitis in subjects aged 5 to 18 years. ClinicalTrials.gov identifier: NCT00538434. Updated September 2, 2016. Accessed October 15, 2021.

[32] Furuta GT, Liacouras CA, Collins MH, Gupta SK, Justinich C, Putnam PE, Bonis P, Hassall E, Straumann A, Rothenberg ME; First International Gastrointestinal Eosinophil Research Symposium (FIGERS) Subcommittees. Eosinophilic esophagitis in children and adults: A systematic review and consensus recommendations for diagnosis and treatment. Gastroenterology. 2007 Oct;133(4):1342–1363. doi: 10.1053/j.gastro.2007.08.017. Epub 2007 Aug 8. PMID: 17919504.

[33] Spergel JM, Rothenberg ME, Collins MH, Furuta GT, Markowitz JE, Fuchs G 3rd, O'Gorman MA, Abonia JP, Young J, Henkel T, Wilkins HJ, Liacouras CA. Reslizumab in children and adolescents with eosinophilic esophagitis: Results of a double-blind, randomized, placebo-controlled trial. J Allergy Clin Immunol. 2012 Feb;129(2):456–463, 463.e1-3. doi: 10.1016/j.jaci.2011.11.044. Epub 2011 Dec 28. PMID: 22206777.

[34] Hirsch FR, McElhinny A, Stanforth D, Ranger-Moore J, Jansson M, Kulangara K, Richardson W, Towne P, Hanks D, Vennapusa B, Mistry A, Kalamegham R, Averbuch S, Novotny J, Rubin E, Emancipator K, McCaffery I, Williams JA, Walker J, Longshore J, Tsao MS, Kerr KM. PD-L1 Immunohistochemistry assays for lung cancer: Results from Phase 1 of the Blueprint PD-L1 IHC assay comparison project. J Thorac Oncol. 2017 Feb;12(2):208–222. doi: 10.1016/j.jtho.2016.11.2228. Epub 2016 Nov 29. PMID: 27913228.

[35] In vitro companion diagnostic devices: Guidance for industry and Food and Drug Administration staff. U.S. Food and Drug Administration. August 6, 2014.

[36] Principles for codevelopment of an in vitro companion diagnostic device with a therapeutic product: Draft guidance for industry and Food and Drug Administration staff. U.S. Food and Drug Administration. July 15, 2016.

[37] Developing and labeling in vitro companion diagnostic devices for a specific group of oncology therapeutic products. U.S. Food and Drug Administration. April 2020.

[38] Pothier KC. *Personalizing Precision Medicine: A Global Voyage from Vision to Reality.* 1st ed. Wiley; 2017.

[39] Kraus VB. Biomarkers as drug development tools: Discovery, validation, qualification and use. Nat Rev Rheumatol. 2018 Jun;14(6):354–362. doi: 10.1038/s41584-018-0005-9. PMID: 29760435.

[40] Holland RL. What makes a good biomarker? Adv Precision Med. 2016;1(1):66–77. doi: 10.18063/APM.2016.01.007.

[41] FDA approves selpercatinib for lung and thyroid cancers with RET gene mutations or fusions. U.S. FDA press release. May 11, 2020. https://www.fda.gov/drugs/drug-approvals-and-databases/fda-approves-selpercatinib-lung-and-thyroid-cancers-ret-gene-mutations-or-fusions. Accessed October 15, 2021. Permalink: https://perma.cc/9SSZ-MY3L.

[42] Sireci A, Hess LM, Han Y, Zhu YE, Bhandari NR, Martinez R. Clinical outcomes between patients with and without RET fusions in advanced/metastatic non-small cell lung cancer in the United States. J Clin Oncol. 2020 May 25;38(15 suppl):e21693. doi: 10.1200/JCO.2020.38.15_suppl.e21693.

4.

STUDY DESIGN

UNTIL ABOUT 2010, most book chapters and articles on evaluating the design of clinical studies had two main sections: randomized controlled trials and everything else. For regulators and practicing physicians, randomized controlled trials (RCTs) have long been the gold standard for evidence-based medicine, while non-RCTs, typically conducted in early stages of drug development, were mainly of interest to R&D insiders and other aficionados.

But in the modern era, there is increased interest in a broader range of trial designs. Particularly in cancer and rare diseases, non-RCTs are increasingly used to assess efficacy in early-stage studies and even to obtain full or accelerated regulatory approval. This makes them of greater relevance to industry watchers and investors as well as to practicing physicians who are increasingly forced to incorporate data from non-RCTs into clinical decision-making.

In this chapter, we group interventional drug trials into three categories based on their main purpose and the presence or absence of randomization and internal controls: RCTs, unblinded studies, and studies without internal controls. We also cover several additional topics related to trial design that cut across multiple study types. Adaptive trials are covered separately in Chapter 15. Note that our focus is on interventional trials, and although observational studies sometimes contribute to drug development after a therapy is already approved for an initial indication, we do not discuss them here.

Randomized controlled trials

Despite evolving standards in drug R&D and regulation, RCTs remain the most common and most widely accepted design for studies intended to demonstrate the efficacy of a new agent. RCTs include three key elements: randomization, blinding, and assignment of some patients to a comparator arm that does not receive the investigational therapy. Although a randomized controlled trial could be run with or without blinding, in this book we use the term "RCT" to refer to blinded studies only, and we discuss unblinded studies separately. For several good reasons, RCTs are still the gold standard for assessing the efficacy of an intervention:

- **Comparator arm:** The inclusion of a comparator arm in a study allows one to isolate the effect of the new treatment and conclude that any observed difference is due solely to the patient having received it as opposed to the alternative. Without this, the only way to evaluate whether the new drug had an effect is to compare it with a so-called external control, such as historical data from prior studies or a matched sample taken from medical records of patients treated in the real world. As discussed later, these are both valid approaches in some clinical scenarios, but they are less precise than internal controls, and they introduce uncertainty in defining the effect size.
- **Randomization:** Randomization between the study arms significantly reduces bias when assessing a novel treatment. Imagine, for example, a trial of a new cancer drug in which half the patients will receive the investigational agent and the others will receive a placebo (an inactive control group). Without random assignment of the subjects, the study physician could—either intentionally or subconsciously—put healthier patients in the active treatment arm and sicker ones in the placebo group. This could lead to finding an apparent efficacy advantage for the new drug even if it actually had no effect.
- **Blinding:** Finally, even if a study includes a comparator and patients are randomly assigned, the most unbiased trials are those in which neither the physicians nor the patients are aware of whether the patient is receiving the experimental drug or the control. If blinding is compromised, either intentionally, accidentally, or subconsciously, the treating

physician might alter the use of ancillary interventions, dosage, or advice to continue the trial based on whether the patient is receiving the new therapy. Unblinding can also affect how endpoints are measured and reported. This is a particular issue with patient-reported outcomes like mood or pain level, but it can also bias the measurement of more "objective" endpoints. For example, the results of pulmonary function tests and the six-minute walk test are highly dependent on effort and thus highly sensitive to the amount of encouragement that the patient receives during the test. This could change if the person administering the test knows the assignment.

Comparator arm

The choice of comparator is one of the most hotly contested aspects of many clinical trials because it has a direct impact on the study's design and execution, the interpretation and impact of the results, and its regulatory and commercial success. For example, the May 2020 approval of olaparib (Lynparza; AstraZeneca) for a subset of prostate cancer patients was based on a study of patients who had progressed after treatment with enzalutamide (Xtandi; Pfizer/Astellas) or abiraterone (Zytiga; Janssen), two commonly used first-line anti-androgen therapies.[1] However, patients in the control arm were permitted to receive only the physician's choice of either enzalutamide or abiraterone, even though they had already been treated with one or both agents. They were not allowed to receive a taxane, which might have been an effective third option. This choice of control was criticized for skewing the study in favor of olaparib and not being relevant to real-world clinical practice.[2]

There are three basic choices of comparators in RCTs, each with its own advantages and challenges:

- **Active comparator:** This is often a sensible and informative choice if there is an approved and at least somewhat effective therapy available. However, the specific choice of comparator is rarely straightforward, and various options may satisfy the needs of physicians and patients, regulators, and commercial sponsors differently. A 2020 analysis found that a quarter of recent U.S. Food and Drug Administration (FDA) approvals of anti-cancer drugs were based on trials that used "suboptimal controls" that excluded potentially beneficial therapies.[3] Not only does this pose an ethical challenge, but it can also make it difficult to interpret the relevance of the results.

From a study design standpoint, an active comparator sets the height of the bar that the new drug needs to surmount, which affects the probability of obtaining a positive result as well as the study size. It can also significantly increase the execution cost of a trial if it needs to be purchased for study participants.

- **Placebo control:** Though often viewed as the sine qua non of RCTs for new drugs, in clinical areas that already have accepted treatments, a placebo-controlled trial does not directly answer the most clinically relevant question of how a new drug's efficacy and safety compare with those of existing options. In addition, placebo controls pose ethical challenges if patients are denied access to an accepted and effective standard of care.[4]

  The so-called placebo effect, in which patients appear to respond to a biologically inert therapy, is often invoked in trials in depression and other psychiatric indications, but this term is frequently misused. A bona fide response to a placebo that exceeds what would have been seen with no treatment at all is extremely uncommon except in assessments of patient-reported outcomes, especially pain.[5] In other clinical areas, a higher-than-expected response rate in the placebo arm is more likely due to the natural variability in disease course or measured parameter, or the use of an imprecise measurement tool.[6,7] Regardless, the takeaway for readers of clinical studies is that one should not automatically assume that the effect in a placebo-control arm will be negligible without first reviewing published results to assess the historical response rate to inert comparators.

- **"Real-world options":** Some trials are designed to test the performance of a new therapy against various existing options for the patients under study, which may include so-called investigator's choice of available agents or, in the case of patients who lack effective treatment options, best supportive care. As noted in the introductory example, however, investigators' options in the control arm are sometimes restricted to a handful of choices, which may affect the study's relevance to clinical practice. On the other hand, allowing a very broad range of active treatments in the control arm may increase variability and uncertainty in the study and compromise the statistical planning.

In late-stage trials, the choice of control may be heavily influenced by policies of regulators and market access authorities. The FDA in principle accepts placebo, other doses of the experimental agent, no treatment, active treatment, and historical results as comparators.[8] But in practice the agency may view certain choices more or less favorably depending on the clinical scenario, the results obtained, and discussions between the sponsor and the agency before the trial. China's National Medical Products Administration recommended in 2021 draft guidance that cancer drugs use best standard of care as a control for registrational studies, but several experts believe this is mainly aimed at explicitly preventing "me-too" competitors from using outdated comparators.[9] And on the pricing front, health technology assessment (HTA) agencies tend to prefer clinically relevant active comparators over other options.

Randomization

Clinical trials of new drugs typically use centralized computer- or phone-based methods to randomly assign patients across all study sites. Most publications of industry-sponsored trials describe the exact randomization method, but detailed information is rarely disclosed in conference proceedings, press releases, or investor presentations.

For readers of clinical trial results, it is impossible to determine whether randomization was undermined. As discussed in Chapter 6 on trial execution, even when apparent imbalances of baseline characteristics between patients in different trial arms are identified, they are assumed to have arisen by chance. Notwithstanding the theoretical risk that investigators could non-randomly assign patients to trial arms in an attempt to influence the study's outcome, we have been unable to identify even a single confirmed example of compromised randomization from an industry-sponsored trial that claimed to be an RCT.

When there are prognostic factors that are known to be highly likely to affect patients' outcomes or adverse events in a trial, RCTs often use **stratified randomization** to ensure that the study arms are balanced with regard to such factors.[10,11] For example, a Phase 2/3 study of Pfizer/BioNTech's COVID-19 vaccine in 2020 stratified enrollees by age into two groups, 18–55 and over 55, which were later revised to three groups, 12–15, 16–54, and 55 and older.[12] This approach maintains randomization between drug and placebo while ensuring that the arms will remain balanced with regard to the parameter of interest. It can also facilitate pre-planned subgroup analyses by allowing sponsors to ensure that subsets of interest are of sufficient size, as Pfizer/BioNTech did by targeting 40% of enrollment in the oldest stratum.

Stratification is particularly helpful in studies that have fewer than 100 patients and trials with planned interim analyses of small groups because the risk of chance imbalances in meaningful characteristics is higher when fewer patients are randomized. But in these cases, investigators need to be judicious in choosing stratification factors as each subgroup needs to have a reasonable number of patients for the analysis to work. Most studies with stratification incorporate fewer than three factors, and trials with five or more are extremely uncommon.

Blinding

Most protocol reports, press releases, meeting presentations, and research papers related to RCTs will explicitly state whether the study was double-blinded, single-blinded, or unblinded. Double blinding means that neither the physician nor the patient knows the treatment arm assignment. Single blinding typically means that the physician is aware, but the patient is not.[13] Although double-blinded studies are more complex and expensive to execute, they are the most rigorous and freest of bias. When blinding is compromised, this may affect how patients respond to therapy due to physiological and psychological factors. It can also change how patients report subjective outcomes like mood or amount of pain, their level of compliance, and their desire to continue participating in the trial. Similarly, unblinding can affect investigators' propensity to administer ancillary treatments, adjust the dose, remove patients from the study, encourage or discourage continuation, and assess outcomes.[14]

Double blinding can be technically challenging in some situations. If a head-to-head study with an active comparator includes agents with different dosing formulations, like an intravenous drug versus an oral one, or a tablet versus a capsule, methods like the double-dummy approach, described later in this chapter, may be needed to prevent physicians or patients from becoming effectively unblinded. Similarly, trials that require patients in one arm to receive an interventional procedure may necessitate requiring the control arm to receive a sham, or inactive, intervention to maintain blinding.[15] Previous studies of percutaneous coronary stenting to reduce patient-reported pain in stable angina yielded positive results, but only one arm received an intervention. When the ORBITA trial explored this question with a sham control as reported in 2017, stenting did not demonstrate an advantage.[16]

Even in a double-blinded RCT of two drugs with the same route of administration, there is a risk of bias from unintentional unblinding if the assignment can be deduced. A relatively common scenario is when one treatment has a characteristic side effect. In trials of first-generation antipsychotics for schizophrenia, it was relatively easy for patients who experienced classic symptoms like involuntary movements of the face, neck, and mouth (tardive dyskinesia) to conclude that they were receiving the active drug.[17] A theoretical concern about trials investigating the effect of a cannabis-based therapy, nabiximols (Sativex; GW Pharmaceuticals), on patient-reported spasticity in multiple sclerosis was that patients in the active therapy arm might know their assignment due to the psychoactive side effects of cannabis and overreport the drug's efficacy. In this case, however, this possibility of bias was formally tested in 2012 by independent investigators and found to be insignificant.[18] Finally, some clinical trial experts have noted that there is an increased incidence of patients using social media to try to determine their treatment assignments.[19]

Unblinded studies

Many studies have control arms and incorporate randomization, but differ from RCTs in their lack of blinding. For sponsors, these "open-label" comparative studies can be much easier to execute. For example, in trials comparing drugs with very different dosage forms, like oral anticoagulants versus subcutaneously injected low-molecular-weight heparin, a blinded RCT requires a double-dummy approach, discussed later in this chapter, which is complicated and expensive. Although some new oral anticoagulants have been tested in this manner, others have been studied in open-label trials.[20]

Unblinding can bias study results, usually in favor of the experimental agent. However, the degree of impact is unpredictable and highly variable. One systematic review that compared studies with blinded and unblinded assessments of the same binary outcome found an average 36% overestimation of the effect size due to unblinding.[21] However, a small analysis of cancer drugs that had been studied both in open-label trials and in RCTs found no difference in the degree of improvement in patient-reported outcomes. This suggests that patients' knowledge of their assignment may not have had as dramatic an effect on how they reported symptoms in those studies as one might have expected.[22]

In general, the best approach to analyzing results from open-label, controlled studies is to keep two considerations in mind. First, one can broadly define the degree of concern about an open-label study by methodically assessing the possible ways unblinding could affect the results. All else being equal, open-label studies with a high degree of patient and physician control over trial execution and endpoint assessment are most concerning. Second, although the magnitude of the effect may vary, there is no denying that open-label studies are more vulnerable to yielding over-exuberant results than blinded RCTs and thus reflect a "best-case" result in virtually all scenarios.

Trials without internal controls

Particularly in rare diseases and oncology, many Phase 2 and 3 studies do not include a control arm. The main rationale commonly given for performing a single-arm efficacy study is that it is too expensive or flatly not feasible to identify and recruit enough patients for an RCT. (We use "single-arm" here to include all studies that lack internal controls, including those that test multiple doses of the experimental therapy in different arms.) As single-arm studies have become more accepted by physicians and regulators, they have become increasingly common. From 2015 to 2017, 17% of FDA approvals were based only on single-arm pivotal trials, mostly in the context of accelerated or conditional pathways,[23] as discussed in more detail below.

In infrequent scenarios, when current outcomes are dismal and an experimental therapy is highly effective, it may be relatively straightforward to conclude that a single-arm study was successful based on a cursory comparison with historical results. In hepatitis C, uncontrolled trials supported approval for several interferon-free regimens based on cure rates of more than 90% compared with documented efficacies below 50% with prior therapies.[24] Similarly, the CAR-T therapy axicabtagene ciloleucel (Yescarta; Kite Pharma [acquired by Gilead]) was approved in 2017 for relapsed or refractory large B-cell lymphoma based on a single-arm trial in which about 80% of patients experienced responses, including more than 50% with complete remissions, compared with historical data showing a response rate of <30% and a complete remission rate of <15%.[25]

But more often, the improvement afforded by a new drug is less dramatic, and it is difficult to evaluate its efficacy from a trial that lacks an internal comparator. A single-arm study in 2014 of the CD19/CD3 bispecific antibody blinatumomab (Blincyto; Amgen) in Philadelphia chromosome-negative precursor B-cell acute lymphoblastic leukemia yielded a 41.6% complete remission rate in relapsed/refractory patients, but this was on par with the best published results with cytotoxic chemotherapy.[26,27] Nonetheless, on the basis of a comparison with a pool of matched historical patients in existing databases, the FDA granted accelerated approval later that year. In this case, possible concerns about the drug's efficacy were alleviated when its superiority over chemotherapy was directly confirmed in 2017 in the head-to-head TOWER trial.[28]

A similar problem arises with uncontrolled trials of combinations of two active therapies, which are particularly common in immuno-oncology studies of new drugs as add-ons to approved checkpoint inhibitors (CPIs). Although many of these trials recruit patients whose tumors recurred after CPI therapy or never responded in the first place, in some analyses as many as 28% of patients who progress on CPIs subsequently respond to continued therapy.[29,30] Thus, it can be hard to know whether promising efficacy of a combination in a single-arm study is due to the new agent or the backbone drug.

The blinatumomab example above illustrates the main solution to the problem of how to evaluate efficacy in single-arm studies: compare the patients on the treatment arm with data from outside the clinical trial.[31] There are three main sources of external comparators that sponsors use to put single-arm data in context:

- **Published comparators:** These are most often derived from examining either the control arms from journal reports of RCTs of other therapies or outcomes from observational case series.
- **Natural history data:** This typically comes from ongoing disease-specific registries or patients identified through electronic medical records.
- **Patient-level data from control arms of completed studies:** Sponsors that have previously run RCTs in a particular therapeutic area can sometimes access such information.

For readers of single-arm studies, it is important to understand the details underlying the external comparator and the analytic methods to determine how much weight to assign to positive findings:

- **Are the comparator data at the level of individual patients?** Published RCTs or case series may include patients who are very different from those in the current single-arm study in terms of baseline characteristics. Without access to patient-level data, it is impossible to correct for this imbalance, and comparisons should be interpreted with caution.

  Conceptually, this is a particular issue for biomarker-defined subsets of oncology indications if published data did not explicitly assess outcomes in this specific sub-population.[32] When first-generation EGFR inhibitors were initially developed, it was not known that patients with EGFR-mutant non-small cell lung cancer live longer even without receiving targeted therapy. Thus, a hypothetical single-arm study in this population at that time would not have been capable of separating a drug's therapeutic value from the inherently better survival odds of these patients. The specific topic of predictive versus prognostic biomarkers is also discussed in Chapter 3 on the patient population. Note that this challenge, while significant, is not necessarily impactful in the modern regulatory environment, where many oncology drugs receive accelerated approval on the basis of single-arm results in biomarker-defined subsets, without any formal patient-level comparison to external data.
- **Have patient-level data been adjusted for baseline imbalances?** Patient-level data derived from another source can be used to generate an external control arm (ECA, also known as "synthetic control arm") that can be analyzed versus the experimental arm using the same basic statistical tools that one would use in an RCT. In contrast to published data, an analysis based on an ECA can—and should—take into account imbalances in baseline characteristics that could potentially affect the outcome. Investigators use methods like matching, covariate adjustment, and stratification to ensure that the ECA population is comparable to the patients included in the single-arm study.
- **How do historical data compare with contemporary data?** Historical findings may not be well suited for comparing to a current single-arm study if treatments and outcomes are ill-defined or evolving. The Phase

3 SIMPLE trial in severe COVID-19 in 2020 included two arms testing different durations of treatment with Gilead's remdesivir but did not include a control.[33] The challenge of assessing the drug's efficacy was compounded by the fact that clinical management of the patients with ventilation and other interventions was evolving in real time. From a practical standpoint, the shortcomings of SIMPLE were rendered moot by a concurrent placebo-controlled RCT, ACTT-1, which yielded positive data a month later[34] and formed the basis of the FDA's approval shortly thereafter.[35]

In addition to evaluating the nature of the comparator population and the analytic approach, readers should consider how the context in which a single-arm study was or is being conducted influences the standards to which it will be held:

- **Single-arm studies for R&D decision-making:** In oncology, multiple analyses in the early 2000s showed that positive results from single-arm Phase 2 studies were poor predictors of success in Phase 3.[36] Most of these historical examples used published articles to contextualize the results seen with the experimental therapy, as opposed to external control arms derived from patient-level data, and even today it is still extremely common to see sponsors deem a single-arm Phase 2 study "successful" and meriting advancement into Phase 3 based on a comparison with published results. As noted above, results from this sort of comparison are difficult to interpret and should generally be viewed as providing weaker evidence of efficacy than either single-arm studies using ECAs or bona fide RCTs.
- **Single-arm studies for regulatory approval:** As enumerated in several recent review articles,[37,38] the FDA and European Medicines Agency (EMA) have granted multiple initial approvals since 2000 based on single-arm studies, often on an accelerated or conditional basis pending the completion of confirmatory RCTs. At the time of writing, there are no examples in oncology where an ECA contributed to a positive regulatory decision, and several cases where a submitted ECA was found lacking. In 2019, sponsors of three cancer drugs—selinexor (Xpovio; Karyopharm), erdafitinib (Balversa; Janssen), and entrectinib (Rozlytrek;

Genentech)—submitted single-arm data to the FDA demonstrating promising response rates, bolstered by comparisons with ECAs. In each case, the drug was granted accelerated approval, but the sponsor was required to conduct confirmatory studies before obtaining full approval because the agency found fault with the methodology employed to compare single-arm results with external data, such as how baseline imbalances were handled.[39]

In non-oncologic rare diseases, regulators have been more permissive and granted many full initial approvals based on single-arm studies with ECAs.[40,41] The FDA granted full approval to onasemnogene abeparvovec-xioi (Zolgensma; AveXis [acquired by Novartis]) in 2019 for spinal muscular atrophy based in part on a comparison between results from a 21-patient single-arm Phase 3 study and 23 patients with similar genetic backgrounds identified from two existing natural history databases.[42,43] It is likely that the FDA required the sponsor to adjust for baseline imbalances between the trial population and the ECA, although this cannot be explicitly confirmed from publicly disclosed documents.

Finally, there may be future options to conduct registration-enabling studies that use control data derived from a combination of both internal and external sources. In 2020, Medicenna reported that it had obtained positive feedback from the FDA on its planned Phase 3 RCT of MDNA55, an IL-4-guided toxin, in recurrent glioblastoma.[44] Under the proposed design, the 200-patient study would randomize patients 3:1 to the experimental therapy or standard of care, and supplement the analysis with a matched ECA to obtain balance between the two arms.[45] The stated intention of the design was to reduce the time and cost of the study and also decrease the number of patients assigned to standard of care. At the time of writing, the Phase 3 study did not appear to have been initiated.

Open-label extensions after Phase 3 RCTs

Many Phase 3 RCTs are followed by an open-label extension, in which patients are permitted to switch from the control to the experimental agent. These unblinded, single-arm studies are typically performed for one or more of three reasons[46]:

- **Provide access to novel, unapproved medicines to all study participants:** This is a commonly invoked rationale in serious indications without effective therapies. The FDA encourages sponsors to consider open-label extensions in rare disease studies.[47]

- **Assess safety and tolerability over a longer time period:** Properly designed open-label extensions can theoretically detect rare but pharmacologically expected adverse events, although they are typically too small to detect unpredictable safety issues that have led to withdrawals of marketed drugs.[48] These trials can also provide data on long-term treatment compliance and discontinuation rates, which can be particularly important for chronic primary care therapies.
- **Assess efficacy over a longer time period:** Some open-label extensions of positive RCTs are intended to demonstrate that efficacy lasts beyond the duration of the original study, which can be particularly important for single-treatment interventions like gene therapy.

Quantifying efficacy from open-label extensions can be extremely problematic. Compared with single-arm studies, these extensions are biased not just due to the lack of blinding but also because enrollment in the extension phase may be non-random and thus skew the characteristics of participating patients.[49] Furthermore, because open-label extensions tend to be long, they often have substantial dropout, which can further complicate the analysis. (See the sections on patient accounting in Chapter 6 and intention-to-treat analyses in Chapter 7.)

Despite these challenges, investigators and sponsors often make efficacy claims based on open-label extensions that may not be fully justified given the limitations of these studies. A Phase 2 RCT of Catabasis's edasalonexent in Duchenne muscular dystrophy (MoveDMD) failed to achieve its primary endpoint, but the sponsor asserted in 2017 that an open-label extension that enrolled 14 of the original 31 patients demonstrated "clinically meaningful evidence" that the drug slowed the rate of clinical decline, based on a qualitative comparison with a hypothetical "projected score."[50,51] The company subsequently initiated a Phase 3 RCT, PolarisDMD, which failed to meet its primary or secondary endpoints.[52]

Finally, open-label extensions create a particular issue for interpreting results from oncology studies that assess overall survival (OS). This topic is discussed in the section on one-way crossover trials.

Non-inferiority studies

Most comparative studies of new drugs are designed to test whether an experimental agent is *superior* to a control agent by more than a given amount. However, non-inferiority trials instead aim to determine whether a new therapy is *not worse* than an active comparator by more than a pre-specified amount. Their interpretation and design have been discussed in several review articles,[53,54,55,56] as well as reports by the U.S. Government Accountability Office[57] and the FDA.[58]

Non-inferiority designs are mainly appropriate in situations where the new drug needs only to be roughly as good as a standard comparator because it offers other benefits that are independent of efficacy. For example:

- **Different mechanism:** In many bacterial infections, a major goal is to develop new agents that are no worse than existing drugs but have a different spectrum of activity or mechanism of action that might allow them to combat resistant strains in the future. Many new antibacterial agents have been approved on the basis of non-inferiority trials in accordance with FDA guidance.[59,60]
- **Improved tolerability or convenience:** Some new therapies may be intended to offer a different profile with regard to tolerability, convenience, or other factors compared with existing options, with equivalent efficacy. For example, a Phase 3 study in complicated urinary tract infections in 2020 showed that the more-conveniently administered oral tebipenem HBr (Spero) was non-inferior to the intravenous standard of care on the primary endpoint of clinical cure plus microbiologic eradication.[61] Non-inferiority designs are particularly common in trials of non-surgical versus surgical interventions, as in a 2016 study showing that an everolimus-eluting cardiovascular stent (XIENCE; Abbott Vascular) could be an acceptable alternative to dramatically more invasive coronary bypass surgery.[62]
- **Effects on additional endpoints:** Some non-inferiority trials are run to further characterize a drug whose superiority has already been established. FDA guidance requires developers to demonstrate that new anti-diabetic agents do not increase cardiovascular risk. To specifically address this concern for semaglutide (Rybelsus; Novo Nordisk), the sponsor ran a non-inferiority trial separately from its efficacy studies,

comparing the drug with a placebo on the primary composite outcome of cardiovascular death, nonfatal myocardial infarction, or nonfatal stroke.[63] The researchers reported in 2016 that for patients with type 2 diabetes who were at high cardiovascular risk, the rates of these events as a group were significantly lower among patients receiving the drug than among those on placebo.

- **Lower cost:** It can also be appropriate to run a non-inferiority study for a drug explicitly designed for comparable efficacy if the new agent is intended to be a lower-cost alternative. It is worth noting, however, that registrational trials of biosimilars are more commonly designed to show equivalence, which is subtly different from non-inferiority, although non-inferiority designs can also be acceptable in some biosimilar development scenarios.[64,65]

In these studies, the "non-inferiority margin" is the window within which the test drug could have lower efficacy than the active comparator, but one would still conclude it is "good enough." For example, the oral tebipenem HBr study cited above set a non-inferiority margin of −12.5% for the primary endpoint of overall response rate. This means that in the head-to-head trial, as long as the 95% confidence interval (CI) for the response rate with tebipenem was not lower than 87.5% of what was seen with intravenous ertapenem, the oral drug would have been deemed non-inferior.

In addition to assessing non-inferiority, one can also learn from the results whether the test agent appears to be objectively superior or inferior to the control, even though this latter comparison is not the objective of the study. Figure 4-1 illustrates five common places that the 95% CI of the difference between the arms can lie relative to the zero point (no difference) and the non-inferiority margin, Δ, and shows how one can use the results to assess two key aspects of the new drug's performance:

- **Non-inferiority:** The cases where the 95% CI for the test drug is entirely to the left of the margin (cases 1 through 3) demonstrate that it is non-inferior to the active control. In cases 4 and 5, the 95% CI crosses the margin, and thus the trial has failed to demonstrate non-inferiority. (If the 95% CI lies entirely to the right of the margin, the interpretation is essentially the same as in case 5.)

- **Relative efficacy:** If the 95% CI lies entirely to the left of the zero point (no risk difference), as in case 1, then the test drug is objectively superior to the active agent. Conversely, if it lies entirely to the right of that point, as in cases 3 and 5, it is inferior to the control. In cases 2 and 4, the 95% CI crosses the zero point, and thus the relative efficacy is inconclusive.

FIGURE 4-1: Illustrative outcomes from a non-inferiority study.

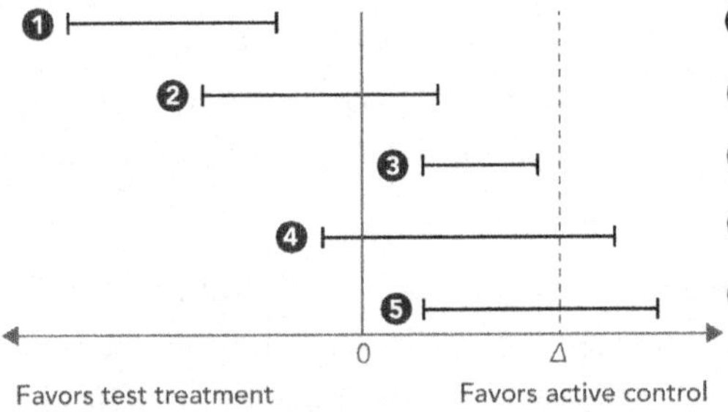

	Positive for non-inferiority?	Relative efficacy
1	Yes	Test superior
2	Yes	Inconclusive
3	Yes	Test inferior
4	No	Inconclusive
5	No	Test inferior

0 Δ

Favors test treatment Favors active control

Figure note: On the x-axis, 0 indicates no difference between the experimental drug and the active comparator, and Δ is the non-inferiority margin. Bars indicate 95% CIs for the difference between the two arms. Cases 1 through 5 are explained in the text.

The most common outcomes of non-inferiority trials are cases 2 and 4 (presence or absence of non-inferiority, with inconclusive relative efficacy). In the oral tebipenem trial discussed above, for example, the 95% CI of –9.7% to +3.2% for the difference in response was entirely better than the non-inferiority margin (–12.5%), so the study demonstrated non-inferiority as in case 2. Even though the study didn't show superiority, because the CI crossed zero, it was still a positive outcome, because it was designed to test for non-inferiority.

Sometimes, however, a drug can outperform and demonstrate not just non-inferiority but also frank superiority, as in case 1. The Phase 3 heiGHt trial was a non-inferiority study designed to test whether a once-weekly human growth hormone (hGH) product, lonapegsomatropin (TransCon hGH; Ascendis Pharma) could improve annualized height velocity to the same degree as daily hGH.[66] The 95% CI for the difference between the two agents was 0.22 to 1.50 cm/year, which did not cross zero and therefore demonstrated superiority.

In case 3, note that although the test drug meets the formal statistical definition of non-inferiority, it is objectively less effective than the active control because the *entire* 95% CI lies to the right of the equivalence line (0). (Case 5 also demonstrates objectively lower efficacy than the control for the same reason.) Besides being linguistically confusing, finding that a drug is technically "non-inferior" but also actually inferior to an active agent may lead to heightened scrutiny by regulators. This situation is extremely uncommon.

Even in appropriate scenarios, non-inferiority trials are extremely difficult to design, execute, and interpret. The most challenging issue involves setting the non-inferiority margin, despite the existence of detailed FDA guidance. The precise selection of the margin is often subjective and relies on expert input to determine the level by which a new drug could fall short of a comparator and still be considered "good enough." Many non-inferiority studies are criticized for having overly permissive margins that inflate the probability of achieving a positive result but are not relevant to practicing physicians. A Phase 3 study in renal cell carcinoma reported in 2013 found that pazopanib (Votrient; GlaxoSmithKline) yielded non-inferior progression-free survival (PFS) compared with sunitinib, with a 25% margin indicating that the test drug had to confer a PFS benefit of only 4.5 months versus the 6 months seen with the control.[67] Some critics questioned the clinical significance of a positive non-inferiority result that could reflect a relative PFS benefit of as little as a month and a half.[68]

Finally, it is important to note that non-inferiority studies are generally more prone to bias toward a positive finding than superiority studies. For example, if patients in both arms of a superiority trial are poorly compliant with the protocol, this will generally tend to make the experimental and control arms seem more equivalent and bias toward a null finding. But in a non-inferiority study, bringing the two arms closer together increases the chance of obtaining a positive result. For this reason, although so-called intention-to-treat (ITT) analyses that include dropouts are standard in most RCTs, it is often considered more appropriate in non-inferiority studies to exclude dropouts.[69] However, some analyses have suggested that the quantitative impact of non-compliance is more complex, and a so-called per-protocol analysis, which excludes dropouts, may not yield a better estimate of the "true" effect in non-inferiority studies.[70,71] More details on ITT and per-protocol analyses are provided in Chapter 7 on analysis.

Other specialized trial designs

Below are brief summaries of some common types of specialized trial designs with key features and situations in which they are commonly used.

- **Add-on and combination trials:** Some clinical studies test a new therapy in combination with a background therapy. This is common in indications such as depression, epilepsy, and heart failure, where there are established and effective therapeutic options, and it would be impractical or unethical to ask patients to discontinue their usual treatments to participate in the trial. It is also common in areas such as immuno-oncology and anti-infectives, where many new agents are not necessarily expected to have superior monotherapy activity versus established agents but instead are thought likely to yield higher efficacy in combination with them.[72] In all these scenarios, a main benefit of the add-on design is that it allows all patients to receive an active therapy.

  In clinical situations with a clearly defined and well-accepted standard of care, like some lines of therapy in particular cancers, it might be appropriate and feasible to explicitly define the background agent in an add-on or combination trial. But in chronic diseases with heterogeneous practice patterns, like epilepsy and heart failure, it might instead be more appropriate to add the new agent to each individual patient's backbone regimen, even though this approach increases the heterogeneity of the patient population, perhaps reducing the odds of detecting a bona fide effect. As shown in one of the examples below, it is important in both scenarios to note the geographies where the combination partners are approved and used.

  Of note, add-on trials in cancer that combine two drugs, each with some degree of monotherapy activity, are generally taken as evidence in favor of the combination. But in oncology, it is often also possible—and untested in a standard add-on trial—that taking the two drugs in sequence could be equally beneficial in prolonging OS.

  Examples: Phase 3 studies published in 2016 and 2017 of the catechol-O-methyltransferase inhibitor opicapone (Ongentys; Neurocrine Biosciences) in Parkinson's disease tested the drug against a placebo as add-ons to the patient's current levodopa-containing regimen.[73,74] This approach was sensible because the drug's mechanism is related to enhancing the potency of levodopa by inhibiting its metabolism.[75] The results were positive and helped form the basis for the drug's approval by the FDA in 2020 as an add-on therapy.

ATTRACTION-4 was a Phase 2/3 RCT conducted in Asia in Her2-negative advanced gastric cancer of nivolumab (Opdivo; Ono) versus placebo in combination with oxaliplatin and either capecitabine or a chemotherapy cocktail (S-1/Teysuno; Taiho) that is approved in Europe and Japan but not the U.S.[76] Ono used the study's positive findings to support a supplemental application for marketing authorization in Japan that was filed in 2020 and was still under review at the time of writing.[77]

- **Crossover studies:** In a two-way crossover study, patients in both arms are required to switch therapies, usually at a defined time point or after a particular event.[78] This design theoretically allows each patient to serve as his or her own matched control, which might be advantageous if one expects high inter-patient variability. It can also reduce the number of patients needed to achieve a given level of statistical power or boost enrollment by making participation more attractive.

  Two-way crossover trials can be appropriate in studies of chronic illnesses with stable symptoms, such as diabetes, asthma, and cancer pain, particularly if there are multiple treatment options and one wants to validate that it is safe and effective to switch between them. They are also used in studies primarily assessing pharmacokinetics, pharmacodynamics, or bioequivalence. They are generally not appropriate for conditions that evolve rapidly, such as acute infection, or conditions with high numbers of expected dropouts due to voluntary withdrawal or death.[79]

  The most significant drawback of two-way crossovers is the risk of a "carryover effect," in which a patient's response to the second treatment may have been altered by having received the first one. Although one can reduce this bias by introducing a washout period between treatments (see below), this adjustment often adds time to the study and complexity to the data analysis and can erase the potential methodologic benefits of the crossover design.[80]

One-way crossovers are typically employed in open-label extensions subsequent to an efficacy trial to give patients on the control arm the opportunity to switch to the new therapy after the main study ends and is unblinded. This design can pose a unique challenge in cancer, where trials with a primary endpoint of PFS commonly allow patients on the control arm to switch to the experimental drug after they progress to aid in recruitment. In these studies, assessment of OS as a secondary endpoint is more difficult: it might be underestimated if both arms of the trial receive a highly active drug,[81] or overestimated if the new drug is only weakly active and patients who cross over forgo access to an alternative later-line therapy with validated efficacy.[82] This situation is very common in oncology, but there are statistical methods available to handle it.[83,84]

Example: The EGALITY study compared the etanercept biosimilar Erelzi (GP2015/etanercept-szzs; Sandoz) with etanercept in plaque psoriasis.[85] It included arms in which patients underwent multiple treatment switches as well as comparator arms that received each individual therapy over the entire trial period. The 2017 trial report demonstrated that patients could switch at will between the originator drug and the biosimilar without any loss of safety or efficacy, which is a critical component of arguing that the two are interchangeable.

- **Double-dummy design:** When an experimental drug and the active control have different formulations, such as tablet versus capsule, or oral versus intravenous, blinding can be compromised unless each patient takes *both* formulations. For example, patients in one arm would take an active tablet and a placebo capsule, while those in the other would take a placebo tablet and an active capsule. Besides the practical issues of manufacturing different placebos, this is no different from a conventional two-armed trial with an active comparator.

  Example: The Phase 3 VARSITY study reported in 2019 used a double-dummy design to demonstrate that the intravenous form of vedolizumab (Entyvio; Takeda) was superior to subcutaneous adalimumab (Humira; AbbVie) in achieving clinical remission and endoscopic improvement in patients with moderately to severely active ulcerative colitis.[86]

- **Randomized discontinuation:** In this design, also sometimes called a "randomized withdrawal" or "maintenance of efficacy" study, all patients are initially treated with the experimental therapy for a short time, after which non-responders, non-compliant patients, and patients with significant adverse reactions are excluded. Then, the remaining patients are randomized to continue receiving the study drug or switch to placebo or an active comparator.[87]

  This enrichment approach is essentially a sub-category of run-in designs (see below) in which all patients initially receive the active drug. The main purported benefit in new-drug development is to reduce the sample size needed to detect a small but clinically important effect compared with a standard RCT, especially in the absence of a plausible patient selection or enrichment strategy based on molecular markers or other clinical characteristics.

  Randomized discontinuation studies can be used for chronic, non-curative drugs. They are unsuitable for potentially curative treatments or therapies that are expected to provide virtually all their benefits acutely instead of during longer-term maintenance. In addition, designs that require patients to respond during the run-in in order to advance into the main study period are poor fits for scenarios in which the short-term endpoint is different from the primary endpoint and a weak predictor of efficacy on the latter measure. This could be due to inherent limitations of the initial surrogate endpoint, the waxing and waning nature of the chronic disease course, or other factors.

  In terms of their interpretation, randomized discontinuation studies generally overestimate the efficacy and underestimate the toxicity of a new therapy compared with a conventional RCT. Although relatively uncommon in new-drug development,[88,89] they have been used in Phase 2 studies in both cancer[90] and non-oncology indications, including rare diseases, to inform both R&D decision-making and regulatory approval.

  Examples: A Phase 3 study of droxidopa (Northera; Chelsea Therapeutics) in neurogenic orthostatic hypertension enrolled 263 patients from 2008 to 2010 in an initial open-label dose optimization period of up to two weeks that identified 162 responders, who were then randomized for a seven-day treatment period.[91] The study met its primary outcome of improvement on a validated patient questionnaire and contributed to the FDA's approval of the drug in 2014.[92]

A Phase 2 study of sorafenib (Nexavar; Bayer) that began in 2002 treated 202 patients with renal cell carcinoma with the drug during a 12-week open-label run-in.[93] Patients with over 25% tumor shrinkage during the run-in were maintained on sorafenib for ethical reasons, and non-responders with over 25% tumor growth were excluded from the rest of the trial. The remaining 69 patients advanced into a placebo-controlled RCT that demonstrated a statistically significant improvement in PFS (50% vs. 18%) after 12 additional weeks. Alongside data from a separate Phase 3 RCT, results from the randomized discontinuation study supported the drug's approval in 2005.[94]

- **Run-in (or lead-in) period:** Some trials impose a delay between consent and randomization in which all patients are either observed or treated with the same therapy, whether placebo or active agent. This run-in period allows investigators to exclude patients who are poorly adherent, have a high response to placebo, or experience an adverse reaction to one of the therapies in the trial. Run-in studies that preferentially include patients who have a short-term positive response to the new drug are also sometimes referred to as randomized discontinuation trials (see above). Note that run-in studies are distinguished from trials with washout periods (see below) in that the pre-treatment in the latter does not affect trial inclusion or exclusion.

  In indications with high placebo response rates, like major depression, the goal of a placebo run-in is usually to increase the ability to detect an efficacy signal versus the control arm. However, there is some evidence that a single-blind placebo run-in may not be very effective in reducing the placebo response rate after randomization and that more sophisticated designs may be needed.[95] The benefits of run-ins have also been questioned in other therapeutic areas like diabetes.[96]

  Although run-ins typically do not decrease the validity of a study, they can complicate the interpretation of the results.[97] If the run-in excludes patients with poor adherence or a high placebo response, then the results may be less relevant to the broader patient population in the real world. Similarly, trials that exclude patients who experience adverse reactions to the experimental drug during the run-in clearly overestimate the true tolerability of the therapy. Additional issues with drug run-ins are discussed above in the section on randomized discontinuation studies. In studies with run-in periods, it is particularly important to scrutinize the accounting of how many patients were initially treated versus how many were randomized after the run-in period to determine how well or poorly the trial reflects likely real-world usage; see Chapter 7 on analysis for details.

In practice, if a trial has a run-in period, one should examine the report in detail to understand the rationale and determine whether it introduces bias that could affect the determination or interpretation of the results.

Examples: The PARADIGM-HF heart failure trial reported in 2014 included two single-blind run-in periods before randomization, one with the control generic agent, enalapril, and the other with the experimental therapy, LCZ696 (Entresto; Novartis). This was done to "ensure an acceptable side-effect profile of the study drugs at target doses," according to the researchers.[98]

The 2014–17 STRATOS-1 and STRATOS-2 trials of tralokinumab (AstraZeneca) in asthma each included a four- to six-week run-in period in which patients were required to demonstrate a threshold response to bronchodilators before being included.[99]

- **Washout period:** Washouts typically refer to periods at the beginning of a study—before treatment with the experimental or control therapy—during which patients are withdrawn from chronic treatment to reduce any carryover effect into the trial. They can also be useful to eliminate persistent effects in later-line studies where a patient may have failed to respond to a therapy that has a long half-life. Although superficially similar to a placebo run-in, a washout period does not have any effect on inclusion or exclusion or randomization, so it does not have the same issues with interpretation of the results.

  Washout periods are also used in crossover studies (see above) to avoid carryover effects from the first treatment to the second.

Example: CONTROL, a Phase 2 RCT reported in 2019, was designed to test whether generic atorvastatin could reverse the increase in lipoproteins induced by treatment of non-alcoholic steatohepatitis (NASH) patients with obeticholic acid (Ocaliva; Intercept Pharmaceuticals).[100] To ensure that observed lipoprotein levels were not affected by prior therapy, each patient underwent a four-week statin washout before initiation of treatment.

Studies with three or more arms

New-drug trials involving three or more arms are most commonly used to either (a) study several doses or dosing regimens of the same experimental agent, or (b) compare the response to a combination of two drugs with the effect of each drug individually.[101,102] A less common scenario is when multiple independent agents are being tested in separate arms that are evaluated periodically over time, as in a "platform" study (discussed in more detail in Chapter 15 on adaptive trials). Another variation, related to the non-inferiority studies described previously, includes an experimental agent, an active control, and a placebo.

For sponsors, this design is more efficient than running multiple two-armed studies because all the experimental groups share the same control arm. In some cases, there is also a theoretical benefit in recruitment speed if one believes that patients will be more likely to enroll in a study in which they have a higher probability of receiving an experimental therapy instead of a control or placebo. However, such trials are typically costlier and more complicated to execute.

From the perspective of readers of clinical trial results, the main challenge of interpreting multi-armed studies that include controls relates to the increased risk of obtaining a false positive result attributable to multiple hypothesis testing. This topic is discussed in more detail in the subgroup section of Chapter 7 on analysis.

Unbalanced assignment to treatment arms

Although most clinical trials randomize patients equally to each of the study arms, sometimes the ratio of patients is uneven, with more patients receiving the experimental therapy. For example, the 2014–17 STRATOS-1 asthma trial randomized patients 2:1 in favor of tralokinumab (AstraZeneca) versus placebo.[103]

Most studies of new drugs or devices with unequal randomization, including STRATOS-1, do not explicitly state their reasoning, but there are several plausible explanations.[104] A common one is that this approach increases the trial's ability to detect adverse events. Assigning more patients to the experimental therapy increases the probability of detecting rare safety events in that arm. It can also help sponsors satisfy regulators' requirements for the minimum size of safety databases available before approval.[105]

Another practical consideration is cost. If the trial budget is fixed, then assigning fewer patients to the more expensive arm may allow for a larger total sample size with the net effect of increasing the statistical power of the study, as discussed more fully in Chapter 13. A common scenario in which this occurs is when the active control needs to be purchased at market price from another company.

Some sponsors believe that unbalanced assignment is needed to boost recruitment in confirmatory studies of agents for which a significant benefit has already been established. Investigators may predict that patients will be more inclined to enroll in the study if they have a higher chance of receiving the new, better therapy. However, this belief is poorly validated, and the practice has been criticized on ethical grounds.[106]

A specific scenario that may favor unbalanced assignment arises in studies with complicated interventions that require operator skill development, like novel surgeries. Here, assigning more patients to the experimental arm can mitigate the impact of the learning curve by increasing the number and fraction of procedures that are performed when the clinicians are maximally skilled in the procedure.

Finally, there can be a theoretical statistical justification for assigning more patients to the experimental arm if a higher variability in the expected outcome with the new treatment could help maintain statistical power. However, the decision to undertake unbalanced assignment is rarely driven by statistical concerns. Under normal circumstances, the power of a study at a given total sample size is almost completely maintained at randomization ratios of 2:1 and 3:2 in favor of the experimental therapy and declines significantly at 3:1 and beyond.[107]

[1] de Bono J, Mateo J, Fizazi K, Saad F, Shore N, Sandhu S, Chi KN, Sartor O, Agarwal N, Olmos D, Thiery-Vuillemin A, Twardowski P, Mehra N, Goessl C, Kang J, Burgents J, Wu W, Kohlmann A, Adelman CA, Hussain M. Olaparib for metastatic castration-resistant prostate cancer. N Engl J Med. 2020 May 28;382(22):2091–2102. doi: 10.1056/NEJMoa1911440. Epub 2020 Apr 28. PMID: 32343890.

[2] Plieth J. Careful label reading reveals more Lynparza doubts. Evaluate Vantage. https://www.evaluate.com/vantage/articles/analysis/vantage-views/careful-label-reading-reveals-more-lynparza-doubts. Accessed October 15, 2021.

[3] Hilal T, Gonzalez-Velez M, Prasad V. Limitations in clinical trials leading to anticancer drug approvals by the U.S. Food and Drug Administration. JAMA Intern Med. 2020 Aug 1;180(8):1108–1115. doi: 10.1001/jamainternmed.2020.2250. PMID: 32539071; PMCID: PMC7296449.

[4] Gupta U, Verma M. Placebo in clinical trials. Perspect Clin Res. 2013 Jan;4(1):49–52. doi: 10.4103/2229-3485.106383. PMID: 23533982; PMCID: PMC3601706.

[5] Hróbjartsson A, Gøtzsche PC. Placebo interventions for all clinical conditions. Cochrane Database Syst Rev. 2010 Jan 20;2010(1):CD003974. doi: 10.1002/14651858.CD003974.pub3. PMID: 20091554; PMCID: PMC7156905.

[6] Colquhoun D. Placebo effects are weak: Regression to the mean is the main reason ineffective treatments appear to work. DC's Improbable Science. December 11, 2015. http://www.dcscience.net/2015/12/11/placebo-effects-are-weak-regression-to-the-mean-is-the-main-reason-ineffective-treatments-appear-to-work/. Accessed October 15, 2021. Permalink: https://perma.cc/X3ZU-4NMY.

[7] Hengartner MP. Is there a genuine placebo effect in acute depression treatments? A reassessment of regression to the mean and spontaneous remission. BMJ Evid Based Med. 2020 Apr;25(2):46–48. doi: 10.1136/bmjebm-2019-111161. Epub 2019 Apr 11. PMID: 30975717.

[8] 21 C.F.R. § 314.126.

[9] Liu A. Is China's drug regulator suddenly raising the bar on cancer med R&D? Not exactly, say experts. FiercePharma. July 8, 2021. https://www.fiercepharma.com/pharma-asia/china-s-drug-regulator-suddenly-raising-bar-cancer-med-r-d-not-exactly-say-experts.

[10] Kernan WN, Viscoli CM, Makuch RW, Brass LM, Horwitz RI. Stratified randomization for clinical trials. J Clin Epidemiol. 1999 Jan;52(1):19–26. doi: 10.1016/s0895-4356(98)00138-3. PMID: 9973070.

[11] Broglio K. Randomization in clinical trials: Permuted blocks and stratification. JAMA. 2018 Jun 5;319(21):2223–2224. doi: 10.1001/jama.2018.6360. PMID: 29872845.

[12] FDA briefing document—Moderna COVID-19 vaccine: Vaccines and related biological products advisory committee meeting. U.S. Food and Drug Administration. December 17, 2020. https://www.fda.gov/media/144434/download. Accessed October 15, 2021. Permalink: https://perma.cc/GM3T-WDV9.

[13] Sedgwick P. What is an open label trial? BMJ. 2014 May 23;348:g3434. doi: 10.1136/bmj.g3434. PMID: 24859904.

[14] Schulz KF, Grimes DA. Blinding in randomised trials: Hiding who got what. Lancet. 2002 Feb 23;359(9307):696–700. doi: 10.1016/S0140-6736(02)07816-9. PMID: 11879884.

[15] Redberg RF. Sham controls in medical device trials. N Engl J Med. 2014 Sep 4; 371(10):892–893. doi: 10.1056/NEJMp1406388. PMID: 25184861.

[16] Kuehn BM. Sham-controlled trial questions benefit of stents for stable angina. Circulation. 2018 Jan 30;137(5):519–520. doi: 10.1161/CIRCULATIONAHA.117.033105. PMID: 29378758.

[17] Leucht S, Heres S, Hamann J, Kane JM. Methodological issues in current antipsychotic drug trials. Schizophr Bull. 2008 Mar;34(2):275–285. doi: 10.1093/schbul/sbm159. Epub 2008 Jan 29. PMID: 18234700; PMCID: PMC2632403.

[18] Wright S, Duncombe P, Altman DG. Assessment of blinding to treatment allocation in studies of a cannabis-based medicine (Sativex) in people with multiple sclerosis: A new approach. Trials. 2012 Oct 9;13:189. doi: 10.1186/1745-6215-13-189. PMID: 23046749; PMCID: PMC3487910.

[19] Lipset CH. Engage with research participants about social media. Nat Med. 2014 Mar;20(3):231. doi: 10.1038/nm0314-231. PMID: 24603786.

[20] Beyer-Westendorf J, Büller H. External and internal validity of open label or double-blind trials in oral anticoagulation: Better, worse, or just different? J Thromb Haemost. 2011 Nov;9(11):2153–2158. doi: 10.1111/j.1538-7836.2011.04507.x. PMID: 21920015.

[21] Hróbjartsson A, Thomsen AS, Emanuelsson F, Tendal B, Hilden J, Boutron I, Ravaud P, Brorson S. Observer bias in randomised clinical trials with binary outcomes: Systematic review of trials with both blinded and non-blinded outcome assessors. BMJ. 2012 Feb 27;344:e1119. doi: 10.1136/bmj.e1119. PMID: 22371859.

[22] Chakravarti PB, Basch EM, Hirshfield KM, King-Kallimanis B, Clark KJ, Strickland PO, Papadopoulos EJ, Demissie K, Kluetz PG. Exploring open-label bias in patient-reported outcome (PRO) emotional domain scores in cancer trials. J Clin Oncol. 2018 Jun 1;36(15 suppl):e18702. doi: 10.1200/JCO.2018.36.15_suppl.e18702.

[23] Zhang AD, Puthumana J, Downing NS, Shah ND, Krumholz HM, Ross JS. Assessment of clinical trials supporting U.S. Food and Drug Administration approval of novel therapeutic agents, 1995–2017. JAMA Netw Open. 2020 Apr 1;3(4):e203284. doi: 10.1001/jamanetworkopen.2020.3284. PMID: 32315070; PMCID: PMC7175081.

[24] Lam BP, Jeffers T, Younoszai Z, Fazel Y, Younossi ZM. The changing landscape of hepatitis C virus therapy: Focus on interferon-free treatment. Therap Adv Gastroenterol. 2015 Sep;8(5):298–312. doi: 10.1177/1756283X15587481. PMID: 26327920; PMCID: PMC4530432.

[25] Summary basis for regulatory action: Yescarta. U.S. Food and Drug Administration. October 19, 2017. https://www.fda.gov/media/108788/download. Accessed October 15, 2021. Permalink: https://perma.cc/9PSC-EE9H.

[26] Summary review for regulatory action: Blincyto. U.S. Food and Drug Administration. December 2, 2014. Available at https://www.accessdata.fda.gov/drugsatfda_docs/nda/2014/125557Orig1s000TOC.cfm. Accessed October 15, 2021. Permalink: https://perma.cc/58XH-UWN6.

[27] Jabbour E, O'Brien S, Ravandi F, Kantarjian H. Monoclonal antibodies in acute lymphoblastic leukemia. Blood. 2015 Jun 25;125(26):4010–4016. doi: 10.1182/blood-2014-08-596403. Epub 2015 May 21. PMID: 25999456; PMCID: PMC4548495.

[28] Kantarjian H, Stein A, Gökbuget N, Fielding AK, Schuh AC, Ribera JM, Wei A, Dombret H, Foà R, Bassan R, Arslan Ö, Sanz MA, Bergeron J, Demirkan F, Lech-Maranda E, Rambaldi A, Thomas X, Horst HA, Brüggemann M, Klapper W, Wood BL, Fleishman A, Nagorsen D, Holland C, Zimmerman Z, Topp MS. Blinatumomab versus chemotherapy for advanced acute lymphoblastic leukemia. N Engl J Med. 2017 Mar 2;376(9):836–847. doi: 10.1056/NEJMoa1609783. PMID: 28249141; PMCID: PMC5881572.

[29] Beaver JA, Hazarika M, Mulkey F, Mushti S, Chen H, He K, Sridhara R, Goldberg KB, Chuk MK, Chi DC, Chang J, Barone A, Balasubramaniam S, Blumenthal GM, Keegan P, Pazdur R, Theoret MR. Patients with melanoma treated with an anti-PD-1 antibody beyond RECIST progression: A U.S. Food and Drug Administration pooled analysis. Lancet Oncol. 2018 Feb;19(2):229–239. doi: 10.1016/S1470-2045(17)30846-X. Epub 2018 Jan 18. PMID: 29361469; PMCID: PMC5806609.

[30] Long GV, Weber JS, Larkin J, Atkinson V, Grob JJ, Schadendorf D, Dummer R, Robert C, Márquez-Rodas I, McNeil C, Schmidt H, Briscoe K, Baurain JF, Hodi FS, Wolchok JD. Nivolumab for patients with advanced melanoma treated beyond progression: Analysis of 2 Phase 3 clinical trials. JAMA Oncol. 2017 Nov 1;3(11):1511–1519. doi: 10.1001/jamaoncol.2017.1588. PMID: 28662232; PMCID: PMC5710191.

[31] Davi R, Mahendraratnam N, Chatterjee A, Dawson CJ, Sherman R. Informing single-arm clinical trials with external controls. Nat Rev Drug Discov. 2020 Dec;19(12):821–822. doi: 10.1038/d41573-020-00146-5. PMID: 32811986.

[32] Saad ED, Paoletti X, Burzykowski T, Buyse M. Precision medicine needs randomized clinical trials. Nat Rev Clin Oncol. 2017 May;14(5):317–323. doi: 10.1038/nrclinonc.2017.8. Epub 2017 Feb 7. PMID: 28169302.

[33] Gilead announces results from Phase 3 trial of investigational antiviral remdesivir in patients with severe COVID-19. Gilead press release. April 29, 2020. https://www.gilead.com/news-and-press/press-room/press-releases/2020/4/gilead-announces-results-from-phase-3-trial-of-investigational-antiviral-remdesivir-in-patients-with-severe-covid-19. Accessed October 15, 2021. Permalink: https://perma.cc/SSM5-K8H6.

[34] Beigel JH, Tomashek KM, Dodd LE, Mehta AK, Zingman BS, Kalil AC, Hohmann E, Chu HY, Luetkemeyer A, Kline S, Lopez de Castilla D, Finberg RW, Dierberg K, Tapson V, Hsieh L, Patterson TF, Paredes R, Sweeney DA, Short WR, Touloumi G, Lye DC, Ohmagari N, Oh MD, Ruiz-Palacios GM, Benfield T, Fätkenheuer G, Kortepeter MG, Atmar RL, Creech CB, Lundgren J, Babiker AG, Pett S, Neaton JD, Burgess TH, Bonnett T, Green M, Makowski M, Osinusi A, Nayak S, Lane HC; ACTT-1 Study Group Members. Remdesivir for the treatment of Covid-19—final report. N Engl J Med. 2020 Nov 5;383(19):1813–1826. doi: 10.1056/NEJMoa2007764. Epub 2020 Oct 8. PMID: 32445440; PMCID: PMC7262788.

[35] FDA approves first treatment for COVID-19. U.S. FDA press release. October 22, 2020. https://www.fda.gov/news-events/press-announcements/fda-approves-first-treatment-covid-19. Accessed October 15, 2021. Permalink: https://perma.cc/K3DY-J9GD.

[36] Grayling MJ, Dimairo M, Mander AP, Jaki TF. A review of perspectives on the use of randomization in Phase II oncology trials. J Natl Cancer Inst. 2019 Dec 1;111(12):1255–1262. doi: 10.1093/jnci/djz126. PMID: 31218346; PMCID: PMC6910171.

[37] Baumfeld Andre E, Reynolds R, Caubel P, Azoulay L, Dreyer NA. Trial designs using real-world data: The changing landscape of the regulatory approval process. Pharmacoepidemiol Drug Saf. 2020 Oct;29(10):1201–1212. doi: 10.1002/pds.4932. Epub 2019 Dec 10. PMID: 31823482; PMCID: PMC7687110.

[38] Hashmi M, Rassen J, Schneeweiss S. Single-arm oncology trials and the nature of external controls arms. J Comp Eff Res. 2021 Aug;10(12):1052–1066. doi: 10.2217/cer-2021-0003. Epub 2021 Jun 22. PMID: 34156310.

[39] Aetion. The role of real-world evidence in FDA approvals. 2021. Available at https://resources.aetion.com/the-role-of-real-world-evidence-in-fda-approvals-ebook. Accessed October 15, 2021.

[40] Baumfeld Andre E, Reynolds R, Caubel P, Azoulay L, Dreyer NA. Trial designs using real-world data: The changing landscape of the regulatory approval process. Pharmacoepidemiol Drug Saf. 2020 Oct;29(10):1201–1212. doi: 10.1002/pds.4932. Epub 2019 Dec 10. PMID: 31823482; PMCID: PMC7687110.

[41] Jahanshahi M, Gregg K, Davis G, Ndu A, Miller V, Vockley J, Ollivier C, Franolic T, Sakai S. The use of external controls in FDA regulatory decision making. Ther Innov Regul Sci. 2021 Sep;55(5):1019–1035. doi: 10.1007/s43441-021-00302-y. Epub 2021 May 20. PMID: 34014439; PMCID: PMC8332598.

[42] Summary basis for regulatory action: Zolgensma. U.S. Food and Drug Administration. May 24, 2019. Available at https://www.fda.gov/vaccines-blood-biologics/zolgensma. Accessed October 15, 2021. Permalink: https://perma.cc/MCP8-EWDZ.

[43] Honig N, Purpura C, Garry L. CBER-approved BLA for Zolgensma (onasemnogene abeparvovec-xioi). Aetion. April 21, 2020. https://aetion.com/evidence-hub/fda-decision-alerts/cder-approved-bla-for-zolgensma-onasemnogene-abeparvovec-xioi/. Accessed October 15, 2021. Permalink: https://perma.cc/Q75F-5RAZ.

[44] Medicenna provides MDNA55 rGBM clinical program update following positive end of Phase 2 meeting with the U.S. Food and Drug Administration (FDA). Medicenna Therapeutics press release. October 15, 2020. https://ir.medicenna.com/news-releases/news-release-details/medicenna-provides-mdna55-rgbm-clinical-program-update-following. Accessed October 15, 2021. Permalink: https://perma.cc/WSM6-3DER.

[45] Miseta E. How an external control arm changed Phase 3 trials for brain cancer. Clinical Leader. August 19, 2021. https://www.clinicalleader.com/doc/how-an-external-control-arm-changed-phase-trials-for-brain-cancer-0001. Accessed October 15, 2021.

[46] Taylor WJ, Weatherall M. What are open-label extension studies for? J Rheumatol. 2006 Apr;33(4):642–643. PMID: 16583468.

[47] Enhancing the diversity of clinical trial populations—eligibility criteria, enrollment practices, and trial designs: Guidance for industry. U.S. Food and Drug Administration. November 2020.

[48] Day RO, Williams KM. Open-label extension studies: Do they provide meaningful

information on the safety of new drugs? Drug Saf. 2007;30(2):93–105. doi: 10.2165/00002018-200730020-00001. PMID: 17253876.

[49] Megan B, Pickering RM, Weatherall M. Design, objectives, execution and reporting of published open-label extension studies. J Eval Clin Pract. 2012 Apr;18(2):209–215. doi: 10.1111/j.1365-2753.2010.01553.x. Epub 2010 Oct 10. PMID: 21040252.

[50] Catabasis Pharmaceuticals reports positive results from open-label extension of Phase 2 MoveDMD trial evaluating edasalonexent in Duchenne muscular dystrophy and plans to initiate Phase 3 clinical trial in first half 2018. Catabasis Pharmaceuticals press release. October 4, 2017. https://ir.catabasis.com/news-releases/news-release-details/catabasis-pharmaceuticals-reports-positive-results-open-label. Accessed October 15, 2021. Permalink: https://perma.cc/MFV9-9VPM.

[51] Catabasis Pharmaceuticals (CATB). Form 10-K for fiscal year ended December 31, 2017. https://www.sec.gov/Archives/edgar/data/0001454789/000104746918001688/a2234670z10-k.htm.

[52] Feuerstein A. Why did this small biotech blow up? Because spinning bad drug data never works. STAT. October 27, 2020. https://www.statnews.com/2020/10/27/why-did-this-small-biotech-blow-up-because-spinning-bad-drug-data-never-works/. Accessed October 15, 2021.

[53] Mauri L, D'Agostino RB Sr. Challenges in the design and interpretation of noninferiority trials. N Engl J Med. 2017 Oct 5;377(14):1357–1367. doi: 10.1056/NEJMra1510063. PMID: 28976859.

[54] Kaul S, Diamond GA. Good enough: A primer on the analysis and interpretation of noninferiority trials. Ann Intern Med. 2006 Jul 4;145(1):62–69. doi: 10.7326/0003-4819-145-1-200607040-00011. PMID: 16818930.

[55] Mulla SM, Scott IA, Jackevicius CA, You JJ, Guyatt GH. How to use a noninferiority trial: Users' guides to the medical literature. JAMA. 2012 Dec 26;308(24):2605–2611. doi: 10.1001/2012.jama.11235. PMID: 23268519.

[56] Wellek S, Blettner M. Establishing equivalence or non-inferiority in clinical trials: Part 20 of a series on evaluation of scientific publications. Dtsch Arztebl Int. 2012 Oct;109(41):674–679. doi: 10.3238/arztebl.2012.0674. Epub 2012 Oct 12. PMID: 23264808; PMCID: PMC3487152.

[57] New drug approval: FDA's consideration of evidence from certain clinical trials (GAO-10-798). U.S. Government Accountability Office. July 2010.

[58] Non-inferiority clinical trials to establish effectiveness: Guidance for industry. U.S. Food and Drug Administration. November 2016.

[59] Antibacterial therapies for patients with an unmet medical need for the treatment of serious bacterial diseases: Guidance for industry. U.S. Food and Drug Administration. August 2017.

[60] Deak D, Outterson K, Powers JH, Kesselheim AS. Progress in the fight against multidrug-resistant bacteria? A review of U.S. Food and Drug Administration–approved antibiotics, 2010–2015. Ann Intern Med. 2016 Sep 6;165(5):363–372. doi: 10.7326/M16-0291. Epub 2016 May 24. PMID: 27239977.

[61] Spero Therapeutics announces positive topline results from its Phase 3 ADAPT-PO clinical trial of oral tebipenem HBr in complicated urinary tract infection and acute pyelonephritis. Spero Therapeutics press release. September 8, 2020. https://www.globenewswire.com/news-release/2020/09/08/2089966/0/en/Spero-Therapeutics-Announces-Positive-Topline-Results-from-its-Phase-3-ADAPT-PO-Clinical-Trial-of-Oral-Tebipenem-HBr-in-Complicated-Urinary-Tract-Infection-and-Acute-Pyelonephritis.html. Accessed October 15, 2021. Permalink: https://perma.cc/6627-KWSP.

[62] Stone GW, Sabik JF, Serruys PW, Simonton CA, Généreux P, Puskas J, Kandzari DE, Morice MC, Lembo N, Brown WM 3rd, Taggart DP, Banning A, Merkely B, Horkay F, Boonstra PW, van Boven AJ, Ungi I, Bogáts G, Mansour S, Noiseux N, Sabaté M, Pomar J, Hickey M, Gershlick A, Buszman P, Bochenek A, Schampaert E, Pagé P, Dressler O, Kosmidou I, Mehran R, Pocock SJ, Kappetein AP; EXCEL Trial Investigators. Everolimus-eluting stents or bypass surgery for left main coronary artery disease. N Engl J Med. 2016 Dec 8;375(23):2223–2235. doi: 10.1056/NEJMoa1610227. Epub 2016 Oct 31. Erratum in: N Engl J Med. 2019 Oct 31;381(18):1789. PMID: 27797291.

[63] Marso SP, Bain SC, Consoli A, Eliaschewitz FG, Jódar E, Leiter LA, Lingvay I, Rosenstock J, Seufert J, Warren ML, Woo V, Hansen O, Holst AG, Pettersson J, Vilsbøll T; SUSTAIN-6 Investigators. Semaglutide and cardiovascular outcomes in patients with type 2 diabetes. N Engl J Med. 2016 Nov 10;375(19):1834–1844. doi: 10.1056/NEJMoa1607141. Epub 2016 Sep 15. PMID: 27633186.

[64] Isakov L, Jin B, Jacobs IA. Statistical primer on biosimilar clinical development. Am J Ther. 2016 Nov/Dec;23(6):e1903–e1910. doi: 10.1097/MJT.0000000000000391. PMID: 26766293; PMCID: PMC5102275.

[65] Scientific considerations in demonstrating biosimilarity to a reference product: Guidance for industry. U.S. Food and Drug Administration. April 2015.

[66] Ascendis Pharma announces once-weekly TransCon growth hormone demonstrated superiority on primary endpoint compared to a daily growth hormone in Phase 3 heiGHt trial for pediatric growth hormone deficiency. Ascendis Pharma press release. March 4,

2019. https://www.globenewswire.com/news-release/2019/03/04/1745793/0/en/Ascendis-Pharma-Announces-Once-weekly-TransCon-Growth-Hormone-Demonstrated-Superiority-on-Primary-Endpoint-Compared-to-a-Daily-Growth-Hormone-in-Phase-3-heiGHt-Trial-for-Pediatric-.html. Accessed October 15, 2021. Permalink: https://perma.cc/64Q3-XTLL.

[67] Motzer RJ, Hutson TE, Cella D, Reeves J, Hawkins R, Guo J, Nathan P, Staehler M, de Souza P, Merchan JR, Boleti E, Fife K, Jin J, Jones R, Uemura H, De Giorgi U, Harmenberg U, Wang J, Sternberg CN, Deen K, McCann L, Hackshaw MD, Crescenzo R, Pandite LN, Choueiri TK. Pazopanib versus sunitinib in metastatic renal-cell carcinoma. N Engl J Med. 2013 Aug 22;369(8):722–731. doi: 10.1056/NEJMoa1303989. PMID: 23964934.

[68] Prasad V. Non-inferiority trials in medicine: Practice changing or a self-fulfilling prophecy? J Gen Intern Med. 2018 Jan;33(1):3–5. doi: 10.1007/s11606-017-4191-y. PMID: 28980180; PMCID: PMC5756169.

[69] Mo Y, Lim C, Watson JA, White NJ, Cooper BS. Non-adherence in non-inferiority trials: Pitfalls and recommendations. BMJ. 2020 Jul 1;370:m2215. doi: 10.1136/bmj.m2215. Erratum in: BMJ. 2020 Jul 10;370:m2692. PMID: 32611541; PMCID: PMC7327542.

[70] Brittain E, Lin D. A comparison of intent-to-treat and per-protocol results in antibiotic non-inferiority trials. Stat Med. 2005 Jan 15;24(1):1–10. doi: 10.1002/sim.1934. PMID: 15532089.

[71] Bai AD, Komorowski AS, Lo CKL, Tandon P, Li XX, Mokashi V, Cvetkovic A, Findlater A, Liang L, Tomlinson G, Loeb M, Mertz D for the McMaster Infectious Diseases Fellow Research Group. Intention-to-treat analysis may be more conservative than per protocol analysis in antibiotic non-inferiority trials: A systematic review. BMC Med Res Methodol. 2021 Apr 19;21:75. doi: 10.1186/s12874-021-01260-7.

[72] Guidance for industry: E10 choice of control group and related issues in clinical trials. U.S. Food and Drug Administration. May 2001.

[73] Ferreira JJ, Lees A, Rocha JF, Poewe W, Rascol O, Soares-da-Silva P; Bi-Park 1 investigators. Opicapone as an adjunct to levodopa in patients with Parkinson's disease and end-of-dose motor fluctuations: A randomised, double-blind, controlled trial. Lancet Neurol. 2016 Feb;15(2):154–165. doi: 10.1016/S1474-4422(15)00336-1. Epub 2015 Dec 23. PMID: 26725544.

[74] Lees AJ, Ferreira J, Rascol O, Poewe W, Rocha JF, McCrory M, Soares-da-Silva P; BIPARK-2 Study Investigators. Opicapone as adjunct to levodopa therapy in patients with Parkinson disease and motor fluctuations: A randomized clinical trial. JAMA Neurol. 2017 Feb 1;74(2):197–206. doi: 10.1001/jamaneurol.2016.4703. PMID: 28027332.

[75] Dingemanse J. Issues important for rational COMT inhibition. Neurology. 2000;55(11 Suppl 4):S24–27; discussion S28–32. PMID: 11147507.

[76] Study of ONO-4538 in gastric cancer. ClinicalTrials.gov identifier: NCT02746796. Updated March 22, 2021. Accessed October 15, 2021.

[77] ONO submits supplemental application for approval for Opdivo (nivolumab) to expand the use for treatment of unresectable advanced or recurrent gastric cancer in Japan. Ono Pharmaceutical press release. December 10, 2020. https://www.ono-pharma.com/sites/default/files/en/news/press/sm_cn201210.pdf. Accessed October 15, 2021. Permalink: https://perma.cc/Q7AR-UFAQ.

[78] Sedgwick P. What is a crossover trial? BMJ. 2014 May 9;348:g3191. doi: 10.1136/bmj.g3191. PMID: 25134118.

[79] Wang T, Malone J, Fu H, Heilmann C, Qu Y, Huster WJ. Crossover design and its application in late-phase diabetes studies. J Diabetes. 2016 Sep;8(5):610–618. doi: 10.1111/1753-0407.12412. PMID: 27100270.

[80] Wellek S, Blettner M. On the proper use of the crossover design in clinical trials: Part 18 of a series on evaluation of scientific publications. Dtsch Arztebl Int. 2012 Apr;109(15):276–281. doi: 10.3238/arztebl.2012.0276. Epub 2012 Apr 13. PMID: 22567063; PMCID: PMC3345345.

[81] Korhonen P, Zuber E, Branson M, Hollaender N, Yateman N, Katiskalahti T, Lebwohl D, Haas T. Correcting overall survival for the impact of crossover via a rank-preserving structural failure time (RPSFT) model in the RECORD-1 trial of everolimus in metastatic renal-cell carcinoma. J Biopharm Stat. 2012;22(6):1258–1271. doi: 10.1080/10543406.2011.592233. PMID: 23075021.

[82] Gyawali B, de Vries EGE, Dafni U, Amaral T, Barriuso J, Bogaerts J, Calles A, Curigliano G, Gomez-Roca C, Kiesewetter B, Oosting S, Passaro A, Pentheroudakis G, Piccart M, Roitberg F, Tabernero J, Tarazona N, Trapani D, Wester R, Zarkavelis G, Zielinski C, Zygoura P, Cherny NI. Biases in study design, implementation, and data analysis that distort the appraisal of clinical benefit and ESMO-Magnitude of Clinical Benefit Scale (ESMO-MCBS) scoring. ESMO Open. 2021 Jun;6(3):100117. doi: 10.1016/j.esmoop.2021.100117. Epub 2021 Apr 20. PMID: 33887690; PMCID: PMC8086024.

[83] Jönsson L, Sandin R, Ekman M, Ramsberg J, Charbonneau C, Huang X, Jönsson B, Weinstein MC, Drummond M. Analyzing overall survival in randomized controlled trials with crossover and implications for economic evaluation. Value Health. 2014 Sep;17(6):707–713. doi: 10.1016/j.jval.2014.06.006. PMID: 25236994.

[84] Ishak KJ, Proskorovsky I, Korytowsky B, Sandin R, Faivre S, Valle J. Methods for adjusting for bias due to crossover in oncology trials. Pharmacoeconomics. 2014 Jun;32(6):533–546. doi: 10.1007/s40273-014-0145-y. PMID: 24595585.

[85] Griffiths CEM, Thaçi D, Gerdes S, Arenberger P, Pulka G, Kingo K, Weglowska J; EGALITY study group, Hattebuhr N, Poetzl J, Woehling H, Wuerth G, Afonso M. The EGALITY study: A confirmatory, randomized, double-blind study comparing the efficacy, safety and immunogenicity of GP2015, a proposed etanercept biosimilar, vs. the originator product in patients with moderate-to-severe chronic plaque-type psoriasis. Br J Dermatol. 2017 Apr;176(4):928–938. doi: 10.1111/bjd.15152. Epub 2017 Mar 1. PMID: 27787890.

[86] Sands BE, Peyrin-Biroulet L, Loftus EV Jr, Danese S, Colombel JF, Törüner M, Jonaitis L, Abhyankar B, Chen J, Rogers R, Lirio RA, Bornstein JD, Schreiber S; VARSITY Study Group. Vedolizumab versus adalimumab for moderate-to-severe ulcerative colitis. N Engl J Med. 2019 Sep 26;381(13):1215–1226. doi: 10.1056/NEJMoa1905725. PMID: 31553834.

[87] Kopec JA, Abrahamowicz M, Esdaile JM. Randomized discontinuation trials: Utility and efficiency. J Clin Epidemiol. 1993 Sep;46(9):959–971. doi: 10.1016/0895-4356(93)90163-u. PMID: 8263581.

[88] Laursen DRT, Paludan-Müller AS, Hróbjartsson A. Randomized clinical trials with run-in periods: Frequency, characteristics and reporting. Clin Epidemiol. 2019 Feb 11;11:169–184. doi: 10.2147/CLEP.S188752. PMID: 30809104; PMCID: PMC6377048.

[89] Collister D, Rodrigues JC, Mbuagbaw L, Devereaux PJ, Guyatt G, Herrington W, Walsh M. Prerandomization run-in periods in randomized controlled trials of chronic diseases: A methodological study. J Clin Epidemiol. 2020 Dec;128:148–156. doi: 10.1016/j.jclinepi.2020.09.035. Epub 2020 Sep 28. PMID: 33002638.

[90] Stadler WM. The randomized discontinuation trial: A Phase II design to assess growth-inhibitory agents. Mol Cancer Ther. 2007 Apr;6(4):1180–1185. doi: 10.1158/1535-7163.MCT-06-0249. PMID: 17431101.

[91] Kaufmann H, Freeman R, Biaggioni I, Low P, Pedder S, Hewitt LA, Mauney J, Feirtag M, Mathias CJ; NOH301 Investigators. Droxidopa for neurogenic orthostatic hypotension: A randomized, placebo-controlled, Phase 3 trial. Neurology. 2014 Jul 22;83(4):328–335. doi: 10.1212/WNL.0000000000000615. Epub 2014 Jun 18. PMID: 24944260; PMCID: PMC4115605.

[92] Northera [package insert]. Chelsea Therapeutics. February 2014. https://www.accessdata.fda.gov/drugsatfda_docs/label/2014/203202lbl.pdf. Accessed October 15, 2021. Permalink: https://perma.cc/Y4AS-585Z.

[93] Ratain MJ, Eisen T, Stadler WM, Flaherty KT, Kaye SB, Rosner GL, Gore M, Desai AA, Patnaik A, Xiong HQ, Rowinsky E, Abbruzzese JL, Xia C, Simantov R, Schwartz B, O'Dwyer PJ. Phase II placebo-controlled randomized discontinuation trial of sorafenib in patients with metastatic renal cell carcinoma. J Clin Oncol. 2006 Jun 1;24(16):2505–2512. doi: 10.1200/JCO.2005.03.6723. Epub 2006 Apr 24. PMID: 16636341.

[94] Nexavar [package insert]. Bayer HealthCare. December 2018. https://www.accessdata.fda.gov/drugsatfda_docs/label/2018/021923s020lbl.pdf. Permalink: https://perma.cc/LDY3-VQF9.

[95] Faries DE, Heiligenstein JH, Tollefson GD, Potter WZ. The double-blind variable placebo lead-in period: Results from two antidepressant clinical trials. J Clin Psychopharmacol. 2001 Dec;21(6):561–568. doi: 10.1097/00004714-200112000-00004. PMID: 11763002.

[96] Fralick M, Avorn J, Franklin JM, Abdurrob A, Kesselheim AS. Application and impact of run-in studies. J Gen Intern Med. 2018 May;33(5):759–763. doi: 10.1007/s11606-018-4344-7. Epub 2018 Feb 15. PMID: 29450684; PMCID: PMC5910356.

[97] Pablos-Méndez A, Barr RG, Shea S. Run-in periods in randomized trials: Implications for the application of results in clinical practice. JAMA. 1998 Jan 21;279(3):222–225. doi: 10.1001/jama.279.3.222. PMID: 9438743.

[98] McMurray JJ, Packer M, Desai AS, Gong J, Lefkowitz MP, Rizkala AR, Rouleau JL, Shi VC, Solomon SD, Swedberg K, Zile MR; PARADIGM-HF Investigators and Committees. Angiotensin-neprilysin inhibition versus enalapril in heart failure. N Engl J Med. 2014 Sep 11;371(11):993–1004. doi: 10.1056/NEJMoa1409077. Epub 2014 Aug 30. PMID: 25176015.

[99] Panettieri RA Jr, Sjöbring U, Péterffy A, Wessman P, Bowen K, Piper E, Colice G, Brightling CE. Tralokinumab for severe, uncontrolled asthma (STRATOS 1 and STRATOS 2): Two randomised, double-blind, placebo-controlled, Phase 3 clinical trials. Lancet Respir Med. 2018 Jul;6(7):511–525. doi: 10.1016/S2213-2600(18)30184-X. Epub 2018 May 20. PMID: 29792288.

[100] Pockros PJ, Fuchs M, Freilich B, Schiff E, Kohli A, Lawitz EJ, Hellstern PA, Owens-Grillo J, Van Biene C, Shringarpure R, MacConell L, Shapiro D, Cohen DE. CONTROL: A randomized Phase 2 study of obeticholic acid and atorvastatin on lipoproteins in nonalcoholic steatohepatitis patients. Liver Int. 2019 Nov;39(11):2082–2093. doi: 10.1111/liv.14209. Epub 2019 Sep 10. PMID: 31402538.

[101] Juszczak E, Altman DG, Hopewell S, Schulz K. Reporting of multi-arm parallel-group randomized trials: Extension of the CONSORT 2010 statement. JAMA. 2019 Apr 23;321(16):1610–1620. doi: 10.1001/jama.2019.3087. PMID: 31012939.

[102] Freidlin B, Korn EL, Gray R, Martin A. Multi-arm clinical trials of new agents: Some design considerations. Clin Cancer Res. 2008 Jul 15;14(14):4368–4371. doi: 10.1158/1078-0432.CCR-08-0325. PMID: 18628449.

[103] Panettieri RA Jr, Sjöbring U, Péterffy A, Wessman P, Bowen K, Piper E, Colice G, Brightling CE. Tralokinumab for severe, uncontrolled asthma (STRATOS 1 and STRATOS 2): Two randomised, double-blind, placebo-controlled, phase 3 clinical trials. Lancet Respir Med. 2018 Jul;6(7):511–525. doi: 10.1016/S2213-2600(18)30184-X. Epub 2018 May 20. PMID: 29792288.

[104] Peckham E, Brabyn S, Cook L, Devlin T, Dumville J, Torgerson DJ. The use of unequal randomisation in clinical trials—an update. Contemp Clin Trials. 2015 Nov;45(Pt A):113–122. doi: 10.1016/j.cct.2015.05.017. Epub 2015 May 28. PMID: 26027788.

[105] Guidance for industry: Premarketing risk assessment. U.S. Food and Drug Administration. March 2005.

[106] Hey SP, Kimmelman J. The questionable use of unequal allocation in confirmatory trials. Neurology. 2014 Jan 7;82(1):77–79. doi: 10.1212/01.wnl.0000438226.10353.1c. Epub 2013 Dec 4. PMID: 24306005; PMCID: PMC3873626.

[107] Pocock SJ. *Clinical Trials: A Practical Approach.* John Wiley & Sons; 1983.

5.

ENDPOINTS

ENDPOINTS ARE THE KEY efficacy or safety outcomes that a study plans to measure. In many situations, trial designers have a great deal of flexibility about which endpoints to assess and how to do so. For readers, it is important to understand how these choices affect the design of the study, the statistical analysis, and the clinical, commercial, and regulatory impact of the results. In this chapter, we discuss key aspects of primary and secondary endpoints, issues with interpreting surrogate endpoints, and other related topics.

Primary endpoints

Most studies explicitly define a "primary" endpoint before the trial is initiated, disclose it in clinical trial databases or corporate press releases, and reference it in presentations of study results. The primary endpoint is the metric by which the sponsor intends readers—including clinicians, investors, journalists, regulators, and R&D decision makers—to evaluate whether the results were "positive" or "negative." Thus, it is important to take the purpose of the study into account when assessing the suitability of a trial's primary endpoint:

- **Primary endpoints intended to support regulatory approval:** In most cases, regulators base approval decisions on the outcome of the primary endpoint analysis. If the primary endpoint of a registration-enabling

---

The Pharmagellan Guide to Analyzing Biotech Clinical Trials, by Frank S. David.

trial is not the same as was used for previously approved therapies, does not fit with guidance issued by the U.S. Food and Drug Administration (FDA) in the specific therapeutic area, or is in an area without historical precedents or clear validation in the scientific literature, there may be significant uncertainty over whether the agency will view a successful trial positively. At a 2017 FDA advisory committee meeting to discuss Spark Therapeutics' gene therapy voretigene neparvovec (Luxturna) for a rare form of inherited blindness, reviewers noted that the primary endpoint—the average vision change across both eyes measured by multi-luminance mobility testing (MLMT)—was likely to mainly reflect function in the better-seeing eye. The agency asked Spark to use MLMT measurements in both eyes and the first treated eye as co-primary endpoints.[1] Spark instead opted to use only a two-eye measurement, which increased the regulatory risk.[2] But an advisory committee nonetheless gave unanimous support to the application,[3] and the drug was approved.

- **Primary endpoints intended to support advancement into Phase 3:** Many Phase 2 studies are intended to generate sufficient evidence for a hypothesis to justify investing in a larger and more expensive Phase 3 trial. When the primary endpoint in Phase 2 is identical to what one would use in a registration-enabling study or uses a highly correlated surrogate endpoint, a positive result could significantly reduce the risks in a subsequent trial.

  In some cases, a Phase 2 study can directly support regulatory approval without another trial. This is true even when the primary endpoint is a surrogate measure of efficacy, provided that regulators believe it has a high degree of correlation with a clinically meaningful outcome. Under its Accelerated Approval Program, the FDA grants market authorization based on a surrogate endpoint but requires sponsors to conduct confirmatory Phase 4 trials (see below) after approval to validate the clinical benefit.[4]
- **Primary endpoints intended to support advancement into Phase 2b:** Many Phase 1 and Phase 2a studies use primary endpoints related to safety, pharmacologic exposure, or "proof of mechanism"—for example, biochemical changes demonstrating that the drug engaged its target. In these scenarios, there may not be a formal, predefined standard for what

would constitute "success," so the impact of the results may be highly subject to interpretation.

- **Primary endpoints in post-approval studies:** Many so-called Phase 4 or post-marketing studies assess primary endpoints that are intended to clinically differentiate a drug from other therapies for commercial or strategic reasons. In others, endpoints are negotiated with regulators because the study was required as part of a post-approval commitment, usually to address an unanswered question about clinical efficacy or gather additional safety data.

Primary endpoint pre-specification and multiple hypothesis testing

When evaluating a planned or completed study, it is important to determine whether a single primary endpoint was explicitly defined and pre-specified as primary before the sponsor analyzed the data. The reason relates to the concept of multiple hypothesis testing: making more comparisons in a trial increases the odds of finding a "positive" result that arose by chance.[5] This is a concern not just for studies that assess several endpoints but also for studies that have other sources of multiplicity, like various doses or patient populations.

Pre-specification of the primary endpoint is particularly important for studies intended for regulatory approval because of the impact that multiple hypothesis testing can have on calculations of statistical significance. Most Phase 3 trials are designed with a significance level, α, of .05, which means that there is less than a 5% chance of observing a difference at least as great as what was seen in a trial if, in fact, the two arms were the same. But when multiple tests are run on the same sample, the odds that at least one of them will generate a significant result can increase dramatically. In an extreme example, if one were to measure 10 endpoints that are completely biologically independent from one another in a typical Phase 3 randomized controlled trial (RCT), there would be about a 40% chance of concluding that one of the results is positive, even if the two arms are in fact completely identical.[6]

In earlier-phase studies there may not be the same regulatory implications of erroneously claiming success because one made too many comparisons, but the same principle still applies. Whatever the odds are that an apparently positive result actually arose by chance, those odds are increased if one assesses multiple independent endpoints. This can lead R&D decision makers and investors astray if they are using the study's outcome to decide whether to invest in further development and how to design follow-up studies.

Assessing multiple independent endpoints in the same trial not only increases the odds of a spurious positive finding but also raises the possibility that the study sponsor or investigator may selectively report just the positive results that arose in the context of a slew of negative findings. This potential for cherry-picking is yet another reason why it is important for readers of clinical study results to confirm that the reported endpoint was declared as primary before the data were analyzed.

Importantly, there are several statistical methods available that allow one to make the appropriate corrections for multiple hypothesis testing and assay several independent endpoints in a single study. These are discussed in more detail in FDA guidance documents[7] and other sources.[8] When it appears that a study may have issues with multiplicity, it is important to review the statistical methods in detail to determine whether appropriate safeguards were employed. Additional issues relevant to this topic are discussed in Chapter 12 on *P* values.

Multiple primary, co-primary, and composite primary endpoints

Although the primary endpoint is often a single variable, some Phase 2b and Phase 3 trials use a combination of two or more clinical readouts. This can be appropriate if a drug is expected to confer benefit along different clinical dimensions or if there is debate about the most important clinical readout. The FDA explicitly defines three distinct terms relevant to this discussion: multiple primary endpoints, co-primary endpoints, and composite endpoints.[9]

- **Multiple primary endpoints:** In a trial with multiple primary endpoints, several independent readouts are measured with the intention to call the trial a success if *any one of them* is positive. For example, a treatment for burns or chronic ulcers could affect the speed of wound closure, the percentage of patients experiencing complete closure, the absence of scarring, or other outcomes that the FDA deems clinically meaningful to patients.[10] Without prior knowledge of how a therapy's clinical activity will manifest itself, one could imagine designing a trial to measure all these outcomes and claim success on whichever ones yield a statistically significant improvement.

One example of a situation in which this might occur is when two regulatory agencies have different endpoint requirements, and the trial is designed to address both issues. The Phase 2 study of cenobamate (Xcopri; SK Life Science) in uncontrolled focal seizures, published in 2020, had two primary endpoints: response rate, required by the FDA, and percent change in seizure frequency from baseline, requested by the European Medicines Agency (EMA).[11]

Of the three scenarios discussed in this section, this is the most potentially problematic because it significantly increases the chances of detecting a false positive result due to multiple hypothesis testing. In other words, if a trial has multiple shots on goal to be successful, then the conventional significance threshold of P=.05 is too lax, and additional statistical corrections need to be made to account for the fact that multiple endpoints were tested. This topic is discussed in more detail in Chapter 12.

Importantly, in this context "multiple primary endpoints" refers to scenarios in which there is more than one *efficacy* endpoint. Although some Phase 1 and Phase 2a studies define both a safety endpoint and an efficacy endpoint as "primary," a single primary efficacy endpoint does not engender statistical problems as noted above. The analysis of safety results is more challenging and is described in more detail in Chapter 9.

- **Co-primary endpoints:** Success in such a situation requires a positive result in *all* of two or more outcomes.[12] In the setting of registration-enabling studies, co-primary endpoints have been used in several scenarios, for example:
  - *Migraine:* Besides pain, migraine patients typically experience one or more other symptoms such as nausea, photophobia, or phonophobia to varying degrees. Updated FDA guidance suggests designing trials of acute migraine therapies with two co-primary endpoints: elimination of headache pain and reduction of the patient's most bothersome non-pain symptom.[13]
  - *Alzheimer's disease:* The FDA historically guided developers to design Alzheimer's studies with co-primary endpoints that separately measured cognition and overall function, in part because it was not

clear whether small cognitive changes were clinically meaningful. Notably, the agency is now moving away from this view, particularly for drug studies in early-stage disease, and is encouraging sponsors to develop, validate, and use integrated scales that assess both cognitive and functional components in the context of a single primary endpoint measurement.[14]

- *Combination vaccines:* The FDA logically requires manufacturers of combination vaccines to demonstrate efficacy against each pathogen separately.[15]

  Because a study with co-primary endpoints still has just one way to be declared successful, there is not an increased risk of false positives. There is, however, a greater chance of obtaining a false negative result because a significant effect on all readouts except one would be considered a failed trial. For this reason, trials with co-primary endpoints tend to be larger than they would have been with just a single endpoint to ensure that they have sufficient statistical power to detect a positive result.

- **Composite endpoint:** A composite endpoint is triggered if *any one* event occurs out of a set of possible outcomes. These are mainly used when several types of serious events are all clinically relevant, but the incidence of each one individually may be too low to allow a reasonably sized study to have adequate power. For example, many cardiovascular drug trials use a composite endpoint of death, myocardial infarction, or stroke. Occurrence of any one of them is an "event," and if the outcome is positive, there is no expectation that any of them alone would yield a statistically significant result. Another example is the Phase 3 Hokusai-VTE study published in 2013 in patients with acute venous thromboembolism, which found that the oral factor Xa inhibitor edoxaban (Savaysa; Daiichi Sankyo) was non-inferior to warfarin using a composite primary endpoint of recurrent deep vein thrombosis, non-fatal pulmonary embolism, or fatal pulmonary embolism.[16] Composite endpoints are used or have been proposed in several other chronic conditions, including pulmonary arterial hypertension and chronic obstructive pulmonary disease (COPD). They can raise several challenges and concerns[17,18]:

- **Are the components equally important?** Composite endpoints typically evaluate a combination of death and severe morbidity such as stroke in cardiovascular disease trials. But if the components have radically different levels of clinical importance, it can be hard to interpret the results. For example, a study of steroids in COPD published in 1999 used a composite endpoint of "first treatment failure" that included both death and increased medication usage,[19] even though the two outcomes are surely not equivalent to patients, physicians, or regulators. Similarly, a Phase 3 study published in 2020 of vericiguat (Verquvo; Merck) in heart failure was designed with a primary outcome of either death from cardiovascular causes or first hospitalization for heart failure.[20]
- **Are the components differentially affected by the treatment?** The vericiguat trial in heart failure was positive, but most of the benefit was due to an effect on the time to first hospitalization, and the lack of a statistically significant improvement in cardiovascular mortality led some analysts to question whether the finding was clinically meaningful.[21] Similarly, in the study of steroids in COPD, although the effect on the composite endpoint was statistically significant, it was almost certainly due to an effect on the less severe component—higher need for medication—rather than mortality.[22] In analyzing results in these types of scenarios, it is critical to see the actual breakdown of how many patients experienced each type of event.

Importantly, many study reports mislabel multiple, co-primary, and composite endpoints, so it is important to scrutinize them in detail. A Phase 3 study published in 2006 of generic decitabine in myelodysplastic syndrome measured (a) overall response rate and (b) the time until either transformation to acute myelogenous leukemia or death.[23] Although these were framed as "co-primary" in the methods, they were actually independent multiple primary outcomes. Despite the inaccurate wording, the authors correctly accounted for multiple hypothesis testing by using the Bonferroni adjustment; see Chapter 12 on *P* values and confidence intervals for further discussion.

Secondary and exploratory endpoints

Besides the primary endpoint, most studies assess several additional clinical, radiographic, pathologic, pharmacologic, or other measures of a drug's effects. These endpoints can yield critical clinical data relevant to practicing physicians, provide evidence of a drug's biological mechanism, guide further R&D, and help physicians and patients make treatment decisions. In some cases, they can also influence regulatory approval.

For registration studies, the FDA classifies non-primary endpoints based on the associated statistical analysis plan. Note that the language in FDA guidance documents[24] and other sources is evolving:

- **Key secondary endpoints:** In such cases, the investigators plan to rigorously interpret the statistical significance of the results—*but only if the primary endpoint is positive.* They are associated with detailed methods for how to prevent the detection of false positives due to multiple hypothesis testing, as discussed in Chapter 7 on analysis. Trials typically have no more than five key secondary endpoints, which must be prespecified like primary endpoints and are chosen for their clinical, regulatory, or commercial relevance. Importantly, most trials define the sample size based on the desired ability to detect a difference in the primary endpoint and therefore may be underpowered to detect differences in key secondary endpoints. For more on this topic, see Chapter 13 on study size and statistical power.
- **Other secondary (or exploratory) endpoints:** These provide ancillary information and suggest hypotheses that could be tested in future studies. From a statistical standpoint, exploratory endpoint analyses do not include any safeguards against multiple hypothesis testing and are thus highly prone to generating false positive results.

Although most journal publications explicitly note which non-primary endpoints are key secondary versus exploratory endpoints, the distinction can be ambiguous in clinical trial registries, company press releases, and other venues. In many scenarios, all non-primary endpoints are lumped together as "secondary endpoints," but they are best considered as exploratory unless explicit mention is made of statistical corrections to mitigate the detection of false positives. In all cases, it is not necessarily true that sponsors' listings of key secondary versus exploratory endpoints on clinicaltrials.gov adhere to the strict definitions above.

Even before examining the results from a study, it is worth assessing whether any of the non-primary endpoints are extremely meaningful to physicians or regulators. Ideally, the primary endpoint is, in fact, primary in terms of having the greatest importance, but in many cases a non-primary endpoint may be as clinically important as the primary one—or more so. The most common example of this is in oncology, where the FDA often approves drugs either fully or conditionally based on large improvements in primary endpoints other than overall survival (OS). The 2019 approval of the androgen receptor inhibitor darolutamide (Nubeqa; Bayer) in non-metastatic castration-resistant prostate cancer was based on a pivotal study that used metastasis-free survival as a primary endpoint.[25] The more crucial secondary endpoint of OS was trending positive at the time the study was analyzed, but the data were immature at that time because not enough deaths had occurred.[26] Longer follow-up confirmed the drug led to a significant improvement in OS,[27] and the FDA approved an update to the label to include these data.[28]

In some registration-enabling studies the primary endpoint is chosen for regulatory reasons, but clinically relevant non-primary endpoints may have important commercial implications. The FDA approved angiotensin II (Giapreza; La Jolla Pharmaceutical) in 2017 for distributive shock on the basis of the ATHOS-3 study, which had a primary endpoint of blood pressure stabilization.[29] The drug's failure to show an improvement on its secondary endpoints of organ failure and overall mortality led some analysts to appropriately question whether physicians would use it.[30] Indeed, net sales in the initial years after approval fell well short of expectations.[31]

A more complete discussion of how to interpret results from secondary and exploratory endpoint analyses, particularly in the setting of failure on the primary endpoint, is in Chapter 8 on efficacy results.

Surrogate endpoints

A surrogate endpoint is an outcome that is meant to be a stand-in for a clinically relevant endpoint of interest.[32] A surrogate endpoint may yield important information about a drug's biological activity or mechanism of action—but it is not necessarily directly impactful to patients and may or may not correlate well with clinically meaningful effects. For example, a trial of a drug for hyperlipidemia might use laboratory levels of low-density lipoprotein (LDL) as a surrogate endpoint instead of hard clinical endpoints like overall or cardiac-specific mortality. A cancer study might use outcomes like total tumor burden measured on radiographic scans or blood markers like CA-125 as surrogates for OS. And trials of drugs for critical care might use the number of days spent on a ventilator, length of stay in the intensive care unit, or the rate of hospital discharge as a surrogate for 90-day mortality.

However, in many cases it is not clear that the surrogate predicts improvement in a clinically meaningful outcome. Although many surrogates have biologically plausible associations with hard endpoints, only a small fraction are supported by correlative data from epidemiologic or post hoc analyses. Even fewer have bona fide trial data demonstrating that treatments that improve the surrogate also improve the clinically relevant outcome. And in some notable cases, improvements in surrogate endpoints can actually be associated with worse outcomes on hard clinical measures, as seen with the sodium channel blockers encainide and flecainide, which reduced ventricular arrhythmias but were associated with increased risk of sudden death.[33]

Although academic statisticians have done considerable work on methods to evaluate predictive power of surrogate endpoints, most clinical areas lack large-enough data sets to make this determination. Cardiology is one of the few clinical areas where this question has been comprehensively assessed.[34] In oncology, although many trials have been run with surrogate endpoints like response rate or progression-free survival (PFS), it appears that their predictive value for OS may depend on the specific tumor type as well as whether the drug being studied operates via an immunologic mechanism.[35,36,37]

In early-stage studies, surrogate endpoints are commonly used to provide some indication of a drug candidate's activity that would justify further investment. In this scenario, a negative or extremely small effect on the surrogate often leads to discontinuation of the program, even if the endpoint's negative predictive value is uncertain. More commonly in biotech, however, companies use positive results on a surrogate endpoint to justify further development, even if evidence for a quantitative relationship between the surrogate and the subsequent trial's hard endpoint is weak or non-existent. For example, outside of advanced colorectal and ovarian cancer, there is continued debate in oncology about the degree to which an improvement in PFS correlates with an effect on OS.[38]

Studies intended for regulatory approval raise a purely practical question: *Will the FDA confer approval based on a positive finding with a surrogate endpoint?* The FDA has defined three categories of surrogate endpoints based on the level of clinical validation.[39]

- **Validated surrogate endpoints:** According to FDA guidance, these are "supported by a clear mechanistic rationale and clinical data providing strong evidence that an effect on the surrogate endpoint predicts clinical benefit." Hemoglobin A1c for diabetes, HIV-RNA for HIV, LDL for LDL-lowering drugs, blood pressure reduction for hypertension, and serum uric acid reduction for gout have all been used extensively to support drug approvals, even though they don't actually measure clinically meaningful outcomes like improved functional performance or reduced risk of death, stroke, or other severe events. Similarly, many vaccines against well-characterized pathogens demonstrate efficacy using surrogate biological measurements, not hard clinical endpoints like infections, illnesses, or deaths. Merck's 15-valent vaccine against *Streptococcus pneumoniae* (Vaxneuvance) was approved by the FDA in 2021 on the basis of assays of how much pneumococcus-specific antibody was present in patients' serum and how well these antibodies killed bacteria in a test tube.[40]
- **Reasonably likely surrogate endpoints:** Such a surrogate marker is "supported by strong mechanistic and/or epidemiologic rationale . . . but without sufficient clinical data to show that it is a validated surrogate endpoint." These include six-month follow-up measures of sputum culture and infection relapse in tuberculosis, response rate and PFS in certain cancers, alkaline phosphatase improvement in primary biliary cirrhosis, and decreased iron stores for non-transfusion-dependent thalassemia. Many of these have been used to support accelerated approvals, but the FDA typically requires a post-approval study with a hard clinical endpoint.
- **Candidate surrogate endpoints:** This category includes all other contenders pending the generation of additional data.

The FDA maintains a list of surrogate endpoints that have previously supported approvals or are explicitly sanctioned based on guidance documents issued by the agency,[41] and several published articles review the historical use of surrogate endpoints to win approval in cancer[42] and pediatric indications,[43] as well as COPD, diabetes, glaucoma, and osteoporosis.[44]

In areas where there is no guidance or precedent, sponsors typically obtain agreement from the FDA in advance of designing Phase 3 studies that intend to use surrogate endpoints to support regulatory approval.[45] Before initiating its Phase 3 HOPE study of voxelotor (Oxbryta) in sickle cell disease, Global Blood Therapeutics announced in 2016 that the FDA had signed off on its proposal to use a surrogate measurement—increase in hemoglobin of >1 g/dL—as its primary endpoint and a new patient-reported outcomes tool as a secondary endpoint.[46] Under the terms of the company's agreement with the agency, success on both measures would have qualified the drug for full approval. The study met its hemoglobin improvement goal but missed the secondary endpoint. The FDA declined to grant full approval but did authorize the drug in 2019 under the Accelerated Approval Program,[47,48] which requires sponsors to run post-marketing confirmatory trials to demonstrate bona fide clinical benefits (in this case, a reduction in stroke risk).[49]

In addition, even if regulators sign off on the use of a surrogate marker as the primary endpoint of a registration-enabling study, the threshold for demonstrating an adequate risk-benefit profile may be more stringent in the absence of a clear clinical improvement. The Phase 3 REGENERATE study of obeticholic acid (Ocaliva; Intercept) in non-alcoholic steatohepatitis (NASH) was designed with two surrogate endpoints, liver fibrosis improvement and resolution of steatohepatitis, so success on either would be scored as trial success.[50] The study showed that Ocaliva improved liver fibrosis but also raised toxicity concerns.[51,52] According to the company, the FDA's rejection of the drug in 2020 was in part because the agency "determined that the predicted benefit . . . based on a surrogate histopathologic endpoint remains uncertain," particularly in light of the adverse safety findings.[53]

Importantly, even for some FDA-validated surrogates, the evidence linking them to hard clinical outcomes is scant. Thus, if a drug is approved based on a surrogate outcome, it is often unclear how physicians will decide whether to use the new therapy in clinical practice.[54]

Endpoint measurement considerations

Endpoints can be loosely grouped into four basic categories:

- **Factual endpoints:** These include endpoints that rely on dates, such as OS or PFS, or counts of the number of clinical events, such as hospitalizations or clinical exacerbations, over a given time period.
- **Objective measurements:** Included in these would mainly be quantitative data from clinical or laboratory tests, such as blood pressure or hemoglobin levels.
- **Clinical assessments:** Scales for depression or performance status, for example, would require a medical professional to administer a test and interpret the results.
- **Patient-reported outcomes:** These assessments of pain or other quality-of-life metrics are reported directly by patients, usually with some structured guidance.

In all these categories, challenges can arise related to an endpoint's accuracy, reproducibility, and potential for bias. For example, when factual endpoints like PFS or clinical exacerbations are assessed in person by physicians, the results are highly dependent on the frequency and regularity of study visits. This topic is explored in more depth in Chapter 11 on time-to-event studies, time-to-event curves, and event curves. Novel biomarkers may be measured with seemingly objective laboratory assays, but issues can arise if these assays have been incompletely vetted for accuracy and reproducibility. And in some disease areas, multiple different clinical assessment and patient-reported outcome tools that are commonly used in trials have different performance characteristics, strengths, and shortcomings due to variability in their components, scales, and other factors.

Several indications use **global assessment variables** as clinical trial endpoints to assess effects on disease severity. Classic examples include the ACR50 score in rheumatoid arthritis, the WOMAC index in osteoarthritis, the PANSS score in schizophrenia, and the MADRS score in major depression. These variables typically incorporate multiple objective, clinical, or patient-reported components across various domains into a single "global" score. Besides the challenges of accuracy, reproducibility, and bias, these variables also raise issues related to the relative clinical importance of the various sub-components, especially if a particular therapy affects only some aspects of the variable. This issue is discussed in more detail in the earlier section on composite endpoints.

In general, when assessing clinical trial endpoints, it is worth understanding their accuracy and reproducibility, the potential for bias, and the possible impact on trial design, statistical analysis, and interpretation. It is also important to be attentive to subtle methodological issues in how the endpoints are defined and measured that could affect the results. Finally, it is important to note that in many clinical areas, consensus is still evolving on the most appropriate endpoints and measurement tools for clinical trials of novel therapies. The COMET (Core Outcome Measures in Effectiveness Trials) Initiative[55] maintains a database of published and unpublished information on core outcome sets in specific indications.

Validation

Laboratory, clinical, and patient-reported measurements vary in the degree to which they have been validated for consistent performance. Those that are components of routine clinical tests, like serum cholesterol and urinary creatinine, are least problematic. Not only are these assays generally extremely well validated, but the labs that perform them are tightly regulated, so one can be more confident that results obtained at different sites are comparable. Similarly, the performance of many well-established clinical scales, like HAM-D in depression, has been extensively analyzed across multiple settings over time.

But if an endpoint is less well vetted, it is important to understand the degree of analytic validation, including sensitivity, specificity, accuracy, and precision. This validation should take into account variation within the population being studied as well as measurement error. For laboratory-based tests, it is also critical to confirm that there is a systematic, well-validated protocol for collecting, handling, storing, and assessing the specimens. And for measurements based on clinical assessments, it is important to verify a high degree of inter-observer agreement, which is typically assessed using kappa values.[56]

Even in well-established areas of drug development, subtle differences in endpoint measurement can lead to differences in accuracy and reproducibility that can affect a trial's outcome and the ability to compare it with other studies. There is notable variability across major hypertension trials in how blood pressure was measured in terms of the types of devices, the type of observer, whether an observer is even present at all, and other parameters, which can make it complicated to compare results across studies.[57] Endpoints that rely on patient-reported measures, like pain intensity scales, may not perform similarly across various geographies due to cultural, educational, and other factors.[58] And emerging home-based digital tools to measure variables like blood pressure, weight, and physical activity may introduce uncertainty if their accuracy and reproducibility have not been vetted and compared with more traditional methods. In cancer, the fact that pivotal trials of approved immunotherapies used different immunohistochemical reagents and cutoff criteria to identify patients with "PD-L1-positive" tumors makes it challenging to compare across trials and has been a persistent challenge for clinicians.[59]

In mid- and late-stage trials, some analytic concerns about lab-based tests can be allayed with the use of standardized collection methods and analysis at a central site. However, these safeguards do not eliminate intrinsic issues with an assay itself. Similarly, clinical and radiographic analyses can be adjudicated at a central site or with multiple independent assessors, with clear protocols to resolve discrepancies.

Potential for bias

Measurements that require clinician assessment or patient reporting are highly subject to bias if there is a possibility of deducing whether the patient is assigned to the experimental treatment or the control. For example, the six-minute walk test is a common endpoint in muscular dystrophy trials, measuring the distance a patient can walk in six minutes. But it is extremely sensitive to the amount of encouragement from the supervising physician, meaning that if blinding is compromised and investigators can deduce which patients are receiving the study drug, then positive results may exaggerate the true effect.

This potential for bias is particularly high in unblinded or single-arm biotech trials. In early-stage cancer studies that measure response rate without a control population, there is a significant risk that despite their best intentions to tamp down their enthusiasm for a potentially impactful new therapy, researchers will overreport the degree of tumor shrinkage.

Importantly, this does not mean that these types of scenarios are irredeemably biased or that the trial outcome is automatically suspect. However, it does highlight the *risk of bias,* which is important to keep in mind when examining and interpreting results.

Comparing primary endpoints between trials

Even in clinical settings with well-worn pathways for drug approval, investigators and sponsors often have many options for defining primary endpoints. It is always worthwhile to carefully compare a trial's primary endpoints with those used by competitors as well as by the same project team in earlier studies because subtle differences can affect a study's outcome and the interpretation of results.

Phase 2 endpoints in the same indication can vary widely, even when the standards for registration trials are fairly consistent. This can make it complicated to compare studies and to predict how an earlier trial's success or failure might affect the outcome of subsequent ones. In asthma, for example, various Phase 2 trials for biologics have used as primary endpoints a decline in one-second forced expiratory volume, the number of clinical exacerbations in a defined period, or improvement in a seven-question survey, the Asthma Control Questionnaire.

In Phase 3, there is typically less variability in endpoints across contemporaneous drug candidates when there are well-established comparators in the market or guidance from the FDA. But in clinical areas that are less mature from a drug development standpoint, there can be substantive differences. Two of the three trials that supported the approval of belimumab (Benlysta; Human Genome Sciences / GlaxoSmithKline) in lupus in 2011 used as the primary endpoint improvement in the SLE Responder Index (SRI), a disease assessment based on patients' performance on three clinical scales.[60] In 2019, anifrolumab (AstraZeneca) failed in the Phase 3 TULIP-1 study that used the SRI responder rate as its primary endpoint.[61] But it was successful in a separate study the following year, TULIP-2, which used a different assessment scheme, the British Isles Lupus Assessment Group-based Composite Lupus Assessment.[62] Both these tools attempt to measure both global and organ-specific disease activity, but they use slightly different criteria.[63] Experts were uncertain about how the discordant findings would be interpreted, but the FDA approved the drug in 2021.[64]

The lupus example highlights a particular challenge in comparing trial endpoints when multiple scales are in common use, or the preferred scale has evolved or is evolving. For example, in major depressive disorder, HAM-D scores patients from zero to 40 based on 17 assessments, whereas the Montgomery–

Åsberg Depression Rating Scale (MADRS) runs from zero to 60 based on 10 independent subscores. Both have been rigorously evaluated in the literature and are commonly assessed numerically as clinical trial endpoints. Furthermore, studies have proposed ways to convert between values obtained using the two scales.[65] In contrast, the appropriate categorical endpoints for COVID-19 therapies were still evolving almost two years into the pandemic. Some Phase 3 trials of inpatient therapies used a 7-point scale from 1 (death) to 7 (not hospitalized),[66] but the World Health Organization proposed an alternative 10-point scale that applies to both inpatients and outpatients.[67] More research would be needed to compare the scales' robustness and determine their interchangeability.

Finally, it is particularly important to examine planned Phase 3 trials for subtle but important changes in primary endpoints compared with their antecedent Phase 2 studies. TC-5214 (Targacept/AstraZeneca) delivered positive results in a Phase 2 trial in depression in 2009 using the HAM-D clinical score as the primary endpoint. But Phase 3 studies conducted over the following three years that used the MADRS scale were negative.[68] Similarly, a Phase 2 study of NicVAX (Nabi), a vaccine for smoking cessation, published positive results in 2011 in a subset of patients on its primary endpoint of continuous abstinence for weeks 19–26 after the start of treatment.[69] But two subsequent Phase 3 studies that reported data later that year, which doubled the assessment period to 16 weeks of continuous abstinence, both failed.[70,71] It is impossible to know in each case exactly why the later studies did not succeed, but it is plausible that changes to the primary endpoints contributed to their increased risk.

Endpoint switching

The terms "outcome switching" and "endpoint switching" are used somewhat interchangeably and haphazardly to refer to two scenarios, each of which has different implications for readers of clinical trial results. One relates to **endpoint switching during trial reporting,** in which a trial fails on its primary endpoint but the sponsor tries to spin the findings to focus attention on secondary or exploratory endpoints.

The second scenario, our focus here, involves **endpoint modification during trial execution or analysis**. In this case, the study's endpoints are changed sometime between when the first patient is enrolled and when the results are reported. This is usually detected by comparing the trial report with its registration record, including the history of changes, in clinicaltrials.gov. Amendments in protocols for new-drug studies are common, but many of these alterations are minor or affect only secondary or exploratory endpoints.

Substantive changes to the primary endpoint after trial initiation, which occur in about 10% of registered studies,[72] raise the risk of bias. As discussed earlier in regard to primary endpoints, the main concern is that the endpoint may have been changed in response to an informal, unplanned interim look at the data that revealed the study was unlikely to succeed with the original endpoints and that the investigators overtly cherry-picked a new endpoint most likely to yield positive findings from among a wide set of possibilities.[73]

It is extremely challenging to learn additional details when one detects or suspects that the endpoints of a study have been changed before the reporting of the results. Although primary and secondary endpoints are among the required elements in clinicaltrials.gov registrations,[74] there is no clear precedent for identifying or sanctioning companies that do not appropriately update this information. Even for Phase 3 studies by publicly traded companies, which are required under law to disclose information materially relevant to investors,[75,76] supporting details about endpoint changes can be scant. On an investor call in 2017, Intercept Pharmaceuticals announced it had changed the two endpoints of its ongoing Phase 3 trial of obeticholic acid (Ocaliva) in NASH from co-primary to multiple,[77] but this change was not reflected in the trial's clinicaltrials .gov listing.[78]

Despite the challenges for readers, whenever possible it is worth seeking answers to several questions:

- **Was the change made independently of data from the trial?** Changes in response to data from other trials or evolving consensus on suitable design are often appropriate. In contrast, changes made based on interim analyses that were not accounted for in the original execution plan are more fraught.
- **Who made the decision?** In Phase 3 trials of new drugs, external data monitoring committees typically have sole authority to authorize protocol changes, and their independence helps ensure that the decision is ethical and maintains the integrity of the study. In earlier-stage trials, however, this responsibility may lie with investigators or sponsors, which introduces the risk of bias.

- **Was the statistical analysis plan updated to account for the change?** For Phase 3 trials intended for regulatory submission, it is particularly important for the sponsor to transparently report the intended statistical approach when endpoints are changed mid-trial to provide reassurance that the subsequent analysis was not manipulated to generate positive results. Companies commonly include this information in press releases, as Spark Therapeutics did in 2015—at a time the database was locked but before analysis had commenced—when the company disclosed that it changed the secondary endpoints in the Phase 3 study of SPK-RPE65 (Luxturna) for RPE-65-mediated inherited retinal dystrophies.[79]

Endpoint changes during a study raise legitimate concerns about bias and analytical shenanigans, and one should always dive into the details to understand why the changes were made. The endpoints of a Phase 3 trial of remdesivir (Veklury; Gilead) for COVID-19 in 2020 were changed in mid-study from binary categories—normalization of fever and oxygen saturation and hospital discharge—to a seven-point clinical assessment scale. Some analysts observed that this change brought the study more into line with similar trials, many of which were launching or reporting data around the same time, while also providing additional statistical power to detect a more modest benefit of the drug.[80] However, when the change was reported, it was not clear whether it was informed by interim data showing the study was unlikely to succeed with its original endpoints, in which case bias may have been introduced.

That said, it is equally important not to reflexively assume that endpoint changes automatically invalidate a trial's findings. The ISCHEMIA trial of upfront cardiac catheterization and revascularization versus medical therapy alone in a subset of patients with ischemia included a possible endpoint change as a contingency plan when recruitment was initiated in 2012.[81] Because of uncertainty around the expected number of events, the original protocol stipulated that the composite primary endpoint could be expanded mid-trial from cardiovascular death or myocardial infarction to include resuscitated cardiac arrest and hospitalization for either unstable angina or heart failure. When it became clear that the event rate was lagging behind the original estimate, an independent advisory panel recommended changing the endpoint as planned. The final analysis showed no difference in outcomes between the two groups.[82]

Finally, it is worth noting that the impact of endpoint changes on regulatory approval can be idiosyncratic. The primary endpoint in the main efficacy trial of tasimelteon (Hetlioz; Vanda Pharmaceuticals) in non-24-hour sleep-wake disorder, an orphan condition, was changed multiple times during the 2010–12 study. The initial plan was to measure just nighttime total sleep, whereas the final co-primary endpoint was composed of a surrogate marker—resetting of the circadian melatonin rhythm as indicated by urinary metabolite measurements—plus a novel, complex composite endpoint that quantified multiple sleep parameters.[83] Although none of the changes was agreed upon with the FDA, an agency advisory committee addressed them only in passing when it overwhelmingly supported approval of the drug, to the surprise of many industry experts.[84,85]

Cause-specific mortality as an endpoint

In studies with death as an endpoint, there is a subtle but important distinction between trials that assess "all-cause mortality," or OS, versus those that count only "cause-specific" fatalities due to the disease under investigation. For example, many studies of drugs to prevent thrombosis count deaths due to heart attack or stroke but not those from cancer or other causes.

The debate over which mortality endpoint is more suitable in an RCT largely hinges on practical considerations. Objectively, all-cause mortality is clearly important to patients and is highly relevant to inform the public health debate around whether to recommend widespread, long-term therapies in chronic indications like hypertension, hyperlipidemia, diabetes, and chronic renal disease. But in these indications, most deaths overall are likely to be unaffected by the treatment, so the therapy's effect on all-cause mortality is likely to be small. A trial designed to detect an improvement in it would need to be impractically large. In heart failure,[86] acute hemorrhage,[87] and critical care,[88] for example, many experts argue that all-cause mortality is an inappropriate primary endpoint for trials of new therapies.

However, there are two considerations to keep in mind when assessing RCTs with cause-specific mortality endpoints. First, in cancer[89] and other indications there is a high risk of misclassification when attempting to assign deaths to particular causes, which could bias the results. This is mostly of significance in single-arm or unblinded trials, but it should be kept in mind even in RCTs when one is trying to put the outcomes in context with historical results. Second, a therapy might improve cause-specific mortality but lead to harms due to other causes, which might reduce the overall net benefit. This was illustrated by the excess cardiac harms that were seen in studies initiated before 1975 of radiotherapy as adjuvant treatment for locoregional breast cancer.[90]

As a final note, there are good arguments for using all-cause mortality as an endpoint in cancer screening studies,[91] but this debate extends beyond trials of therapeutics and is thus beyond our scope here.

---

[1] BLA 125610 (voretigene neparvovec; Spark Therapeutics, Inc.): Cellular, tissue, and gene therapies advisory committee meeting (OTAT/CBER/FDA). U.S. Food and Drug Administration. October 12, 2017. https://www.fda.gov/media/108598/download. Accessed October 15, 2021. Permalink: https://perma.cc/6T9M-LBFP.

[2] Carroll J. Spark Therapeutics faces a grilling as FDA ponders a pioneering OK for gene therapy. Endpoints News. October 10, 2017. https://endpts.com/spark-therapeutics-faces-a-grilling-as-fda-ponders-a-pioneering-ok-for-gene-therapy/. Accessed October 15, 2021.

[3] Carroll J. FDA experts offer a unanimous endorsement for Spark's pioneering AAV gene therapy for blindness. October 12, 2017. https://endpts.com/fda-experts-offer-a-unanimous-endorsement-for-sparks-pioneering-aav-gene-therapy-for-blindness/. Accessed October 15, 2021.

[4] Accelerated approval. U.S. Food and Drug Administration. https://www.fda.gov/patients/fast-track-breakthrough-therapy-accelerated-approval-priority-review/accelerated-approval. Updated January 4, 2018. Accessed October 15, 2021. Permalink: https://perma.cc/3JUR-9D6X.

[5] Dmitrienko A, D'Agostino RB Sr. Multiplicity considerations in clinical trials. N Engl J Med. 2018 May 31;378(22):2115–2122. doi: 10.1056/NEJMra1709701. PMID: 29847757.

[6] Bender R, Lange S. Adjusting for multiple testing—when and how? J Clin Epidemiol. 2001 Apr;54(4):343–349. doi: 10.1016/s0895-4356(00)00314-0. PMID: 11297884.

[7] Multiple endpoints in clinical trials: Guidance for industry (draft guidance). U.S. Food and Drug Administration. January 2017.

[8] Dmitrienko A, Tamhane AC, Bretz F, eds. *Multiple Testing Problems in Pharmaceutical Statistics.* 1st ed. Chapman and Hall/CRC; 2010.

[9] Multiple endpoints in clinical trials: Guidance for industry (draft guidance). U.S. Food and Drug Administration. January 2017.

[10] Guidance for industry: Chronic cutaneous ulcer and burn wounds—developing products for treatment. U.S. Food and Drug Administration. June 2006.

[11] Krauss GL, Klein P, Brandt C, Lee SK, Milanov I, Milovanovic M, Steinhoff BJ, Kamin M. Safety and efficacy of adjunctive cenobamate (YKP3089) in patients with uncontrolled focal seizures: A multicentre, double-blind, randomised, placebo-controlled, dose-response trial. Lancet Neurol. 2020 Jan;19(1):38–48. doi: 10.1016/S1474-4422(19)30399-0. Epub 2019 Nov 14. Erratum in: Lancet Neurol. 2020 Mar;19(3):e3. PMID: 31734103.

[12] Hamasaki T, Evans SR, Asakura K. Design, data monitoring, and analysis of clinical trials with co-primary endpoints: A review. J Biopharm Stat. 2018;28(1):28–51. doi: 10.1080/10543406.2017.1378668. Epub 2017 Oct 30. PMID: 29083951; PMCID: PMC6135538.

[13] Migraine: Developing drugs for acute treatment: Guidance for industry. U.S. Food and Drug Administration. February 2018.

[14] Early Alzheimer's disease: Developing drugs for treatment: Guidance for industry (draft guidance). U.S. Food and Drug Administration. February 2018.

[15] Guidance for industry for the evaluation of combination vaccines for preventable diseases: Production, testing, and clinical studies. U.S. Food and Drug Administration. April 1997.

[16] Büller HR, Décousus H, Grosso MA, Mercuri M, Middeldorp S, Prins MH, Raskob GE, Schellong SM, Schwocho L, Segers A, Shi M, Verhamme P, Wells P; Hokusai-VTE Investigators. Edoxaban versus warfarin for the treatment of symptomatic venous thromboembolism. N Engl J Med. 2013 Oct 10;369(15):1406–1415. doi: 10.1056/NEJMoa1306638. Epub 2013 Aug 31. Erratum in: N Engl J Med. 2014 Jan 23; 370(4):390. PMID: 23991658.

[17] Irony TZ. The "utility" in composite outcome measures: Measuring what is important to patients. JAMA. 2017 Nov 14;318(18):1820–1821. doi: 10.1001/jama.2017.14001. PMID: 29136430.

[18] Kleist P. Composite endpoints for clinical trials. Int J Pharm Med 2007 Jun;21:187–198. doi: 10.2165/00124363-200721030-00001.

[19] Niewoehner DE, Erbland ML, Deupree RH, Collins D, Gross NJ, Light RW, Anderson P, Morgan NA; Department of Veterans Affairs Cooperative Study Group. Effect of systemic glucocorticoids on exacerbations of chronic obstructive pulmonary disease. N Engl J Med. 1999 Jun 24;340(25):1941–1947. doi: 10.1056/NEJM199906243402502. PMID: 10379017.

[20] Armstrong PW, Pieske B, Anstrom KJ, Ezekowitz J, Hernandez AF, Butler J, Lam CSP, Ponikowski P, Voors AA, Jia G, McNulty SE, Patel MJ, Roessig L, Koglin J, O'Connor CM; VICTORIA Study Group. Vericiguat in patients with heart failure and reduced ejection fraction. N Engl J Med. 2020 May 14;382(20):1883–1893. doi: 10.1056/NEJMoa1915928. Epub 2020 Mar 28. PMID: 32222134.

[21] Mast J. The $1B Merck-Bayer drug that divided cardiologists in March gets priority review. Endpoints News. July 16, 2020. https://endpts.com/the-1b-merck-bayer-drug-that-divided-cardiologists-in-march-gets-priority-review/. Accessed October 15, 2021.

[22] McCoy CE. Understanding the use of composite endpoints in clinical trials. West J Emerg Med. 2018 Jul;19(4):631–634. doi: 10.5811/westjem.2018.4.38383. Epub 2018 Jun 4. PMID: 30013696; PMCID: PMC6040910.

[23] Kantarjian H, Issa JP, Rosenfeld CS, Bennett JM, Albitar M, DiPersio J, Klimek V, Slack J, de Castro C, Ravandi F, Helmer R 3rd, Shen L, Nimer SD, Leavitt R, Raza A, Saba H. Decitabine improves patient outcomes in myelodysplastic syndromes: Results of a Phase III randomized study. Cancer. 2006 Apr 15;106(8):1794–1803. doi: 10.1002/cncr.21792. PMID: 16532500.

[24] Multiple endpoints in clinical trials: Guidance for industry (draft guidance). U.S. Food and Drug Administration. January 2017.

[25] FDA approves darolutamide for non-metastatic castration-resistant prostate cancer. U.S. FDA press release. July 31, 2019. https://www.fda.gov/drugs/resources-information-approved-drugs/fda-approves-darolutamide-non-metastatic-castration-resistant-prostate-cancer. Accessed October 15, 2021. Permalink: https://perma.cc/HBW2-BH72.

[26] Fizazi K, Shore N, Tammela TL, Ulys A, Vjaters E, Polyakov S, Jievaltas M, Luz M, Alekseev B, Kuss I, Kappeler C, Snapir A, Sarapohja T, Smith MR; ARAMIS Investigators. Darolutamide in nonmetastatic, castration-resistant prostate cancer. N Engl J Med. 2019 Mar 28;380(13):1235–1246. doi: 10.1056/NEJMoa1815671. Epub 2019 Feb 14. PMID: 30763142.

[27] Fizazi K, Shore N, Tammela TL, Ulys A, Vjaters E, Polyakov S, Jievaltas M, Luz M, Alekseev B, Kuss I, Le Berre MA, Petrenciuc O, Snapir A, Sarapohja T, Smith MR; ARAMIS Investigators. Nonmetastatic, castration-resistant prostate cancer and survival with darolutamide. N Engl J Med. 2020 Sep 10;383(11):1040–1049. doi: 10.1056/NEJMoa2001342. PMID: 32905676.

[28] U.S. FDA approves addition of overall survival and other secondary endpoint data to Nubeqa (darolutamide) prescribing information. Bayer press release. January 8, 2021. https://www.biospace.com/article/releases/u-s-fda-approves-addition-of-overall-survival-and-other-secondary-endpoint-data-to-nubeqa-darolutamide-prescribing-information/. Accessed October 15, 2021. Permalink: https://perma.cc/S2UV-9YFC.

[29] Senatore F, Jagadeesh G, Rose M, Pillai VC, Hariharan S, Liu Q, McDowell TY, Sapru MK, Southworth MR, Stockbridge N. FDA approval of angiotensin II for the treatment of hypotension in adults with distributive shock. Am J Cardiovasc Drugs. 2019 Feb;19(1):11–20. doi: 10.1007/s40256-018-0297-9. Erratum in: Am J Cardiovasc Drugs. 2019 Apr;19(2):227. PMID: 30144016.

[30] Feuerstein A. Mixed outcomes for La Jolla Pharma shock drug fuels debate over sales potential. TheStreet. May 22, 2017. https://www.thestreet.com/investing/stocks/mixed-outcomes-for-la-jolla-pharma-shock-drug-fuels-debate-over-sales-potential-14144059. Accessed October 15, 2021.

[31] Van Voorhis S. La Jolla stock plummets 44% after disappointing drug sales projections. TheStreet. January 7, 2019. https://www.thestreet.com/markets/la-jolla-stock-plummets-44-after-disappointing-drug-sales-projections-14826657. Accessed October 15, 2021.

[32] Bucher HC, Guyatt GH, Cook DJ, Holbrook A, McAlister FA; Evidence-Based Medicine Working Group. Users' guides to the medical literature: XIX. Applying clinical trial results. A. How to use an article measuring the effect of an intervention on surrogate end points. JAMA. 1999 Aug 25;282(8):771–778. doi: 10.1001/jama.282.8.771. PMID: 10463714.

[33] Shi Q, Sargent DJ. Meta-analysis for the evaluation of surrogate endpoints in cancer clinical trials. Int J Clin Oncol. 2009 Apr;14(2):102–111. doi: 10.1007/s10147-009-0885-4. Epub 2009 Apr 24. PMID: 19390940.

[34] Weintraub WS, Lüscher TF, Pocock S. The perils of surrogate endpoints. Eur Heart J. 2015 Sep 1;36(33):2212–2218. doi: 10.1093/eurheartj/ehv164. Epub 2015 May 13. PMID: 25975658; PMCID: PMC4554958.

[35] Blumenthal GM, Karuri SW, Zhang H, Zhang L, Khozin S, Kazandjian D, Tang S, Sridhara R, Keegan P, Pazdur R. Overall response rate, progression-free survival, and overall survival with targeted and standard therapies in advanced non-small-cell lung cancer: U.S. Food and Drug Administration trial-level and patient-level analyses. J Clin Oncol. 2015 Mar 20;33(9):1008–1014. doi: 10.1200/JCO.2014.59.0489. Epub 2015 Feb 9. PMID: 25667291; PMCID: PMC4356710.

[36] Ye J, Ji X, Dennis PA, Abdullah H, Mukhopadhyay P. Relationship between progression-free survival, objective response rate, and overall survival in clinical trials of PD-1/PD-L1 immune checkpoint blockade: A meta-analysis. Clin Pharmacol Ther. 2020 Dec;108(6):1274–1288. doi: 10.1002/cpt.1956. Epub 2020 Jul 18. PMID: 32564368; PMCID: PMC7689755.

[37] Solomon BJ, Loong HHF, Summers YJ, Thomas ZM, French PP, Lin BK, Sashegyi A, Wolf J, Yang JC, Drilon AE. Correlation between overall response rate and progression-free survival/overall survival in comparative trials involving targeted therapies in molecularly enriched populations. J Clin Oncol. 2020 May 20;38(15 suppl):3558. doi: 10.1200/JCO.2020.38.15_suppl.3588.

[38] Booth CM, Eisenhauer EA. Progression-free survival: Meaningful or simply measurable? J Clin Oncol. 2012 Apr 1;30(10):1030–1033. doi: 10.1200/JCO.2011.38.7571. PMID: 22370321.

[39] FDA-NIH Biomarker Working Group. BEST (Biomarkers, EndpointS, and other Tools) Resource. U.S. Food and Drug Administration and U.S. National Institutes of Health; 2016. Available at https://www.ncbi.nlm.nih.gov/books/NBK326791/. Accessed October 15, 2021.

[40] Merck announces U.S. FDA approval of Vaxneuvance (pneumococcal 15-valent conjugate vaccine) for the prevention of invasive pneumococcal disease in adults 18 years and older caused by 15 serotypes. Merck press release. July 16, 2021. https://www.merck.com/news/merck-announces-u-s-fda-approval-of-vaxneuvance-pneumococcal-15-valent-conjugate-vaccine-for-the-prevention-of-invasive-pneumococcal-disease-in-adults-18-years-and-older-caused-by-15-serot/. Accessed October 15, 2021. Permalink: https://perma.cc/NE72-LN5Y.

[41] Table of surrogate endpoints that were the basis of drug approval or licensure. U.S. Food and Drug Administration. https://www.fda.gov/drugs/development-resources/table-surrogate-endpoints-were-basis-drug-approval-or-licensure. Updated September 16, 2021. Accessed October 15, 2021. Permalink: https://perma.cc/Y4GX-6SNN.

[42] Kim C, Prasad V. Strength of validation for surrogate end points used in the U.S. Food and Drug Administration's approval of oncology drugs. Mayo Clin Proc. 2016 May 10:S0025-6196(16)00125-7. doi: 10.1016/j.mayocp.2016.02.012. Epub ahead of print. PMID: 27236424; PMCID: PMC5104665.

[43] Green DJ, Sun H, Burnham J, Liu XI, van den Anker J, Temeck J, Yao L, McCune SK, Burckart GJ. Surrogate endpoints in pediatric studies submitted to the U.S. FDA. Clin Pharmacol Ther. 2019 Mar;105(3):555–557. doi: 10.1002/cpt.1117. Epub 2018 Aug 9. PMID: 30094815; PMCID: PMC6481930.

[44] Yu T, Hsu YJ, Fain KM, Boyd CM, Holbrook JT, Puhan MA. Use of surrogate outcomes in U.S. FDA drug approvals, 2003–2012: A survey. BMJ Open. 2015 Nov 27;5(11):e007960. doi: 10.1136/bmjopen-2015-007960. PMID: 26614616; PMCID: PMC4663404.

[45] Lai R. Early engagement with FDA to discuss novel surrogate endpoints. CDER SBIA Chronicles, U.S. Food and Drug Administration. November 27, 2018. https://www.fda.gov/media/118871/download. Accessed October 15, 2021. Permalink: https://perma.cc/KYA2-DY3X.

[46] Global Blood Therapeutics announces pivotal study for GBT440 in sickle cell disease with primary hemoglobin endpoint. Global Blood Therapeutics press release. October 24, 2016. https://ir.gbt.com/news-releases/news-release-details/global-blood-therapeutics-announces-pivotal-study-gbt440-sickle. Accessed October 15, 2021. Permalink: https://perma.cc/KC7F-P3CS.

[47] FDA approves voxelotor for sickle cell disease. U.S. FDA press release. November 25, 2019. https://www.fda.gov/drugs/resources-information-approved-drugs/fda-approves-voxelotor-sickle-cell-disease. Accessed October 15, 2021. Permalink: https://perma.cc/7REK-EXUM.

[48] Lehrer-Graiwer J, Yokoshima L, Tong B, Love TW. Accelerated approval of Oxbryta (voxelotor): A case study on novel endpoint selection in sickle cell disease. Contemp Clin Trials. 2020 Nov;98:106161. doi: 10.1016/j.cct.2020.106161. Epub 2020 Sep 30. PMID: 33010428.

[49] Guidance for industry: Expedited programs for serious conditions—drugs and biologics. U.S. Food and Drug Administration. May 2014.

[50] Adams B. Intercept jumps on NASH Phase 3 protocol changes. Intercept press release. February 10, 2017. https://www.fiercebiotech.com/biotech/intercept-jumps-nash-phase-3-protocol-change. Accessed October 15, 2021.

[51] Younossi ZM, Ratziu V, Loomba R, Rinella M, Anstee QM, Goodman Z, Bedossa P, Geier A, Beckebaum S, Newsome PN, Sheridan D, Sheikh MY, Trotter J, Knapple W, Lawitz E, Abdelmalek MF, Kowdley KV, Montano-Loza AJ, Boursier J, Mathurin P, Bugianesi E, Mazzella G, Olveira A, Cortez-Pinto H, Graupera I, Orr D, Gluud LL, Dufour JF, Shapiro D, Campagna J, Zaru L, MacConell L, Shringarpure R, Harrison S, Sanyal AJ; REGENERATE Study Investigators. Obeticholic acid for the treatment of non-alcoholic steatohepatitis: Interim analysis from a multicentre, randomised, placebo-controlled phase 3 trial. Lancet. 2019 Dec 14;394(10215):2184–2196. doi: 10.1016/S0140-6736(19)33041-7. Epub 2019 Dec 5. Erratum in: Lancet. 2020 Aug 1;396(10247):312. Erratum in: Lancet. 2021 Jun 19;397(10292):2336. PMID: 31813633.

[52] Plieth J, Armstrong M. Intercept's Nash hopes rest on Ocaliva's borderline hit. Evaluate Vantage. February 19, 2019. https://www.evaluate.com/vantage/articles/news/trial-results/intercepts-nash-hopes-rest-ocalivas-borderline-hit. Accessed October 15, 2021.

[53] Intercept receives complete response letter from FDA for obeticholic acid for the treatment of fibrosis due to NASH. Intercept Pharmaceuticals press release. June 29, 2020. https://ir.interceptpharma.com/news-releases/news-release-details/intercept-receives-complete-response-letter-fda-obeticholic-acid. Accessed October 15, 2021. Permalink: https://perma.cc/59P8-Z45A.

[54] Bucher HC, Guyatt GH, Cook DJ, Holbrook A, McAlister FA; Evidence-Based Medicine Working Group. Users' guides to the medical literature: XIX. Applying clinical trial results. A. How to use an article measuring the effect of an intervention on surrogate end points. JAMA. 1999 Aug 25;282(8):771–778. doi: 10.1001/jama.282.8.771. PMID: 10463714.

[55] COMET (Core Outcome Measures in Effectiveness Trials) Initiative home page. http://www.comet-initiative.org/. Accessed October 15, 2021. Permalink: https://perma.cc/EA2H-JG7W.

[56] McHugh ML. Interrater reliability: The kappa statistic. Biochem Med (Zagreb). 2012;22(3):276–282. PMID: 23092060; PMCID: PMC3900052.

[57] Chen Y, Lei L, Wang JG. Methods of blood pressure assessment used in milestone hypertension trials. Pulse (Basel). 2018 Jul;6(1-2):112-123. doi: 10.1159/000489855. Epub 2018 Jul 18. PMID: 30283753; PMCID: PMC6140594.

[58] Pathak A, Sharma S, Jensen MP. The utility and validity of pain intensity rating scales for use in developing countries. Pain Rep. 2018 Aug 6;3(5):e672. doi: 10.1097/PR9.0000000000000672. PMID: 30534623; PMCID: PMC6181466.

[59] Wang M, Wang S, Trapani JA, Neeson PJ. Challenges of PD-L1 testing in non-small cell lung cancer and beyond. J Thorac Dis. 2020 Aug;12(8):4541–4548. doi: 10.21037/jtd-2019-itm-010. PMID: 32944371; PMCID: PMC7475552.

[60] Benlysta [package insert]. Human Genome Sciences / GlaxoSmithKline. March 2012. https://www.accessdata.fda.gov/drugsatfda_docs/label/2012/125370s016lbl.pdf. Permalink: https://perma.cc/GGA5-SSJ4.

[61] Furie RA, Morand EF, Bruce IN, Manzi S, Kalunian KC, Vital EM, Ford TL, Gupta R, Hiepe F, Santiago M, Brohawn PZ, Berglind A, Tummala R. Type I interferon inhibitor anifrolumab in active systemic lupus erythematosus (TULIP-1): A randomised, controlled, phase 3 trial. Lancet Rheumatol. 2019 Dec;1(4):e208–e219. doi: 10.1016/S2665-9913(19)30076-1.

[62] Grover N. AstraZeneca sets stage for marketing application with promising pivotal lupus drug data. Endpoints News. November 13, 2019. https://endpts.com/astrazeneca-sets-stage-for-marketing-application-with-promising-pivotal-lupus-drug-data/. Accessed October 15, 2021.

[63] Mikdashi J, Nived O. Measuring disease activity in adults with systemic lupus erythematosus: The challenges of administrative burden and responsiveness to patient concerns in clinical research. Arthritis Res Ther. 2015 Jul 20;17(1):183. doi: 10.1186/s13075-015-0702-6. PMID: 26189728; PMCID: PMC4507322.

[64] Tong A. Watch out GlaxoSmithKline: AstraZeneca's once-failed lupus drug is now approved. August 2, 2021 (updated August 4, 2021). https://endpts.com/watch-out-glaxosmithkline-astrazenecas-once-failed-lupus-drug-is-now-approved/. Accessed October 15, 2021.

[65] Leucht S, Fennema H, Engel RR, Kaspers-Janssen M, Szegedi A. Translating the HAM-D into the MADRS and vice versa with equipercentile linking. J Affect Disord. 2018 Jan 15;226:326–331. doi: 10.1016/j.jad.2017.09.042. Epub 2017 Sep 27. PMID: 29031182.

[66] Desai A, Gyawali B. Endpoints used in Phase III randomized controlled trials of treatment options for COVID-19. EClinicalMedicine. 2020 Jun 2;23:100403. doi: 10.1016/j.eclinm.2020.100403. PMID: 32632415; PMCID: PMC7265861.

[67] WHO Working Group on the Clinical Characterisation and Management of COVID-19 infection. A minimal common outcome measure set for COVID-19 clinical research. Lancet Infect Dis. 2020 Aug;20(8):e192–e197. doi: 10.1016/S1473-3099(20)30483-7. Epub 2020 Jun 12. Erratum in: Lancet Infect Dis. 2020 Oct;20(10):e250. PMID: 32539990; PMCID: PMC7292605.

[68] Levin J. AstraZeneca and Targacept announce remaining TC-5214 Phase 3 efficacy studies do not meet primary endpoint, regulatory filing will not be pursued. FierceBiotech. March 20, 2012. https://www.fiercebiotech.com/r-d/astrazeneca-and-targacept-announce-remaining-tc-5214-phase-3-efficacy-studies-do-not-meet. Accessed October 15, 2021.

[69] Hatsukami DK, Jorenby DE, Gonzales D, Rigotti NA, Glover ED, Oncken CA, Tashkin DP, Reus VI, Akhavain RC, Fahim RE, Kessler PD, Niknian M, Kalnik MW, Rennard SI. Immunogenicity and smoking-cessation outcomes for a novel nicotine immunotherapeutic. Clin Pharmacol Ther. 2011 Mar;89(3):392–399. doi: 10.1038/clpt.2010.317. Epub 2011 Jan 26. PMID: 21270788; PMCID: PMC4106715.

[70] Nabi Biopharmaceuticals announces results of first NicVAX Phase III clinical trial. Nabi Pharmaceuticals press release. July 18, 2011. https://www.globenewswire.com/news-release/2011/07/18/451456/226731/en/Nabi-Biopharmaceuticals-Announces-Results-of-First-NicVAX-R-Phase-III-Clinical-Trial.html. Accessed October 15, 2021. Permalink: https://perma.cc/4AYA-E7LF.

[71] Nabi Biopharmaceuticals announces results of second NicVAX Phase III clinical trial. Nabi Biopharmaceuticals press release. November 7, 2011. https://www.globenewswire.com/news-release/2011/11/07/460749/237357/en/Nabi-Biopharmaceuticals-Announces-Results-of-Second-NicVAX-R-Phase-III-Clinical-Trial.html. Accessed October 15, 2021. Permalink: https://perma.cc/R3EE-AYXV.

[72] Ramagopalan S, Skingsley AP, Handunnetthi L, Klingel M, Magnus D, Pakpoor J, Goldacre B. Prevalence of primary outcome changes in clinical trials registered on ClinicalTrials.gov: A cross-sectional study. F1000Res. 2014 Mar 26;3:77. doi: 10.12688/f1000research.3784.1. PMID: 25075294; PMCID: PMC4032105.

[73] Evans S. When and how can endpoints be changed after initiation of a randomized clinical trial? PLoS Clin Trials. 2007 Apr 13;2(4):e18. doi: 10.1371/journal.pctr.0020018. PMID: 17443237; PMCID: PMC1852589.

[74] 42 CFR § 11.28.

[75] Matrixx Initiatives, Inc. v. Siracusano, 563 U.S. 27 (2011).

[76] Eckstein L. Assessing the legal duty to use or disclose interim data for ongoing clinical trials. J Law Biosciences. 2019 Oct;6(1):51–84. doi: 10.1093/jlb/lsz012.

[77] Adams B. Intercept jumps on NASH Phase 3 protocol changes. FierceBiotech. February 10, 2017. https://www.fiercebiotech.com/biotech/intercept-jumps-nash-phase-3-protocol-change. Accessed October 15, 2021.

[78] Randomized global Phase 3 study to evaluate the impact on NASH with fibrosis of obeticholic acid treatment (REGENERATE). ClinicalTrials.gov identifier: NCT02548351. Updated September 9, 2021. Accessed October 15, 2021.

[79] Spark Therapeutics announces database lock for SPK-RPE65 Phase 3 clinical trial and expected release of top-line data in October. Spark Therapeutics press release. September 9, 2015. https://sparktx.com/press_releases/spark-therapeutics-announces-database-lock-for-spk-rpe65-phase-3-clinical-trial-and-expected-release-of-top-line-data-in-october/. Accessed October 15, 2021. Permalink: https://perma.cc/WNM3-6956.

[80] Carroll J. Did Gilead just lower the bar on crucial remdesivir trials for Covid-19? Switching endpoints, amping up trial size stir analysts' fears—and hopes. Endpoints News. April 8, 2020. https://endpts.com/did-gilead-just-lower-the-bar-on-crucial-remdesivir-trials-for-covid-19-switching-endpoints-amping-up-trial-size-raises-analysts-doubts/. Accessed October 15, 2021.

[81] Bangalore S, Maron DJ, Reynolds HR, Stone GW, O'Brien SM, Alexander KP, Hochman JS. ISCHEMIA: Establishing the primary end point. Circ Cardiovasc Qual Outcomes. 2018 May;11(5):e004791. doi: 10.1161/CIRCOUTCOMES.118.004791. PMID: 29752391; PMCID: PMC5967873.

[82] Maron DJ, Hochman JS, Reynolds HR, Bangalore S, O'Brien SM, Boden WE, Chaitman BR, Senior R, López-Sendón J, Alexander KP, Lopes RD, Shaw LJ, Berger JS, Newman JD, Sidhu MS, Goodman SG, Ruzyllo W, Gosselin G, Maggioni AP, White HD, Bhargava B, Min JK, Mancini GBJ, Berman DS, Picard MH, Kwong RY, Ali ZA, Mark DB, Spertus JA, Krishnan MN, Elghamaz A, Moorthy N, Hueb WA, Demkow M, Mavromatis K, Bockeria O, Peteiro J, Miller TD, Szwed H, Doerr R, Keltai M, Selvanayagam JB, Steg PG, Held C, Kohsaka S, Mavromichalis S, Kirby R, Jeffries NO, Harrell FE Jr, Rockhold FW, Broderick S, Ferguson TB Jr, Williams DO, Harrington RA, Stone GW, Rosenberg Y; ISCHEMIA Research Group. Initial invasive or conservative strategy for stable coronary disease. N Engl J Med. 2020 Apr 9;382(15):1395–1407. doi: 10.1056/NEJMoa1915922. Epub 2020 Mar 30. PMID: 32227755; PMCID: PMC7263833.

[83] Feuerstein A. Vanda's sleep disorder drug is a nightmare. TheStreet. June 19, 2013. https://www.thestreet.com/investing/stocks/vandas-sleep-disorder-drug-is-a-nightmare-11954365. Accessed October 15, 2021.

[84] Plieth J. Despite shock adcom vote, Vanda will struggle to remain relevant. Evaluate Vantage. November 15, 2013. https://www.evaluate.com/vantage/articles/news/despite-shock-adcom-vote-vanda-will-struggle-remain-relevant. Accessed October 15, 2021.

[85] Meeting minutes: Peripheral and central nervous system drugs advisory committee. U.S. Food and Drug Administration. November 14, 2013. Permalink: https://wayback.archive-it.org/7993/20170404154523/https://www.fda.gov/downloads/AdvisoryCommittees/CommitteesMeetingMaterials/Drugs/PeripheralandCentralNervousSystemDrugsAdvisoryCommittee/UCM386061.pdf.

[86] Zanolla L, Zardini P. Selection of endpoints for heart failure clinical trials. Eur J Heart Fail. 2003 Dec;5(6):717–723. doi: 10.1016/s1388-9842(03)00101-6. PMID: 14675849.

[87] Brenner A, Arribas M, Cuzick J, Jairath V, Stanworth S, Ker K, Shakur-Still H, Roberts I. Outcome measures in clinical trials of treatments for acute severe haemorrhage. Trials. 2018 Oct 1;19(1):533. doi: 10.1186/s13063-018-2900-4. PMID: 30285839; PMCID: PMC6167881.

[88] Farkas J. It's insane to keep using mortality as a primary endpoint in critical care trials. EMCrit blog. February 19, 2020. https://emcrit.org/pulmcrit/mortality-2/. Accessed October 15, 2021. Permalink: https://perma.cc/THK9-XQYW.

[89] Bright CJ, Brentnall AR, Wooldrage K, Myles J, Sasieni P, Duffy SW. Errors in determination of net survival: Cause-specific and relative survival settings. Br J Cancer. 2020 Mar;122(7):1094–1101. doi: 10.1038/s41416-020-0739-4. Epub 2020 Feb 10. PMID: 32037401; PMCID: PMC7109046.

[90] Cuzick J, Stewart H, Rutqvist L, Houghton J, Edwards R, Redmond C, Peto R, Baum M, Fisher B, Host H, et al. Cause-specific mortality in long-term survivors of breast cancer who participated in trials of radiotherapy. J Clin Oncol. 1994 Mar;12(3):447–453. doi: 10.1200/JCO.1994.12.3.447. PMID: 8120544.

[91] Penston J. Should we use total mortality rather than cancer-specific mortality to judge cancer screening programmes? Yes. BMJ. 2011 Oct 13;343:d6395. doi: 10.1136/bmj.d6395. PMID: 21998347.

6.

EXECUTION

DESPITE THE BEST INTENTIONS of sponsors and investigators, drug trials never follow the textbook perfectly. Patients drop out at various points along the path from initial screening to final analysis, and the ones who are enrolled are never *exactly* comparable between study arms, even with the most robust randomization.

The question for readers is how these imperfections might affect interpretation of the results. Dropouts and imbalances are usually part of the statistical noise, but they can occasionally introduce bias into the trial or raise questions about the experimental drug's efficacy or safety.

In this chapter, we discuss how to assess patient accounting and randomization and provide some guidelines for putting the findings in context. We also include a brief discussion of how to interpret studies that are stopped prematurely.

Patient accounting

To understand how many patients withdrew from a study and why, it's important to know how many patients were screened for, enrolled in, and completed a clinical trial. Depending on when and why dropouts occurred, they can affect the assessment of the drug's efficacy and provide important information about how patients experienced side effects and adverse events, even ones that were ostensibly mild.

Most journal articles reporting clinical trial results include a detailed flow chart that describes how many patients were included and excluded in each arm during enrollment, allocation, follow-up, and analysis, and the reasons for exclusions, in accordance with the CONSORT publication guidelines, as in Figure 6-1.[1] But in other materials such as press releases and medical meeting abstracts, the presentation is typically more limited and variable. Figure 6-2 shows a typical example, from a Phase 3 study of two doses of topical diltiazem cream (VEN 307; Ventrus Biosciences) versus placebo for the treatment of anal fissures.[2]

FIGURE 6-1: Recommended patient flow diagram for a randomized controlled trial from the CONSORT Group.

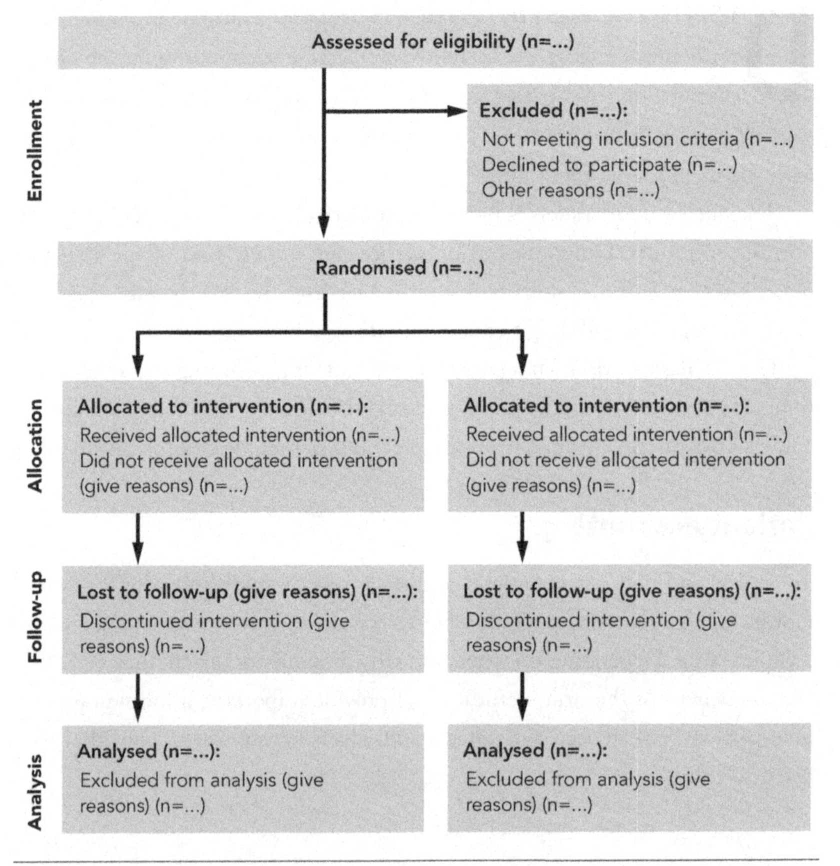

Figure note: Adapted from the original; see text for source information.

FIGURE 6-2: Example of patient flow diagram.

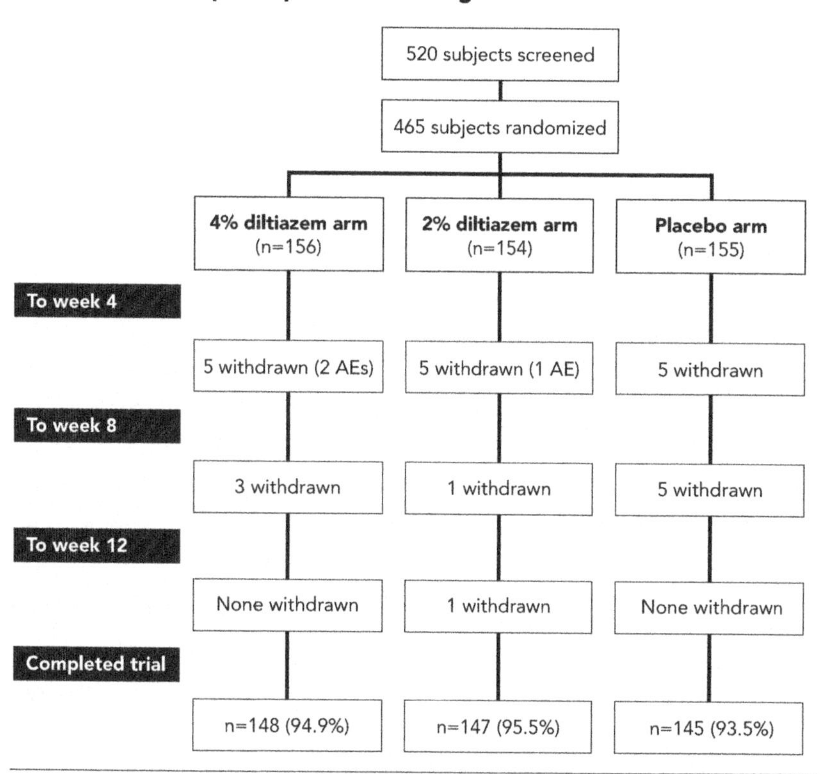

Figure note: Adapted from the original; see text for source information. AE, adverse event.

Regardless of the level of detail provided, readers should try to extract the following information[3]:

- **Enrollment:** Number of patients screened; how many were excluded due to failure to meet enrollment criteria, refusal to enroll, or other reasons; and the net number enrolled and randomized.
- **Allocation and treatment:** Number of patients assigned to each arm, how many did or did not receive the assigned intervention, and how many discontinued participation, including dropouts due to inefficacy or adverse events, withdrawal of consent, logistical issues, or other factors.
- **Analysis:** Number of patients in each arm of the final data analysis and how many were excluded from each arm and why.

To assess the patient accounting, it is helpful to consider the data in two groups: before and after randomization. Exclusions before randomization are often due to failure to meet certain entry criteria related to biomarkers or laboratory findings. These may be appropriate and expected based on what is known about the indication, but a high pre-randomization screen failure rate relative to prior studies in an identical or closely related indication could suggest that the entry criteria are rarer than expected or that there is some other barrier that prevents potentially eligible patients from being included, such as refusing to submit to an additional tumor biopsy or other invasive procedure during screening. In these situations, trial participants may not be reflective of the broader patient population, which could make the trial findings less broadly applicable.

A more common and worrisome scenario is when patients discontinue participation after randomization but before completion of the trial. Here, the key question is whether the reason patients dropped out is somehow associated with what they expected the outcome to be if they completed the trial. That could introduce bias into the results. To detect this potential bias, it is important to assess how frequent the dropouts were and whether they were balanced between the arms:

- **Frequency:** The proportion of trial dropouts after randomization varies depending on the indication and type of intervention. Some experts have proposed as a rule of thumb that dropout rates greater than 20% should be viewed with concern, although rates of 30% or more are not uncommon in Phase 3 studies.[4] Dropout rates tend to be higher across both arms for studies of less severe conditions or prevention of rare events, particularly if they last for long periods. It is worth comparing a trial's dropout rate with rates of similar studies in the same indication.
- **Balance across study arms:** A higher-than-expected dropout rate after randomization that is roughly balanced across treatment arms could suggest that the trial protocol is particularly onerous for patients or indicate poor execution by the study sponsor. This is less likely to bias the results because the dropouts should be unrelated to patients' underlying characteristics or outcomes. However, even balanced dropouts are worth noting if they occur at a high frequency, because they may affect how one interprets the relevance of the study findings to real-world practice.

Unbalanced dropouts that are substantially more frequent in one arm than another often reflect adverse safety or tolerability effects. Up to 20% of patients who received the highest dose of gefapixant (Merck) in two Phase 3 studies for chronic cough reported in 2020 withdrew from the studies compared with fewer than 5% of patients treated with placebo.[5] This imbalance did not affect the efficacy analysis per se, but it could affect the drug's reception by regulators, prescribers, or patients.

Modern analytic methods are reasonably adept at handling dropouts in mid-trial even if they are unbalanced. In most contemporary cases, the assessment of efficacy is not compromised, although some approaches that used to be more popular (like "last observation carried forward") are more problematic.[6] However, if the total fraction of dropouts is quite high or the imbalance is pronounced, then there is a theoretical risk that the results could mis-specify the true treatment effect. This concern has been raised for placebo-controlled randomized controlled trials (RCTs) of anti-psychotics, where patients in the control arm tend to withdraw at higher rates, presumably because they fail to experience symptomatic relief.[7] There are no strict definitions for what level of imbalance in dropout rates is concerning. In most cases, the best a reader can do is note the imbalance and consider all possible ways that it could skew one's interpretation of the trial's results.

Characteristics of participating patients

Virtually all journal articles reporting clinical trials and most other presentations of results provide a summary table describing key baseline characteristics of patients who participated in the study.[8] The example in Figure 6-3 was prepared by the U.S. Food and Drug Administration (FDA) to summarize patient characteristics from four trials executed starting in 2014 of cannabidiol oral solution (Epidiolex; GW Pharmaceuticals) in Dravet syndrome and Lennox-Gastaut syndrome[9]:

FIGURE 6-3: Example of table of baseline characteristics.

			Cannabidiol				Placebo
			5	10	20	All	
		n	10	75	238	323	227
Dravet	**GWEP1332 Part A**	n (%)	10 (100%)	8 (11%)	9 (4%)	27 (8%)	7 (3%)
	GWEP1332 Part B	n (%)	0 (0%)	0 (0%)	61 (26%)	61 (19%)	59 (26%)
Lennox-Gastaut	**GWEP1414**	n (%)	0 (0%)	67 (89%)	82 (34%)	149 (46%)	76 (33%)
	GWEP1423	n (%)	0 (0%)	0 (0%)	86 (36%)	86 (27%)	85 (37%)
	Patient-years	Total	0.8	18.8	58.4	78.1	60.4
	Age	Mean±SD	7.2±1.9	14.0±8.6	14.1±9.2	13.9±9.0	13.6±8.8
		Median	6.7	11.9	11.8	11.5	11.4
		Min;Max	5;11	3;38	3;48	3;48	2;45
	Age categories, n (%)	2-5	2 (20%)	10 (13%)	39 (16%)	51 (16%)	38 (17%)
		6-11	8 (80%)	28 (37%)	81 (34%)	117(36%)	79 (35%)
		12-17	0 (0%)	18 (24%)	62 (26%)	80 (25%)	57 (25%)
		18-45	0 (0%)	19 (25%)	53 (22%)	72 (22%)	53 (23%)
		46-55	0 (0%)	0 (0%)	3 (1%)	3 (1%)	0 (0%)
		≥56	0 (0%)	0 (0%)	0 (0%)	0 (0%)	0 (0%)
	Sex, n (%)	Male	5 (50%)	39 (52%)	132 (55%)	176 (54%)	119(52%)
		Female	5 (50%)	36 (48%)	106 (45%)	147 (46%)	108(48%)
	Race, n (%)	White	9 (90%)	60 (80%)	200 (84%)	269 (83%)	201 (89%)
		Black	0 (0%)	7 (9%)	8 (3%)	15 (5%)	8 (4%)
		Asian	0 (0%)	1 (1%)	6 (3%)	7 (2%)	5 (2%)
		Other	1 (10%)	7 (9%)	24 (10%)	32 (10%)	13 (6%)
	Location, n (%)	US	8 (80%)	62 (83%)	170 (71%)	240 (74%)	171 (75%)
		Spain	0 (0%)	9 (12%)	11 (5%)	20 (6%)	12 (5%)
		France	0 (0%)	1 (1%)	12 (5%)	13 (4%)	6 (3%)
		UK	2 (20%)	3 (4%)	15 (6%)	20 (6%)	11 (5%)
		Netherlands	0 (0%)	0 (0%)	3 (1%)	3 (1%)	2 (1%)
		Poland	0 (0%)	0 (0%)	27 (11%)	27 (8%)	25(11%)
	Weight (kg)	Mean±SD	28±9	41±26	40±21	40±22	41±22
		Median	17.0	18.2	17.7	17.7	18.5
		Min;Max	14;26	11;50	10;94	10;94	10;51
	Number of current AEDs, n (%)	0	0 (0%)	0 (0%)	0 (0%)	0 (0%)	0 (0%)
		1	2 (20%)	3 (4%)	15 (6%)	20 (6%)	11 (5%)
		2	2 (20%)	19 (25%)	48 (20%)	69 (21%)	54 (24%)
		3	4 (40%)	29 (39%)	94 (39%)	127 (39%)	83 (37%)
		≥4	2 (20%)	24 (32%)	81 (34%)	107 (33%)	79 (35%)
	Valproate/ Clobazem use, n (%)	Valproate	2 (20%)	18 (24%)	59 (25%)	79(24%)	52 (23%)
		Clobazem	1 (10%)	31(41%)	70 (29%)	102 (32%)	76 (33%)
		Both	5 (50%)	10 (13%)	55 (23%)	70 (22%)	47 (21%)
		Neither	2 (20%)	16 (21%)	54 (23%)	72 (22%)	52 (23%)

Figure note: Adapted from the original; see text for source information. AEDs, anti-epileptic drugs.

Examining the baseline characteristics allows one to compare the patients in a study with one's expectations based on the inclusion and exclusion criteria as well as with external reference points. In 2015, Geron Corp. initiated a 107-patient uncontrolled study of the effect of two dose levels of its telomerase inhibitor, imetelstat, on patients with myelofibrosis. The trial, known as IMbark, enrolled patients whose disease had progressed during or after treatment with the first-line agent, ruxolitinib (Jakafi; Incyte), making them second-line patients.[10] An interim analysis in early 2018 reported a median overall survival (OS) of at least 19 months across both dose arms,[11] which Geron compared favorably with the seven-month OS recorded in second-line patients in a real-world outcomes study reflecting results from everyday clinical treatments.[12] However, one analyst noted that in the real-world study, most of the patients who received ruxolitinib in first-line treatment (77% according to the abstract) were too sick to receive any other treatments,[13] suggesting that even though the two populations appeared superficially similar, the patients in IMbark may have actually been far healthier than those in the real-world study. The table of baseline characteristics from IMbark was disclosed later in 2018,[14] but the data were insufficient to address Feuerstein's concern. However, the sponsor later showed in a post hoc analysis that the high-dose imetelstat patients survived longer than matched controls from the real-world study[15] and initiated a Phase 3 RCT in 2020 that is still ongoing.[16]

Tables of baseline patient data typically include a list of variables and the value for each arm of the study. Values for continuous variables are reported as mean and standard deviation or median and interquartile range, and those for categorical variables are reported as the number of patients in each group.

A common misconception about these tables is that their main utility is to quantify differences between study arms. In fact, baseline data provide at most only directional guidance about imbalances between the arms, and although statistical comparisons are commonly reported, they are not meaningful. This issue is discussed in more detail in the next section.

How to interpret the table of baseline data

1. Examine the list of characteristics/variables

As a first step, you should ensure that the list of clinical variables in the baseline data table includes all variables you might expect to influence the outcome of the study or your interpretation of the results. These commonly include demographics such as age, gender, and race; measures of disease severity; current and prior therapies; and key clinical or laboratory parameters. Many of these might be invoked later in the report for subgroup or covariate analyses.

Almost any patient attribute could *potentially* affect the results and implications of a trial. But in practice, for a given indication and study design, there are usually a few key parameters that are most likely to have an impact, and others are considered minor possible contributors to the outcome. For example, results of a study of a new drug for chronic pain are probably highly dependent on the baseline analgesic usage of patients and probably less so on a difference in the ages of the patients between the two arms.

It's particularly important at this stage to note any patient characteristics that *should* be described but aren't—particularly in press releases, abstracts, and investor presentations, which often report skimpy baseline data or none at all. When this table is incomplete, there is a risk that positive results could be due to inclusion of a narrow subset of patients or biased by imbalances between the study arms. For example, after disclosing data in 2009 from an apparently successful Phase 2 trial of enobosarm for cancer cachexia across a mix of tumor types,[17] GTx launched two Phase 3 studies of the drug in lung cancer.[18] When the full Phase 2 results were published in 2013,[19] however, one analyst observed that an imbalance in the fraction of lung cancer patients with advanced disease in each arm (60% on placebo vs. 38% on enobosarm) could have biased the results to favor the study drug.[20] As it turned out, the two Phase 3 trials in lung cancer cachexia subsequently failed.[21]

2. Examine the aggregate characteristics of participating patients

The baseline data table provides important information about how generalizable the results are likely to be. In contrast to the inclusion and exclusion criteria, which define which patients *can* be part of a trial, the table of baseline characteristics shows who actually *did* participate. This may be a narrower and skewed subset compared with the target recruitment population. Determining the characteristics of the patients in the entire study typically requires some extra work by the reader because results are typically presented separately across the arms.

If the participating patients are not as planned on key parameters, this could affect not only the outcome of the study and how you interpret the results but also how you compare the findings with other trials that have superficially similar inclusion and exclusion criteria. For example, many adult cancer trials fail to enroll many patients over age 70, even though elderly patients are technically eligible.[22] Similarly, a study that is open to patients with a broad range of disease severities may primarily enroll patients at the mildest or the most severe end of the spectrum. In addition, some trials may primarily include patients with a skewed distribution of a particular physiologic parameter, like renal or liver function, that is not intimately related to the indication being studied.

Whether a trial succeeds or fails, the results need to be interpreted based on the types of patients who actually enrolled—which can in some cases be very different from the intended population. For example, an asthma study found that a triple therapy combining steroids and two other drug classes reduced the incidence of moderate or severe exacerbations compared with a dual therapy, which for some of the control patients excluded steroids.[23] However, more than 70% of patients enrolled in the trial were already on inhaled steroids and thus would have been expected to have a high rate of exacerbations if assigned to the steroid-free control arm. This may have biased the study toward a more positive result for the triple therapy.[24]

3. Compare patient characteristics between the study arms

Because both arms of a study are selected randomly from the same patient population, there will almost always be some degree of difference between the arms that is statistical "noise." The disparity between arms can be particularly noteworthy if the study is small. The baseline data table provides *directional* guidance as to whether there are imbalances in key variables that could either introduce bias into the interpretation of the results or highlight the need to adjust for confounding, as discussed below. In scanning the characteristics across the two arms, one should ask three questions:

- **Is the variable likely to affect the outcome?** In a study of a new drug for metastatic melanoma with an endpoint of OS, the gender balance between the arms is probably somewhat less important than whether patients in the two arms received a similar number of lines of prior therapy.
- **How big is the difference between the arms?** This is extremely subjective and depends on how much influence you think the variable is likely to be. If it is a particularly powerful determinant of response, then even a small imbalance could have a large impact on the results. In a Phase

2 trial published in 2016 of the dual anti-VEGF/anti-PDGF therapy E10030 (Fovista; Ophthotech) in age-related macular degeneration, control arm patients had slightly more-severe disease at baseline (1.8 disc areas) compared with those in the dose group that yielded a statistically significant positive effect (1.5 disc areas).[25] In retrospect, some experts argued that even this slight bias toward the experimental therapy may partly explain why several subsequent Phase 3 studies failed.[26]

- **What is the potential effect of the imbalance?** In the example above, the worrisome finding was that the imbalance favored the experimental therapy; if the E10030-treated patients had more-severe disease at baseline than those in the control arm, the slight difference would not have been a concern. In cases where there are several imbalances, they might sometimes be expected to qualitatively cancel each other out, but it is more problematic if they are all likely to favor the experimental arm of the trial.[27]

Although many reports provide *P* values for each of the variables in tables of baseline characteristics, experts explicitly discourage this practice, and readers should not give credence to these results.[28,29] The reason is that in this scenario, the *P* value assesses the probability of obtaining a given difference or greater *if* the two sets of patients were selected from the same pool. But here we *know* that the patients were selected from a common pool. Because there is no hypothesis being tested when one compares the two arms in this way, it is illogical to calculate a *P* value for differences between them. Assuming proper blinding and randomization, any differences between the arms by definition must have arisen by chance. The correct approach for readers is to qualitatively assess whether imbalance is a potential concern, and then determine whether the investigators used appropriate methods to handle it, as discussed below.[30,31]

Finally, although it may seem that one could use the baseline data table to deduce whether patients were inappropriately assigned to specific arms due to unblinding, it is virtually impossible to detect compromised or illegitimate randomization in practice.

4. Correlate with the statistical analysis plan

It is crucial to examine the methods to see whether appropriate and robust statistical methods were used to correct for imbalances in potentially influential baseline variables. In large Phase 2 and 3 studies, the most common and appropriate way to handle potential baseline imbalances is to adjust for them in a multivariate analysis.[32] This needs to be pre-specified in the analysis plan to avoid increasing the likelihood of spurious positive results.[33]

In practice, however, many RCTs do not control for all baseline variables that one might plausibly hypothesize to have an effect. Particularly in small trials, such adjustments may be unfeasible. In other scenarios, investigators may eschew these methods due to legitimate differences in opinion about methodology, ignorance, willful malfeasance to increase the chances of a positive finding, or some combination thereof.

For readers of clinical study results, there are three main takeaways. First, if a study has apparent imbalances in baseline characteristics that are highly unlikely to influence the outcome, then these can be safely ignored. Second, if there are imbalances in potentially influential variables but they are accounted for with appropriate statistical methods, then they are not of any particular concern. And third, if an apparently positive trial seemingly has imbalances between the arms in a characteristic that might favor the experimental therapy—as in the enobosarm and E10030 examples above—and appropriate methods were not employed to adjust for the imbalances during analysis, this raises the risk that at least some of the positivity may be less than reported.

Early termination

The three main reasons a study might be ended before reaching its planned enrollment are (a) early evidence of efficacy or lack thereof, (b) early evidence of harm, and (c) practical considerations, of which slow or inefficient recruitment is probably the most common.

The *only* reason that results from a prematurely terminated study should be taken at face value is if the trial was stopped due to *pre-specified* criteria. This could include preset stopping rules based on the occurrence of a given number of events. This often occurs in studies of cardiovascular drugs intended to prevent death or stroke. Or a pre-planned interim analysis could result in the trial's cessation due to meeting pre-set thresholds for efficacy or futility. Studies with interim analyses that lead to a change in the trial's design or execution are a subtype of adaptive trials, the topic of Chapter 15. These sorts of scenarios will always be outlined in the description of methods and will be accompanied by a statistical plan to ensure that the analysis is appropriate.

Although there are historical examples of studies stopped based on unplanned early analyses that purportedly showed efficacy, in the modern era the main reasons drug trials are stopped *unexpectedly* are an unanticipated adverse safety/tolerability signal or poor recruitment. In the recruitment case, any analysis of the treatment's efficacy should be interpreted very cautiously because of their insufficient power and the significantly heightened risk of a false positive result. This risk can be illustrated with a coin-flipping example. If one plans a 100-flip test of whether a quarter is "fair," but one's thumb tires after five flips, the fact that 4/5 of those flips were heads is almost certainly a random and non-significant finding. Although some academic studies failed to reach their recruitment goals but still attempted to salvage positive results by showing that the smaller trial was still appropriately powered,[34] this situation is rare to nonexistent in biopharma.

---

[1] Schulz KF, Altman DG, Moher D; CONSORT Group. CONSORT 2010 statement: Updated guidelines for reporting parallel group randomised trials. Trials. 2010 Mar 24;11:32. doi: 10.1186/1745-6215-11-32. PMID: 20334632; PMCID: PMC2857832.

[2] Presentation to Bank of America Merrill Lynch 2012 Health Care Conference. Ventrus Biosciences. May 16, 2012. https://www.sec.gov/Archives/edgar/data/1426800/000114420412030103/v313620_ex99-1.htm. Accessed October 15, 2021.

[3] Andrade C. Examination of participant flow in the CONSORT diagram can improve the understanding of the generalizability of study results. J Clin Psychiatry. 2015 Nov;76(11):e1469–1471. doi: 10.4088/JCP.15f10436. PMID: 26646042.

[4] U.S. National Research Council Panel on Handling Missing Data in Clinical Trials. The prevention and treatment of missing data in clinical trials. U.S. National Academies Press; 2010. Available at https://www.ncbi.nlm.nih.gov/books/NBK209904/. doi: 10.17226/12955. Accessed October 15, 2021.

[5] Merck's gefapixant (45 mg twice daily) significantly decreased cough frequency compared to placebo at week 12 and 24 in patients with refractory or unexplained chronic cough. Merck press release. September 8, 2020. https://www.merck.com/news/mercks-gefapixant-45-mg-twice-daily-significantly-decreased-cough-frequency-compared-to-placebo-at-week-12-and-24-in-patients-with-refractory-or-unexplained-chronic-cough/. Accessed October 15, 2021. Permalink: https://perma.cc/LL66-G9RR.

[6] Vickers AJ, Altman DG. Statistics notes: Missing outcomes in randomised trials. BMJ. 2013 Jun 6;346:f3438. doi: 10.1136/bmj.f3438. PMID: 23744649.

[7] Kemmler G, Hummer M, Widschwendter C, Fleischhacker WW. Dropout rates in placebo-controlled and active-control clinical trials of antipsychotic drugs: A meta-analysis. Arch Gen Psychiatry. 2005 Dec;62(12):1305–1312. doi: 10.1001/archpsyc.62.12.1305. PMID: 16330718.

[8] Pocock SJ, Assmann SE, Enos LE, Kasten LE. Subgroup analysis, covariate adjustment and baseline comparisons in clinical trial reporting: Current practice and problems. Stat Med. 2002 Oct 15;21(19):2917–2930. doi: 10.1002/sim.1296. PMID: 12325108.

[9] NDA 210395 (cannabidiol; GW Pharmaceuticals): Peripheral and central nervous systems drugs advisory committee meeting briefing document. U.S. Food and Drug Administration. April 19, 2018. https://www.fda.gov/media/112565/download. Accessed October 15, 2021. Permalink: https://perma.cc/W4ZP-FTDT.

[10] Study to evaluate activity of 2 dose levels of imetelstat in participants with intermediate-2 or high-risk myelofibrosis (MF) previously treated with Janus kinase (JAK) inhibitor. ClinicalTrials.gov identifier: NCT02426086. Updated September 14, 2021. Accessed October 15, 2021.

[11] Geron Corporation reports fourth quarter and annual 2017 financial results and recent events. Geron Corporation press release. March 16, 2018. http://ir.geron.com/investors/press-releases/press-release-details/2018/Geron-Corporation-Reports-Fourth-Quarter-and-Annual-2017-Financial-Results-and-Recent-Events/default.aspx. Accessed October 15, 2021. Permalink: https://perma.cc/QG4K-DX3K.

[12] Mehra M, Potluri R, He J, Wang G, Mundle S, Bussolari J. Characterization of disease, treatment patterns, and outcomes of patients with myelofibrosis: Analysis of 2 United States commercial claims databases. Blood. 2016 Dec 2;128(22):4769. doi: 10.1182/blood.V128.22.4769.4769.

[13] Feuerstein A. The top-performing biotech stock this year has surged on flimsy data. STAT. March 27, 2018. https://www.statnews.com/2018/03/27/geron-stock-price-surge/. Accessed October 15, 2021.

[14] Mascarenhas J, Komrokji RS, Cavo M, Martino B, Niederwieser D, Reiter A, Scott BL, Baer MR, Hoffman R, Odenike O, Bussolari J, Zhu E, Huang F, Rose E, Sherman L, Dougherty S, Feller FM, Kiladjian JJ. Imetelstat is effective treatment for patients with intermediate-2 or high-risk myelofibrosis who have relapsed on or are refractory to Janus kinase inhibitor therapy: Results of a Phase 2 randomized study of two dose levels (abstract 685). ASH oral presentation. November 29, 2018. https://www.geron.com/file

.cfm/53/docs/imetelstat_IMbark_ASH%202018_FINAL.pdf. Accessed October 15, 2021. Permalink: https://perma.cc/4F4R-7HU9.

[15] Kuykendall A, Wan Y, Mascarenhas J, Kiladjian JJ, Vannuchi A, Wang J, Xia Q, Zhu E, Feller F, Rizo A, Bussolari J, Komrokji R. Favorable overall survival of imetelstat-treated relapsed/refractory myelofibrosis patients compared with closely matched real-world data (abstract 1456). ASH poster presentation. 2019. https://library.ehaweb.org/eha/2019/24th/267073/andrew.kuykendall.favorable.overall.survival.of.imetelstat-treated.relapsed.html. Accessed October 15, 2021. Permalink: https://perma.cc/W7PU-KZM5.

[16] A study comparing imetelstat versus best available therapy for the treatment of intermediate-2 or high-risk myelofibrosis (MF) who have not responded to Janus kinase (JAK)-inhibitor treatment. ClinicalTrials.gov identifier: NCT04576156. Updated October 8, 2021. Accessed October 15, 2021.

[17] GTx presents Phase II Ostarine (MK-2866) cancer cachexia clinical trial results at Endocrine Society annual meeting. GTx press release. June 12, 2009. https://www.fiercebiotech.com/biotech/gtx-presents-phase-ii-ostarine-mk-2866-cancer-cachexia-clinical-trial-results-at-endocrine/. Accessed October 15, 2021. Permalink: https://perma.cc/U52R-J69T.

[18] Crawford J, Prado CM, Johnston MA, Gralla RJ, Taylor RP, Hancock ML, Dalton JT. Study design and rationale for the Phase 3 clinical development program of enobosarm, a selective androgen receptor modulator, for the prevention and treatment of muscle wasting in cancer patients (POWER trials). Curr Oncol Rep. 2016 Jun;18(6):37. doi: 10.1007/s11912-016-0522-0. PMID: 27138015; PMCID: PMC4853438.

[19] Dobs AS, Boccia RV, Croot CC, Gabrail NY, Dalton JT, Hancock ML, Johnston MA, Steiner MS. Effects of enobosarm on muscle wasting and physical function in patients with cancer: A double-blind, randomised controlled phase 2 trial. Lancet Oncol. 2013 Apr;14(4):335–345. doi: 10.1016/S1470-2045(13)70055-X. Epub 2013 Mar 14. PMID: 23499390; PMCID: PMC4898053.

[20] Feuerstein A. The GTx cancer muscle-wasting drug studies will fail. Here's why. TheStreet. July 10, 2013. https://www.thestreet.com/investing/stocks/the-gtx-cancer-muscle-wasting-drug-studies-will-fail-heres-why-11974668. Accessed October 15, 2021.

[21] Gardner J. Cachexia drug failure falls heavily on GTx. Evaluate Vantage. August 20, 2013. https://www.evaluate.com/vantage/articles/news/cachexia-drug-failure-falls-heavily-gtx. Accessed October 15, 2021.

[22] Hutchins LF, Unger JM, Crowley JJ, Coltman CA Jr, Albain KS. Underrepresentation of patients 65 years of age or older in cancer-treatment trials. N Engl J Med. 1999 Dec 30;341(27):2061–2067. doi: 10.1056/NEJM199912303412706. PMID: 10615079.

[23] Lipson DA, Barnhart F, Brealey N, Brooks J, Criner GJ, Day NC, Dransfield MT, Halpin DMG, Han MK, Jones CE, Kilbride S, Lange P, Lomas DA, Martinez FJ, Singh D, Tabberer M, Wise RA, Pascoe SJ; IMPACT Investigators. Once-daily single-inhaler triple versus dual therapy in patients with COPD. N Engl J Med. 2018 May 3;378(18):1671–1680. doi: 10.1056/NEJMoa1713901. Epub 2018 Apr 18. PMID: 29668352.

[24] Suissa S, Drazen JM. Making sense of triple inhaled therapy for COPD. N Engl J Med. 2018 May 3;378(18):1723–1724. doi: 10.1056/NEJMe1716802. Epub 2018 Apr 18. PMID: 29669218.

[25] Jaffe GJ, Ciulla TA, Ciardella AP, Devin F, Dugel PU, Eandi CM, Masonson H, Monés J, Pearlman JA, Quaranta-El Maftouhi M, Ricci F, Westby K, Patel SC. Dual antagonism of PDGF and VEGF in neovascular age-related macular degeneration: A Phase IIb, multicenter, randomized controlled trial. Ophthalmology. 2017 Feb;124(2):224–234. doi: 10.1016/j.ophtha.2016.10.010. Epub 2016 Oct 28. PMID: 28029445.

[26] Rosenfeld PJ, Feuer WJ. Lessons from recent Phase III trial failures: Don't design Phase III trials based on retrospective subgroup analyses from Phase II trials. Ophthalmology. 2018 Oct;125(10):1488–1491. doi: 10.1016/j.ophtha.2018.06.002. PMID: 30243330.

[27] Estellat C, Torderson DJ, Ravaud P. How to perform a critical analysis of a randomized controlled trial. Best Pract Res Clin Rheumatol. 2009 Apr;23(2):291–303. doi: 10.1016/j.berh.2009.03.003. PMID: 19393572.

[28] Roberts C, Torgerson DJ. Understanding controlled trials: Baseline imbalance in randomised controlled trials. BMJ. 1999 Jul 17;319(7203):185. doi: 10.1136/bmj.319.7203.185. PMID: 10406763; PMCID: PMC1116277.

[29] Altman DG. Comparability of randomised groups. J Royal Stat Soc: Series D (The Statistician). 1985;34(1):125–136. doi: 10.2307/2987510.

[30] Senn S. Testing for baseline balance in clinical trials. Stat Med. 1994 Sep 15;13(17):1715–1726. doi: 10.1002/sim.4780131703. PMID: 7997705.

[31] Roberts C, Torgerson DJ. Understanding controlled trials: Baseline imbalance in randomised controlled trials. BMJ. 1999 Jul 17;319(7203):185. doi: 10.1136/bmj.319.7203.185. PMID: 10406763; PMCID: PMC1116277.

[32] Senn S. Baseline balance and valid statistical analyses: Common misunderstandings. Applied Clinical Trials. March 1, 2005. http://www.appliedclinicaltrialsonline.com/baseline-balance-and-valid-statistical-analyses-common-misunderstandings. Accessed October 15, 2021.

[33] Pocock SJ, McMurray JJV, Collier TJ. Statistical controversies in reporting of clinical trials: Part 2 of a 4-part series on statistics for clinical trials. J Am Coll Cardiol. 2015 Dec 15;66(23):2648–2662. doi: 10.1016/j.jacc.2015.10.023. PMID: 26670066.

[34] Karthikeyan G, Guzic Salobir B, Jug B, Devasenapathy N, Alexanderson E, Vitola J, Kraft O, Ozkan E, Sharma S, Purohit G, Dolenc Novak M, Meave A, Trevethan S, Cerci R, Zier S, Gotthardtová L, Jonszta T, Altin T, Soydal C, Patel C, Gulati G, Paez D, Dondi M, Kashyap R. Functional compared to anatomical imaging in the initial evaluation of patients with suspected coronary artery disease: An international, multi-center, randomized controlled trial (IAEA-SPECT/CTA study). J Nucl Cardiol. 2017 Apr;24(2):507–517. doi: 10.1007/s12350-016-0664-3. Epub 2016 Oct 28. PMID: 27796852; PMCID: PMC5413523.

7.

ANALYSIS

IN THIS CHAPTER, we address two significant issues related to analytic methods that readers of clinical trial reports should evaluate: whether the analysis includes all randomized patients, and whether the analysis plan including studies of subsets was pre-specified.

As we will discuss, there are scenarios in which it may be appropriate to exclude some patients from analysis or to examine several patient subgroups in an overall negative trial. But both these practices increase the odds of finding a positive result that either is spurious or should be viewed with extreme caution, so the analytic approach needs to be closely examined. This is particularly critical when evaluating results from clinical studies performed by small biotechs, which are often under enormous pressure to use encouraging results to justify further development even if they were derived using suboptimal analytic methods.

Intention-to-treat analyses

Imagine a six-month randomized, controlled trial of a drug for severe asthma in which the outcome being measured is decreased hospitalizations during that period. As previously discussed, some of the patients who are randomized to one of the arms will probably drop out before they complete six months of therapy. Some may withdraw very close to the end of the trial, and a few may withdraw before receiving even a single dose of medicine. Who, then, should be analyzed to determine whether the treatment had an effect?

There are two schools of thought on this. One could argue that only the patients who completed the entire course of therapy dictated in the trial should be analyzed. After all, the relevant question is whether six full months of treatment with the experimental drug reduces the hospitalization rate compared with six full months of the comparator agent. But one could also argue that including all the patients who entered the study would provide a more relevant real-world estimate of the new drug's effects. If a third of the patients in the experimental arm failed to complete the trial, this could be because the new drug caused clinical deterioration or had serious side effects that caused patients to withdraw. In this case, an analysis of all the randomized patients would provide a more complete estimate of the net treatment effect that is meaningful to physicians and patients, taking into account the agent's tolerability issues. In contrast, analyzing only the patients who completed the full course of therapy could give an inflated view of the drug's benefits.

The most widely accepted and conservative approach is an **intention-to-treat (ITT) analysis**, which can be described simply as "once randomized, always analyzed."[1] This means that every patient is included in the final analysis, regardless of the level of compliance during the course of the study. In almost all cases, regulatory agencies strongly favor ITT.[2]

Some trials report using a **modified ITT (mITT)** analytic approach. Although this term is not strictly defined, in practice it most often refers to scenarios in which a small number of patients were excluded after randomization because they were found to be ineligible or withdrew before receiving even a single dose of therapy. These situations are generally unconcerning, and guidance documents from the FDA explicitly permit such exclusions provided they are appropriately enumerated and justified.[3] Obviously, patients who leave a study before receiving any treatment have no post-baseline data that could be analyzed.

In contrast, **per-protocol (PP)** analyses (sometimes called "as treated" or "evaluable") omit patients if they failed to complete the full regimen, typically because they withdrew from the study, refused a procedure, missed visits, skipped doses, or were lost to follow-up. This approach can introduce substantial bias into the findings, especially if the number of excluded patients is large or imbalanced across the study arms.[4] It is impossible to know without an ITT analysis whether the results were biased in favor of greater efficacy or tolerability in the treatment arm. And although FDA guidance does not completely exclude the possibility of approving a drug based on a PP analysis, this is unheard-of except in the context of non-inferiority studies, described in Chapter 4. In 2021, Otonomy's Phase 3 study of OTO-104 (Otvidex) in Ménière's disease failed to achieve statistical significance in the ITT population but was positive in a PP analysis.[5] The company promptly announced it was ceasing development of the drug candidate and refocusing its assets and attention on other programs.

In some cases, a sponsor's description of the patient population can be ambiguous. In 2021, Inovio reported on its Phase 3 REVEAL-1 study of the cancer immunotherapy VGX-3100 in patients with high-grade cervical pre-cancers. The trial randomized 201 patients, but seven of those in the experimental arm and one who received the placebo were excluded because they did not receive all three planned doses.[6] The sponsor called the remaining 193 patients an mITT population, but it would have been more accurate to call them a PP group because the excluded patients did receive some doses. Although the non-ITT results favored Inovio's drug, the ITT analysis failed to hit statistical significance, and journalists appropriately questioned whether the FDA would accept the non-ITT data for approval.[7] At the time of writing, a second trial was in progress, and a regulatory filing had not been made.

Analyses of patient subgroups

Many Phase 2 and Phase 3 studies of new drugs report positive findings in a small group of the patients who enrolled in the trial. The main issue that arises with interpreting these subgroup analyses relates to multiplicity: unless the appropriate statistical safeguards are employed, performing many comparisons increases the odds of observing a "positive" result in a subgroup that actually arose by chance. Thus, readers should generally interpret subgroup results with a high degree of skepticism before evaluating both the statistical methods employed and the purpose of the study.

Generally speaking, there are two main uses for patient subgroup analyses in drug trials: regulatory and non-regulatory. This distinction affects the stringency with which one should view the methods and the results. Regulators' bar for granting approval in a population identified via a subgroup analysis is quite high, whereas sponsors and investors often have laxer standards for using positive results in a subset of patients to support R&D decision-making, inform the design of subsequent studies, or justify additional internal or external investment in an R&D program.

Although we cover several key elements of evaluating subgroup analyses here, readers are strongly advised to review European regulatory guidance on this topic,[8] which largely mirrors current practice in the U.S., as well as a 2018 review article that considers this issue in the broader context of multiplicity issues that arise in clinical trials.[9] These sources are a crucial starting point for thinking about how to interpret subgroup results in both regulatory and non-regulatory settings.

Definition of patient subgroups

Regardless of the intention of a subgroup analysis, it is important that the subsets are identified by baseline characteristics that can be measured at the start of the trial before randomization and treatment. The alternative, so-called outcome-based subgroups, can be affected by the treatment itself and are thus highly prone to bias. The most common of such improper subgroups are those that compare responders with non-responders, or fully compliant with partially compliant patients. In both cases, the factor that defines the subgroup may result from the outcome rather than determining it.[10]

Plausibility of results from subgroup analyses

Independent of issues related to trial design or statistical methods, it is important to be skeptical of scientifically or clinically illogical results from subgroup analyses, particularly as their number increases. Biotech journalist Adam Feuerstein wasn't so far off when he parodied a typical press release: "Our drug didn't prolong survival compared to a placebo, except in a subset of left-handed patients who ate meatloaf three days prior to enrolling."[11]

The most infamous published case of an implausible subgroup was a study that found that the combination of streptokinase and aspirin for acute myocardial infarction led to fewer deaths than either therapy alone, but the subset of patients born under the astrological signs of Libra or Gemini actually appeared to die more frequently with the two-drug regimen.[12] This is an obviously absurd result that arose due to a statistical fluke, but more subtle cases are widespread.

A more realistic example comes from the development of vandetanib (AstraZeneca) in advanced non-small cell lung cancer. A Phase 2 study in previously treated patients reported in 2007 that the drug combined with docetaxel failed to improve progression-free survival (PFS), but an exploratory analysis suggested that female patients had a more pronounced benefit.[13] Despite the lack of an obvious biological rationale for this result, this observation plus similar findings in other studies led the sponsor to design the Phase 3 ZODIAC trial to analyze PFS in women as a co-primary endpoint.[14] Contrary to the prior results, the pivotal study found a median PFS improvement of 0.8 months in all patients but only 0.4 months in women; neither population demonstrated a statistically significant improvement in the secondary endpoint of OS. The sponsor submitted the drug to regulators for consideration in 2009 but withdrew the applications later that year after receiving feedback that approval was unlikely.[15]

Any analysis that appears to show *opposite* effects of a treatment between two subgroups should be scrutinized particularly carefully.[16] The 15,000-patient CHARISMA trial reported in 2006 tested whether a combination of clopidogrel and low-dose aspirin prevented clotting events in high-risk patients better than aspirin alone.[17] Although the overall study was negative, the authors conducted 20 pre-planned subgroup analyses, of which two were statistically significant at $P<.05$. The combination arm was superior in symptomatic patients but actually inferior in asymptomatic ones. These results sowed confusion in the field, in part because of questions about their statistical validity,[18] and it was not until several additional studies were conducted that the appropriate population for so-called dual anti-platelet therapy was more clearly defined.

A more insidious example of medical or biological implausibility occurs when subgroups are defined by artificial cutoffs of continuous variables. This is particularly common with age groups such as 65 and older versus younger than 65. There is no reason in most trials why a 64-year-old and a 66-year-old should respond differently to treatment, so this dichotomization inherently raises the risk that a positive result will be spurious.[19]

Subgroup analyses intended to support regulatory approval

Regulators generally require that sponsors clearly predefine the subgroups they intend to evaluate for possible approval and what statistical tools they intend to use to account for multiplicity. This information is often reported in the methods section of articles in high-quality journals,[20] but press releases and other non-journal reports can be more challenging to evaluate.

If a subgroup analysis is intended for regulatory submission, the specific subgroups for evaluation typically need to have been clearly articulated before the data were analyzed. As the number of comparisons increases, the positive predictive value of a significant subgroup finding declines dramatically, even if the ingoing odds of efficacy in the particular subgroup was quite strong.[21] Pre-specifying the analytic approach eliminates the possibility that the sponsor tested the efficacy in many groups and "cherry-picked" one that came up positive by chance.

Another key component of evaluating subgroup analyses intended for drug approval involves the statistical methods. Credible reports of pivotal trials that analyze patient subsets typically limit their analysis to no more than two key groups,[22] and they clearly explain the investigators' strategy for preserving the overall type I error rate, which refers to splitting the standard significance level (α) of .05 across various subgroups. (Statistical significance is discussed in more detail in Chapter 12 on *P* values.) It is impractical for non-experts to attempt to vet the specific methods in most scenarios, but common approaches include defining a predefined, hierarchical sequence of population testing and employing statistical tools developed by Bonferroni, Hochberg, Holm, and Hommel, among others.[23]

If a subset analysis approach was predefined and used the appropriate methods, and all other aspects of the study were also acceptable, then a positive result is typically permissive for approval. Conversely, if in this same scenario the pre-specified subset fails but the study yields a positive result in the entire population, this should not jeopardize the drug's approval with a broad label unless there are other significant issues with the study.

Analyses of subsets that were not pre-specified are almost always excluded from consideration by regulators. Many overall negative Phase 3 studies report positive findings in a subset that was not pre-specified, but this is generally considered to be extremely weak, "hypothesis-generating" evidence at best, and its impact in virtually all cases is to inform a subsequent trial to test the drug in the specific patient population of interest. This is the basis of the strategy that Alzheon is undertaking with its amyloid-modifying drug, ALZ-801 (tramiprosate), which it acquired in 2013 from Bellus Health (formerly Neurochem).[24] The drug previously failed two large Phase 3 trials in mild to moderate Alzheimer's disease, but a subsequent post hoc analysis suggested that it might be effective in patients who were homozygous carriers of the APOE4 allele.[25] A follow-up pivotal placebo-controlled trial of 300 patients with that particular genetic background is currently underway.[26]

We are unaware of any examples of full regulatory approval being granted on the basis of a negative overall result and a positive finding in a subset that was not pre-specified, although some sort of conditional approval is theoretically possible in this scenario. Similarly, it is theoretically possible that if a study's results were positive both overall and in a subset that was not pre-planned, regulators might allow the less-valid subset findings to be incorporated into the label for marketing purposes, but here, too, we do not know of any historical examples.

Subgroup analyses in non-pivotal trials

Most Phase 2 studies of new drugs do not explicitly pre-specify key subgroups or employ appropriate statistical safeguards against spurious positive results due to multiplicity. Thus, positive subset results in these trials are by definition solely exploratory and need to be confirmed in follow-up studies.

For readers, determining the degree to which positive subset results in Phase 2 justify further investment and clinical development is highly subjective. As discussed, a major consideration is typically the scientific and clinical plausibility of the finding. Positive subgroup results that fit poorly with prior knowledge have high odds of having arisen by chance and generally should be viewed skeptically. Readers should take into account not just the specific trial under consideration, but also the broader context of what is known about the drug's mechanism and the underlying pathophysiology of the disease, as well as successes and failures of prior therapies in similar settings. A more complete discussion of these issues is presented in Chapter 8 on efficacy results in the section on interpreting positive results.

---

[1] Gupta SK. Intention-to-treat concept: A review. Perspect Clin Res. 2011 Jul;2(3):109–112. doi: 10.4103/2229-3485.83221. PMID: 21897887; PMCID: PMC3159210.

[2] Good review practice: Clinical review of investigational new drug applications. U.S. Food and Drug Administration. December 2013.

[3] Guidance for industry: E9 statistical principles for clinical trials. U.S. Food and Drug Administration. September 1998.

[4] Ellenberg S. Avoiding bias and random error in data analysis. FDA Clinical Investigator Course, November 13, 2013. https://www.fda.gov/media/87420/download. Permalink: https://perma.cc/H4P9-5XFN.

[5] Ontomy announces top-line results for the Phase 3 clinical trial of Otividex in patients with Ménière's disease. Ontonomy press release. February 22, 2021. https://investors.otonomy.com/news-releases/news-release-details/otonomy-announces-top-line-results-phase-3-clinical-trial. Accessed October 15, 2021. Permalink: https://perma.cc/2V4L-AE3Z.

[6] Inovio announces positive results from REVEAL 1, a Phase 3 pivotal trial evaluating VGX-3100, its DNA-based HPV immunotherapy for the treatment of high-grade precancerous cervical dysplasia caused by HPV-16 and/or HPV-18. Inovio press release. March 1, 2021. https://ir.inovio.com/news-releases/news-releases-details/2021/INOVIO-Announces-Positive-Results-from-REVEAL-1-a-Phase-3-Pivotal-Trial-Evaluating-VGX-3100-its-DNA-based-HPV-Immunotherapy-for-the-Treatment-of-High-grade-Precancerous-Cervical-Dysplasia-Caused-by-HPV-16-andor-HPV-18/default.aspx. Accessed October 15, 2021. Permalink: https://perma.cc/P5KP-8GWN.

[7] Armstrong M. Inovio's reinvention falls flat. Evaluate Vantage. March 2, 2021. https://www.evaluate.com/vantage/articles/news/trial-results/inovios-reinvention-falls-flat. Accessed October 15, 2021.

[8] Guideline on the investigation of subgroups in confirmatory clinical trials, EMA/CHMP/539146/2013. European Medicines Agency. January 31, 2019.

[9] Dmitrienko A, D'Agostino RB Sr. Multiplicity considerations in clinical trials. N Engl J Med. 2018 May 31;378(22):2115–2122. doi: 10.1056/NEJMra1709701. PMID: 29847757.

[10] Yusuf S, Wittes J, Probstfield J, Tyroler HA. Analysis and interpretation of treatment effects in subgroups of patients in randomized clinical trials. JAMA. 1991 Jul 3;266(1):93–98. PMID: 2046134.

[11] Feuerstein A. Biotech stock mailbag: How to spot red flags in clinical trial data. TheStreet. March 24, 2016. https://www.thestreet.com/investing/stocks/biotech-stock-mailbag-how-to-spot-red-flags-in-clinical-trial-data-13506801. Accessed October 15, 2021.

[12] ISIS-2 (Second International Study of Infarct Survival) Collaborative Group. Randomised trial of intravenous streptokinase, oral aspirin, both, or neither among 17,187 cases of suspected acute myocardial infarction: ISIS-2. Lancet. 1988 Aug 13;2(8607):349–360. PMID: 2899772.

[13] Heymach JV, Johnson BE, Prager D, Csada E, Roubec J, Pesek M, Spásová I, Belani CP, Bodrogi I, Gadgeel S, Kennedy SJ, Hou J, Herbst RS. Randomized, placebo-controlled Phase II study of vandetanib plus docetaxel in previously treated non small-cell lung cancer. J Clin Oncol. 2007 Sep 20;25(27):4270-4277. doi: 10.1200/JCO.2006.10.5122. Erratum in: J Clin Oncol. 2008 Jan 1;26(1):165–166. PMID: 17878479.

[14] Herbst RS, Sun Y, Eberhardt WE, Germonpré P, Saijo N, Zhou C, Wang J, Li L, Kabbinavar F, Ichinose Y, Qin S, Zhang L, Biesma B, Heymach JV, Langmuir P, Kennedy SJ, Tada H, Johnson BE. Vandetanib plus docetaxel versus docetaxel as second-line treatment for patients with advanced non-small-cell lung cancer (ZODIAC): A double-blind, randomised, Phase 3 trial. Lancet Oncol. 2010 Jul;11(7):619–626. doi: 10.1016/S1470-2045(10)70132-7. PMID: 20570559; PMCID: PMC3225192.

[15] Hirschler B. AstraZeneca pulls submissions for lung cancer drug. Reuters. October 28, 2009. https://www.reuters.com/article/astrazeneca-zactima/update-2-astrazeneca-pulls-submissions-for-lung-cancer-drug-idUSLS62629120091028. Accessed October 15, 2021.

[16] Pocock SJ, McMurray JJV, Collier TJ. Statistical controversies in reporting of clinical trials: Part 2 of a 4-part series on statistics for clinical trials. J Am Coll Cardiol. 2015 Dec 15;66(23):2648–2662. doi: 10.1016/j.jacc.2015.10.023. PMID: 26670066.

[17] Bhatt DL, Fox KA, Hacke W, Berger PB, Black HR, Boden WE, Cacoub P, Cohen EA, Creager MA, Easton JD, Flather MD, Haffner SM, Hamm CW, Hankey GJ, Johnston SC, Mak KH, Mas JL, Montalescot G, Pearson TA, Steg PG, Steinhubl SR, Weber MA, Brennan DM, Fabry-Ribaudo L, Booth J, Topol EJ; CHARISMA Investigators. Clopidogrel and aspirin versus aspirin alone for the prevention of atherothrombotic events. N Engl J Med. 2006 Apr 20;354(16):1706–1717. doi: 10.1056/NEJMoa060989. Epub 2006 Mar 12. PMID: 16531616.

[18] Lagakos SW. The challenge of subgroup analyses—reporting without distorting. N Engl J Med. 2006 Apr 20;354(16):1667–1669. doi: 10.1056/NEJMp068070. Erratum in: N Engl J Med. 2006 Aug 3;355(5):533. PMID: 16625007.

[19] Naggara O, Raymond J, Guilbert F, Altman DG. The problem of subgroup analyses: An example from a trial on ruptured intracranial aneurysms. AJNR Am J Neuroradiol. 2011 Apr;32(4):633–636. doi: 10.3174/ajnr.A2442. Epub 2011 Mar 24. PMID: 21436333; PMCID: PMC7965892.

[20] Wang R, Lagakos SW, Ware JH, Hunter DJ, Drazen JM. Statistics in medicine—reporting of subgroup analyses in clinical trials. N Engl J Med. 2007 Nov 22;357(21):2189–2194. doi: 10.1056/NEJMsr077003. PMID: 18032770.

[21] Burke JF, Sussman JB, Kent DM, Hayward RA. Three simple rules to ensure reasonably credible subgroup analyses. BMJ. 2015 Nov 4;351:h5651. doi: 10.1136/bmj.h5651. PMID: 26537915; PMCID: PMC4632208.

[22] Burke JF, Sussman JB, Kent DM, Hayward RA. Three simple rules to ensure reasonably credible subgroup analyses. BMJ. 2015 Nov 4;351:h5651. doi: 10.1136/bmj.h5651. PMID: 26537915; PMCID: PMC4632208.

[23] Victor A, Elsässer A, Hommel G, Blettner M. Judging a plethora of p-values: How to contend with the problem of multiple testing: Part 10 of a series on evaluation of scientific publications. Dtsch Arztebl Int. 2010 Jan;107(4):50–56. doi: 10.3238/arztebl.2010.0050. Epub 2010 Jan 29. PMID: 20165700; PMCID: PMC2822959.

[24] Alzheon launches with veteran team and funding to accelerate drug development in Alzheimer's disease and other neurodegenerative disorders. Alzheon press release. October 23, 2013. https://alzheon.com/alzheon-launches-with-veteran-team-and-funding-to-accelerate-drug-development-in-alzheimers-disease-and-other-neurodegenerative-disorders/. Accessed October 15, 2021. Permalink: https://perma.cc/H5N7-6FLW.

[25] Abushakra S, Porsteinsson A, Vellas B, Cummings J, Gauthier S, Hey JA, Power A, Hendrix S, Wang P, Shen L, Sampalis J, Tolar M. Clinical benefits of tramiprosate in Alzheimer's disease are associated with higher number of APOE4 alleles: The "APOE4 gene-dose effect." J Prev Alzheimer's Dis. 2016;3(4):219–228. doi: 10.14283/jpad.2016.115. PMID: 29199323.

[26] An efficacy and safety study of ALZ-801 in APOE4/4 early AD subjects (APOLLOE4). ClinicalTrials.gov identifier: NCT04770220. Updated October 6, 2021. Accessed October 15, 2021.

8.

RESULTS–EFFICACY

IT IS TEMPTING to reduce a biotech clinical trial to the simple question of whether it was "positive" or "negative," but this is an oversimplification and a mistake. Nominally positive studies always come with caveats and qualifiers, and most negative studies leave some wiggle room to argue that the development program isn't yet completely, irredeemably dead.

In this chapter, we provide guidance on factors to consider before reaching definitive conclusions about positive and negative clinical trial results, including specific considerations related to early-stage studies. We also provide some related guidance on how to predict success or failure in late-stage trials as opposed to interpreting the results after they are complete.

Interpreting positive results

Positive outcomes from drug trials should be viewed with an appropriate degree of skepticism and should lead readers to carefully examine several factors before accepting them at face value.[1] These include inherent believability, robustness and consistency, and impact.

Inherent believability

It is now well known that many experimental results are difficult to reproduce. One contributor to this phenomenon is that every clinical study has some intrinsic **false positive rate (FPR)**,[2] even if the drug does not have an effect. The FPR

---

is sometimes referred to as the false discovery rate,[3] but this can create confusion because false discovery rate was originally defined in relation to massive multiplicity in preclinical testing,[4] and it has different implications in that context.

A crucial component of the FPR is the intrinsic likelihood that the scientific hypothesis is valid. Before reviewing the results from a clinical trial of whether homeopathic doses of apple juice can treat tuberculosis, one would surely bet that any positive finding that might be eked out of the study is highly likely to be a false positive. In contrast, a similar study of an improved version of rifampin, which is already approved and has proved effective in this indication, probably has an extremely low FPR. Most biotech trials obviously fall somewhere between these two cases.

Without diving too deeply into the underlying statistics, the relationship between the inherent believability of the hypothesis and the FPR can be illustrated for a study that uses a binary primary endpoint, such as alive versus dead or symptomatic versus asymptomatic. Assuming this trial has typical statistical parameters of power (1-β) of .8 and significance level (α) of .05, if one thinks that the drug intrinsically has 50/50 odds of being active, the FPR is 6%. That is, 6% of positive findings will, in fact, be false positives. But if the intrinsic odds that the drug is active drop from 50% to 10%—that is, if the evidence base from preclinical and prior clinical results is weak—then the FPR increases to 36%, so more than a third of positive findings will be false positives. (Power and significance are discussed in more detail in Chapter 12 on *P* values and confidence intervals and in Chapter 13 on study size and statistical power, and the mathematical relationship between FPR, β, and α is explored in more detail in the references cited above.)

A mathematically precise estimate of the intrinsic odds of success of a drug is difficult to define. Qualitatively it depends on the amount and quality of supporting data, the degree to which prior preclinical or early clinical studies are thought to predict clinical outcomes in the patient population being studied, and one's perception of how well the disease pathophysiology, the drug's mechanism of action, and the relationship between the two are understood.

In Alzheimer's disease, for example, the absence of preclinical models with good predictive power, translational biomarkers linked to meaningful clinical endpoints, convincing human genetic data, or well-supported patient selection hypotheses based on underlying biology all contribute to a historically high likelihood that many promising Phase 2 results were, in fact, false positive findings. Similarly, it is difficult to be as confident about a positive clinical trial result for a drug with a pleiotropic or poorly understood mechanism, even if the rationale is buttressed with supporting data from preclinical and early clinical experiments, as one would be for a therapy with a well-defined pharmacologic activity that fits well with one's understanding of the cause of the disease.

Robustness and consistency

Several aspects of positive trials increase the odds that the results may have arisen by chance. These aren't deal-killers per se, but they are worth considering, particularly if the positive study is being used as the justification for further R&D investment:

- **Fragility:** In small positive studies, it is more likely that a single responder or non-responder could have swayed the results. One way to assess the robustness of positive trial results is to calculate the "fragility index," which is the minimum number of patients whose results would have to change for the overall finding to switch from positive ($P<.05$) to negative ($P>.05$).[5] Intuitively, a trial of 50 patients that detects a given effect size with $P=.04$ is less robust than an identical trial of 500 patients with the same effect size and *P* value; the fragility index provides a relative assessment of how much less robust the smaller study is compared with the larger one.

  As with the FPR, one can calculate the fragility index for any study that measures a dichotomous endpoint and generate an approximate value for time-to-event studies by treating the event as a dichotomous outcome. It is calculated by successively using a test suitable for dichotomous endpoints, such as Fisher's exact test, to assess the effect on the *P* value of changing patients' outcomes; an online calculator is available.[6] An illustrative example, analyzed in a review of Phase 3 oncology studies,[7] is a trial of the ability of ixazomib (Ninlaro; Millennium/Takeda) versus placebo, in combination with lenalidomide and dexamethasone, to extend progression-free survival (PFS) in patients with multiple myeloma.[8] The study, reported in 2016, yielded a positive result (median PFS 20.6 months versus 14.7 months; hazard ratio [HR, see Chapter 11 on time-to-event studies] 0.74; $P=.01$). At the time of analysis, 129 of 360 patients in the experimental arm had progressed, compared with 157 of 362 patients on placebo, corresponding to a nominal *P* value of .040. The analysis revealed that if just two additional patients had progressed on ixazomib (131 instead of 129 of 360), the nominal *P* value would have been non-significant (.058). The opposite situation arose in the Phase 3 APEX trial of betrixaban (Bevyxxa; Portola) to prevent thromboembolic events in hospitalized patients, published in 2016. The *P* value in the primary cohort would have shifted from .054 (non-significant) to below .05 (significant) if just two of the 3,870 patients had different clinical outcomes.[9]

The best use of the fragility index is to provide a "gut check" on the robustness of trial results, particularly in comparison with similar studies. There is nothing inherently suspicious or nefarious about a study with a fragility index of two patients, but one might be more confident in the reproducibility of the findings if the endpoint had been overall survival (OS), which is inherently less subjective to assess than PFS.

- **Idiosyncratic dose-response relationship:** A somewhat common and particularly concerning situation in biopharma trials related to consistency is when a study tests multiple doses of the experimental drug but observes significant effects only at low or intermediate doses. Normally a therapy's effect should either increase or stabilize as the dose increases, but if it declines at high levels, this could indicate that there are aspects of the disease or the drug that are poorly understood.

  A Phase 2 trial completed in 2012 studied the ability of RAD1901 (elacestrant; Radius Health) to treat postmenopausal vasomotor symptoms ("hot flashes"), as assessed by several exploratory endpoints.[10] RAD1901 elicited a statistically significant change in the frequency of moderate and severe hot flashes at the 10 mg dose compared with placebo, but three higher doses up to 50 mg failed to yield positive results. Development of the drug in that indication was discontinued. Additional preclinical studies later clarified key aspects of RAD1901's complex pharmacology, and studies in breast cancer were subsequently initiated.[11]

  A similar scenario occurred in the BLAZE-1 Phase 2 clinical trial of Lilly's neutralizing antibody to SARS-CoV-2, bamlanivimab (LY-CoV555), in recently diagnosed outpatients with mild to moderate

COVID-19. The results were reported in 2020.[12] A significant improvement in the primary outcome—change in viral load at day 11 after initiation of therapy—was seen at the middle dose of 2,800 mg, but not at the lower or higher doses of 700 mg or 7,000 mg. The company discontinued development of the monotherapy and at time of writing was instead pursuing studies in combination with other therapies, including another Lilly anti-SARS-CoV-2 antibody, etesevimab (LY-CoV016). No explanation for the idiosyncratic dose-response finding in BLAZE-1 was disclosed to date.

Impact

Finally, even if positive results appear to be believable and robust, there is a final question: Do they matter? Particularly in later-phase trials, a statistically significant finding may be necessary but insufficient to sway the opinions of regulators, physicians, payers, and patients. There are several scenarios in which results with $P<.05$ are less meaningful than they may appear at first glance:

- **Effect is statistically significant but not clinically significant:** Because power can be boosted with increased trial size, it is often possible to obtain a statistically significant positive result with a weakly effective therapy if one studies enough patients. This concept is discussed in more detail in Chapter 12 on *P* values and in Chapter 13 on study size and statistical power. A Phase 3 trial of ramucirumab (Cyramza; Lilly) versus placebo in combination with docetaxel in second-line lung cancer yielded an OS of 10.5 months versus 9.1 months (HR 0.86, 95% CI 0.75–0.98, P=.023).[13] The REVEL study, published in 2014, was clearly statistically positive, but at the time the data were disclosed, it was not clear on first principles whether the absolute improvement in life span of 1.4 months (5–6 weeks) would be considered clinically meaningful for the drug's approval, reimbursement, or use. The U.S. Food and Drug Administration (FDA) in fact did grant a label extension for the indication based on REVEL later that year.[14]

  Another factor that commonly arises with regard to the clinical insignificance of the effect is the choice of comparator. An academic study found that 17% of oncology drugs approved by the FDA on the basis of randomized controlled trials (RCTs) used "suboptimal" comparators that were already known to be inferior to other marketed alternatives, inappropriately limited the investigator's choice of therapy, forbade combination treatments, or consisted of re-administration of a therapy already known to have no benefit upon re-exposure.[15] In this scenario, a sponsor presumably chooses to use a suboptimal comparator to try to boost the trial's odds of success, knowing that regulators routinely approve drugs tested in this way as long as the control arm is at least somewhat plausible and the data demonstrate appropriate safety and efficacy. Once a drug is on the market, critiques of the control arm may or may not have a significant effect on its commercial success.

- **Endpoint is irrelevant or poorly predictive:** In late-stage studies, a trial's endpoint may have little relevance to clinical care and thus have a low impact on the drug's perceived efficacy. This is a chronic issue in oncology, where there is an ongoing debate about whether the surrogate endpoint of PFS is clinically meaningful in the absence of a demonstrated improvement in length or quality of life,[16] and it arises in other therapeutic areas as well. Patients with vasodilatory shock have low blood pressures that are life-threatening, and a synthetic angiotensin II drug (Giapreza; La Jolla Pharmaceuticals) was approved for the condition based on a single Phase 3 study, ATHOS-3, published in 2017.[17] The trial was designed to measure the proportion of patients whose blood pressure was successfully increased within three hours of receiving the drug without the need for additional vasopressors. The primary endpoint was positive (69.9% vs. 23.4%, $P<.001$), but there was no improvement in 28-day mortality, which was a secondary endpoint (46% vs. 54%, $P=.12$). The FDA approved the drug, but intensive care physicians have remained equivocal about its therapeutic utility, given that the clinically relevant endpoint is bona fide survival, not blood pressure response over a short time period.[18] Similarly, as discussed in more detail in Chapter 5 on endpoints, positive results on a surrogate endpoint in early-phase trials may not predict a drug's performance on measures that will eventually be needed for regulatory approval and commercial success.
- **Effect is inconsistent across key subgroups or endpoints:** Even when a drug is likely to be approvable based on a positive primary outcome, findings in key secondary endpoints or sub-populations that are incon-

sistent, weak, or downright contradictory can make it commercially unattractive, especially in light of the profiles of competitors' products. The Phase 3 trial of the selective estrogen receptor modulator arzoxifene (Lilly) was positive on its primary endpoints of lessening the three-year incidence of new vertebral fractures in patients with osteoporosis (HR 0.059, 95% CI 0.45–0.77, *P*<.001) as well as the incidence of invasive breast cancer in women with either osteoporosis or low bone mass (HR 0.44, 95% CI 0.26–0.76, *P*<.001).[19] However, results reported in 2009 were negative on many clinically important secondary efficacy endpoints, including prevention of non-vertebral fractures and cardiovascular events, suggesting it was inferior to tamoxifen on key measures. Based on these data, the sponsor discontinued development.[20] A similar situation arose with the cholesterol-lowering CETP inhibitor anacetrapib, which Merck abandoned in 2017 after disclosing that the Phase 3 REVEAL study yielded a positive outcome but missed a key secondary endpoint.[21]

A related but less common scenario is when the primary endpoint is a composite that includes two or more types of events with different levels of clinical importance and a drug's positive effect is mainly conferred by an improvement in the less meaningful component. This topic is discussed in more detail in Chapter 5 on endpoints.

- **Positive effect comes with trade-offs:** The importance of the efficacy-safety balance typically depends on the specific clinical scenario, but in all cases it is important to dispassionately assess it. In the study of ramucirumab in lung cancer mentioned earlier, the improvement in OS was associated with an increased risk of neutropenia and other side effects. And the published results of the ATHOS-3 trial of angiotensin II in shock discussed previously did not report meaningful differences in safety or tolerability, but the product insert indicates the drug conferred a higher risk of thrombotic and thromboembolic events (13% versus 5%), mostly due to deep vein thromboses.[22] Even in rare diseases with high mortality rates, where patients may be willing to tolerate significant levels of discomfort and risk in exchange for longer life, there is typically a point at which the perceived risks and harms exceed the benefits.

Interpreting negative results

Just as it is tempting but overly simplistic to accept a "positive" study report on face value, it can also be a mistake to automatically dismiss all "failed" therapeutic trials without further analysis. In early stages of drug development, negative trials can often provide justification for further studies, especially if earlier failures inform the design of subsequent trials. In later stages, it can be important to assess negative studies to determine the likelihood that a repeat or follow-up study will be positive.

To be clear: when evaluating negative results, one needs to be extremely vigilant for companies and investigators that attempt to "spin" negative results as positive. In almost all cases, the value of carefully interpreting failed trials is *not* to find a way to re-interpret them as positive. Instead, the main utility is to suggest hypotheses and approaches for future studies.

With this caveat in mind, there are several issues to consider when assessing negative clinical trial results. Many of these were covered in an excellent article by Stuart J. Pocock and Gregg W. Stone published in 2016 in the *New England Journal of Medicine*.[23] The factors most relevant to studies of drugs that have not yet been approved are summarized below:

- **Signs of possible clinical benefit:** One problem with using "positive" as a shorthand for $P<.05$ is that barely non-significant results are often incorrectly dismissed without further consideration. As one commentator asked: What is the material difference between two studies with a relative risk of 0.75, one with a 95% CI of 0.57 to 0.99 ($P=.048$) and the other with a 95% CI of 0.55 to 1.03 ($P=.07$)?[24]

  In fact, the answer depends on whether one believes the point estimate of the effect size is just barely clinically meaningful, or whether a somewhat smaller effect of the experimental drug might still be important. A 492-patient Phase 3 trial published in 2008 tested whether the addition of etoposide to a standard chemotherapy regimen improved event-free survival (EFS) of high-risk patients with Ewing's sarcoma. The study was powered to detect a 15% improvement in the fraction of event-free patients at three years.[25] In fact, the primary analysis was negative, with an HR of 0.83 (95% CI, 0.65 to 1.05). Given that the CI just barely crosses 1.0, one could argue that the study provides at least some suggestion that the drug is effective around the level of the middle of the outcome distribution (HR=0.83), and perhaps failed to reach statistical significance because the trial was too small. (This topic is addressed in more depth in Chapter 13 on study size and statistical power.) Whether an EFS improvement of less than 15% would be deemed clinically beneficial is a separate question that requires more in-depth clinical investigation.

- **Evidence of comparable efficacy to an active control:** Even if a new therapy does not demonstrate superiority versus one that is known to be active, the study may provide explicit or suggestive evidence that it has meaningful clinical activity. A Phase 3 study of vandetanib (AstraZeneca) in advanced non-small cell lung cancer reported in 2011 that the drug had failed to beat the already-approved agent erlotinib (Tarceva; Roche) head-to-head.[26] However, a pre-planned non-inferiority analysis validated that the two drugs yielded equivalent PFS and OS. Although the sponsor decided not to continue developing the drug in this indication, this type of outcome could possibly justify additional investment in some scenarios.
- **Insights from subset analyses:** A common scenario in drug development is that a drug fails to demonstrate efficacy in a broadly defined population, but there is reason to believe it works in a subset of patients. In fact, many Phase 2 studies (particularly those denoted by sponsors as "Phase 2a") are intentionally designed to suggest subsets for further analysis. In these cases, the hypothesis-generating subset analyses are typically either defined post hoc or pre-planned but inadequately sized to detect a clinically significant effect size. Despite their lack of statistical power, these subset analyses can be valuable for informing the design of follow-up studies.
- **Insights from secondary endpoint analyses:** Although some clinical settings have well-defined endpoints for advancing R&D projects and garnering regulatory approval, in others the path may be less clear. In these situations, a study that fails in its primary analysis but appears to provide a benefit on a secondary endpoint may suggest that a follow-up study should use the secondary endpoint as its primary one. This is a particularly common scenario in rare diseases, in which there may be little

precedent for regulatory approval of new therapies, and the definition of appropriate endpoints evolves through ongoing discussions between sponsors and regulators.[27]

- **Issues with trial design or execution:** Some trial failures provide evidence to suggest modifications to the design that could improve the odds of success in a future study. From a statistical perspective, if the outcomes of patients on the control arm, or the degree of variability in patients' outcomes in one or both arms, were not as predicted, this may have led trial planners to err in calculating the optimal size of the study. In other cases, negative results can suggest modifications to the dose or length of treatment, the timing of endpoint assessment, specific inclusion or exclusion criteria, or other factors in a follow-up trial. Or enrollment may have been halted before the target trial size was reached, leaving the trial underpowered for the difference it sought to detect. Notably, many sponsors employ adaptive trial designs precisely to avoid these sorts of challenges, as discussed in Chapter 15.

  One of the co-primary endpoints in the Phase 2/3 study of VTS-270 (Mallinckrodt) in the rare genetic disorder Niemann-Pick type C, reported in 2018, was the change from baseline in a composite clinical score, NPC-SS.[28,29] The investigators expected that all patients would progress over the course of the 52-week study but that those in the treatment arm would progress less than those receiving the sham therapy. In fact, neither group progressed significantly by NPC-SS over the course of the study, suggesting that the suboptimal choice of patients, endpoint, or other factors may have contributed to the trial's failure.

  Other specialized situations need to be evaluated on a case-by-case basis. Dermira ran two Phase 3 trials for DRM04/glycopyrronium (Qbrexza) in primary axillary hyperhidrosis with the co-primary endpoints of improvement from baseline in a patient-reported Axillary Sweating Daily Diary (ASDD) and gravimetrically measured sweat production.[30] One study missed on the second outcome, but in reporting the findings the company maintained in 2016 that excluding an outlier trial center, as agreed in advance with the FDA, yielded a positive result.[31] The FDA subsequently approved the drug.[32]

Finally, in some cases the analysis of biological or pharmacologic factors can help explain a negative finding and possibly justify a follow-up study with a different design. The ESCAPE-NA1 Phase 3 trial of nerinetide (NoNO Therapeutics) for the treatment of acute ischemic stroke was designed to detect an 8.7% difference in the share of patients who achieved a favorable neurologic outcome, with 80% power and a two-sided α of .05.[33] When the study failed, as published in 2020, the investigators concluded that due to an unforeseen pharmacologic interaction, nerinetide was inactivated in patients who had received thrombolytics (~60% of the participants). A post hoc analysis of the non-thrombolysed group suggested that nerinetide led to a 9.6% improvement in the primary outcome. In this case, there is no evidence that the study was underpowered. Not unsurprisingly, a follow-up study that is ongoing at the time of writing is powered essentially identically to the original one, except that it excludes patients who received prior thrombolytics.[34]

From a regulatory standpoint, drugs with "negative" top-line findings can sometimes support approval, but this is extremely rare. A notable recent example was aducanumab (Aduhelm; Biogen), which failed to meet its primary objectives in pivotal studies in Alzheimer's disease but was granted accelerated approval by the FDA in 2021 based largely on a post hoc subset analysis of the drug's effect on a surrogate efficacy marker.[35,36] As a condition of approval under this special pathway, Biogen was required to conduct a new RCT to validate the drug's benefit. Similarly, although the FDA acknowledges that "the suggestion of a favorable result on a major outcome such as mortality may be difficult to ignore," even if mortality was a secondary outcome and the effect on the primary endpoint was not statistically significant,[37] success on a secondary measure in the setting of primary outcome failure rarely influences a drug's approval, especially in clinical areas with well-defined endpoints. The main historical example of this scenario is the agency's 1996 approval of the alpha- and beta-adrenergic signaling blocker carvedilol (Coreg; SmithKline Beecham) for patients with left ventricular dysfunction following an acute myocardial infarction despite the failure of the CAPRICORN trial.[38] But in the modern era of mandatory endpoint prespecification, we have not identified any drugs that gained full, unconditional regulatory approval, outside of a special pathway and without a requirement for confirmatory studies, based on trials that failed on their primary outcomes but yielded positive data in secondary endpoint analyses.

Results of small, early-stage trials

Many small, early-stage studies measure some aspect of efficacy, either as a primary goal in Phase 2 or as an ancillary intention of Phase 1 studies of pharmacokinetics and short-term safety. Results from these trials are extremely difficult to evaluate and prone to overinterpretation and overenthusiasm. Many of the main concerns and challenges are covered elsewhere but are worth revisiting in this context:

- **Comparator:** Many early-stage studies are single-arm, and results are compared with historical or natural history data. In these cases, as discussed in Chapter 4 on study design, it is important to assess the quality and consistency of the comparator data. This is a particular issue in chronic, progressive diseases, in which it may be difficult to determine from a small study whether a new therapy meaningfully slows the rate of decline due to uncertainties around both the observed results and the assumed slope in untreated patients.
- **Endpoints:** Many early trials use surrogate endpoints that are not clearly linked to clinical outcomes. Changes in biomarkers can often provide initial evidence that a drug gets to the right place and has the expected molecular or cellular effect, but in many scenarios, there are scant data correlating those changes with quantitative clinical responses. And in unblinded or uncontrolled early studies, clinical surrogate endpoints that involve subjective measurements by physicians or patients are particularly prone to bias.
- **Fragility:** In a small study, even one additional responder or non-responder can often make the difference between a nominally positive result and a negative one. Similarly, when a small study has a notable number of patients who withdrew from the trial prematurely or were lost to follow-up, the results need to be interpreted extremely cautiously.
- **Population:** Many early trials in oncology and rheumatology that treat "later-line" patients who have failed to respond to many other therapies are interpreted as positive if even a handful of patients show drug activ-

ity. However, unless there is a clear mechanistic hypothesis why those particular patients responded to guide more explicit patient selection in subsequent studies, it may be difficult to reproduce initially promising results.

- **Statistics:** Many early-stage trials present data on statistical significance (confidence intervals or *P* values), even though few of them pre-specify the analytic approach. Although these statistics tend to capture attention in top-line summaries, they are almost always suspect due to the risk of multiple hypothesis testing and therefore are useful only as hypothesis generators.
- **Threshold effect size:** Many early-stage studies do not pre-specify a minimum outcome that would warrant further development, so readers need to make their own assessments. This is a particular issue in small, single-arm oncology trials; for example, it is not clear a priori how to interpret a single-arm study of 20 patients that reports two partial responses and three patients with stable disease.

In general, apparent efficacy signals from small, early-stage studies, especially those that are single-arm or unblinded, are highly prone to being overvalued and overinterpreted. Although the *absence* of a credible signal of potential efficacy in such a study can often inform a decision to abandon development, positive results from these trials should typically be viewed with caution and at most as being permissive of investing in further studies.

Finally, as discussed in Chapter 9 on safety results, most clinical trials are not formally powered to detect adverse events, and this issue is even more salient in small studies. A pooled analysis by Novartis researchers published in 2018 found that across 77 first-in-human studies, mild increases in liver enzymes, heart rate, and blood pressure each occurred in over 5% of healthy volunteers treated with placebo, suggesting that for these readouts a modest incidence in a small trial may not be particularly concerning.[39] However, adverse events that are more idiosyncratic or fit with known concerns related to the biology of the disease or the pharmacology of the drug may merit closer examination, even in small studies.

Predictors of failure of Phase 3 studies

Why do fully a third[40] of new-drug candidates fail even after getting all the way to Phase 3 trials? Part of the reason is simply that drug development is complicated and difficult, and we understand far less about how to safely manipulate disease biology than we think we do. Other failures reflect the "Proteus phenomenon," also known as the "winner's curse," in which initial trials showing positive results are often followed by replication attempts that show less compelling or frankly opposite findings.[41]

But some failures are clearly "own goals" by drug developers that even outside observers could see coming a mile away. Several factors can portend failure in late-stage development, based on analyses by pharmaceutical companies[42,43,44] and other experts.[45,46,47] Many of these can be detected in preclinical research findings, early- and mid-stage trial results, and Phase 3 protocols. They include:

- **Poor biologic rationale:** As discussed in the context of false positive rates, the chances that a positive Phase 2 result represents a bona fide finding are higher if the pretest likelihood of success was also high. Conversely, positive Phase 2 results should be viewed skeptically if there is scant supporting evidence from robust preclinical models or early clinical studies.
- **Justified by low-quality clinical data:** All other factors being equal, encouraging Phase 2 studies that suffer from flaws in design, execution, or analysis provide weak comfort that a subsequent Phase 3 trial will succeed. Common scenarios include overly permissive statistical criteria, like low power or a *P* value threshold above .05; small studies that are overly fragile and prone to false positive findings; trial designs that fall short of the RCT standard such as single-arm or open-label; non-ITT analyses that bias the findings in favor of the experimental agent; studies that test several doses of a drug and claim "success" if any one of them yields statistically significant positive results without any accounting for type I error; and issues with allocation, randomization, or blinding that compromise the integrity of the study. For example, in a Phase 2 trial reported in 2017 in age-related wet macular degeneration, lampalizumab (Genentech/Roche) demonstrated a 20% reduction in disease progression compared with the control group, but with a *P* value of .117. The

researchers nonetheless claimed success based on their pre-specified threshold of $P<.2$, which "was selected given that this was a proof-of-concept, hypothesis-generating clinical study."[48] Two subsequent Phase 3 studies failed.[49]

In addition, Phase 1 and 2 trials often lack explicit, pre-specified thresholds for defining success, giving investigators broad latitude to interpret efficacy results as "positive" and justifying advancement to Phase 3. One analysis found that almost three-quarters of oncology drugs that failed in Phase 3 after supposedly succeeding in earlier studies had failed to surmount a relatively low bar such as 20% response rate in Phase 2.[50] Not surprisingly, most of those paltry Phase 2 findings were characterized as positive by investigators or sponsors.

- **Over-exuberant assumption of effect size:** Sponsors may sometimes design clinical trials to detect large differences so that they can make the study smaller and thus increase execution feasibility. However, it is possible in some of these cases that a smaller difference would have still been clinically meaningful, but the study was too small to detect it. This phenomenon of "underpowering" is discussed in more detail in Chapter 13 on study size and statistical power.
- **Inconsistent dose or formulation:** A significant source of risk in late-stage studies is the use of a dose that has been inadequately vetted in earlier trials. A Phase 1 study reported in 2016 of tabalumab (Lilly), an anti-BAFF monoclonal antibody, evaluated the pharmacokinetics and safety of intravenous doses in patients with systemic lupus erythematosus and rheumatoid arthritis (RA), as well as subcutaneous doses in RA patients.[51] Subcutaneous dosing was subsequently shown to be effective in Phase 2 studies in RA,[52,53] but in lupus, the same formulation was taken straight into two Phase 3 trials without any additional confirmation of its efficacy. Both trials failed.[54,55]

Another risk related to dose selection, discussed earlier in the section on interpreting positive results, occurs when a drug appears to work at lower doses but not at higher doses, thus raising the risk that future studies could fail due to idiosyncratic biological or pharmacologic factors. In a Phase 2 study reported in 2018, the dual PI3K/mTor inhibitor RTB101 (Restorbio) reduced the incidence of respiratory tract infections in high-risk elderly patients at a dose of 10 mg daily but not at 10 mg twice daily.[56] Although a dose-response curve does not have to be strictly linear, inconsistencies like this call into question the causal relationship between the therapy and the clinical effect and indicate there is additional risk to further development. In this case, a subsequent Phase 3 trial, which used the apparently effective dose from the prior study, failed.[57]

- **Change in endpoints:** Many positive Phase 2 trials measure surrogate endpoints that are faster and cheaper to measure than "hard" regulatory endpoints. Even though many of these surrogate endpoints may appear logical and predictive on first principles, the data linking them to Phase 3 outcome measures are often scant. This is a particular issue when the surrogate endpoint is more of a biological measurement than a clinical one. For example, the anti-inflammatory agent darapladib (GlaxoSmithKline) significantly stabilized atherosclerotic plaques in a 330-patient Phase 2 study published in 2008.[58] But subsequent trials that measured cardiovascular death and other clinically meaningful cardiology endpoints rather than atherosclerotic plaques were negative.[59,60]
- **Change in patient population:** A common setup for Phase 3 failure is when a late-stage trial targets a patient subset that was identified post hoc as part of an earlier, failed study. The multi-kinase inhibitor motesanib (Takeda/Amgen) failed a Phase 3 study in lung cancer in 2012,[61] but a subsequent "exploratory subgroup analysis" found a positive result in Asian patients.[62] Based on the post hoc findings, the sponsors ran a second Phase 3 trial restricted to patients in Japan, Korea, Taiwan, and Hong Kong. The drug flopped in that study as well.[63]

  In other cases, the variance in population can be quite subtle. A positive Phase 2 study in Crohn's disease of a Smad7 antisense oligonucleotide (GED-0301; Celgene) published in 2015 used a clinical score to identify patients with moderate to severe disease.[64] The subsequent Phase 3 trial was run in ostensibly the same patient population, but actually had a more stringent requirement for endoscopy-proven mucosal disease.[65] It seems plausible that the sponsor made this change due to a belief that enriching for high-severity patients might boost the odds of success or the magnitude of the observed effect. Unfortunately, this strategy was unsuccessful, and the trial failed.[66]

Red flags in press releases and investor presentations

Although most drug developers plainly report whether a clinical trial succeeded or failed, companies sometimes puff up negative or inconclusive results. This behavior can range from hyperbolic "spin" to accentuate the positive aspects of borderline data all the way to frank deception that's intended to bury suspicious findings or overt failures.

Press releases and investor presentations issued to announce study results are particularly hard to assess because unlike full journal articles, these short reports often lack key details about the trial's protocol, execution, and analysis. That means the most common red flags in them are sins of omission that raise questions about whether the supposedly good outcome is as good as advertised, and not outright deal-killers. That said, occasionally a smoking gun in a company's PR or PowerPoint deck demonstrates clearly that the data are much more worrisome than the sponsor is making it appear.

Besides the caveats and challenges related to positive findings described previously, a few common shenanigans that companies sometimes pull in press releases and investor presentations warrant particular mention:

- **Any top-line statement except "met primary endpoint":** Some sponsors bury the lede when results are not quite positive. The first bullet of ImmuPharma's 2018 news release on top-line results from its Phase 3 study of regiremod (Lupuzor) in lupus touted a "superior response rate over placebo" on the primary endpoint (52.5% response rate vs. 44.6%), but the next sentence disclosed that the finding was not statistically significant.[67] Similarly, Raptor said in the sub-headline to its 2014 press release that the Phase 2/3 study of its delayed-release cysteamine drug RP103 in Huntington's disease "showed significantly slower progression" with the study drug. But a few sentences later, the company disclosed that this was a "positive trend,"[68] which is a term with no statistical meaning: a study either succeeded or it failed. And sure enough, the study was a bust, with a *P* value of .19 on the primary endpoint.
- **Misdirection toward non-primary endpoints:** Positive secondary endpoints can yield interesting and important information to inform future development, but if a sponsor pushes them to the fore to divert attention from a negative primary outcome, that's cause for concern. Mesoblast

claimed in a 2020 press release that in the Phase 3 DREAM-HF trial of its cell therapy rexlemestrocel-L, patients "had 60% reduction in incidence of heart attacks or strokes and 60% reduction in death from cardiac causes" compared with placebo.[69] But then came the caveat: "there was no reduction in recurrent non-fatal decompensated heart failure events, which was the trial's primary endpoint."

It's often advisable to confirm the primary endpoint when a company releases top-line data. Clicking "history of changes" near the bottom of a record on clinicaltrials.gov enables one to compare all the archived versions word-for-word and establish when changes were made. Industry watchers were correct in 2020 to question top-line results from Gilead's positive ACTT-1 trial of remdesivir (Veklury) in COVID-19 when it became clear that the primary endpoint was changed in midstream.[70] In this case, experts generally agreed that there were good reasons for the change, and it didn't materially change the results.

- **Over-emphasis on positive results in a subset of patients:** When a trial fails, sponsors can almost always find a subset of patients that appears to have responded. Sometimes the subgroup may involve an arbitrary threshold of age, levels of a biomarker, or some other continuous variable, when there's no a priori justification for the cutoff. But even if the definition is extremely logical and scientifically valid, such as when patients are divided based on disease severity or expression of a genetic mutation linked to the drug's mechanism, subset analyses are prone to a form of "*P*-hacking" where a company tests many patient groups until it lands on one that yields a positive result. Unless the analysis was pre-planned and included appropriate controls for multiple hypothesis testing, it should be viewed as an intriguing hypothesis at best until it's explicitly validated in a new study. In 2021, CytoDyn headlined a press release about its Phase 3 study with the finding that its CCR5 antagonist, leronlimab, caused a 24% reduction in all-cause mortality versus placebo in critically ill COVID-19 patients.[71] However, further down the page the company revealed that this group represented a small subset of enrolled patients, and it later disclosed that the trial failed on all measures in the full study population.[72]

- **Non-standard statistical methods:** It's impossible to list all the statistical tricks drug companies play in biotech PR, but a particular one that's important to note is the use of one-sided *P* values. Most industry watchers know that "$P<.05$" is the generally accepted threshold for statistical significance, but this assumes that the analysis was two-sided, meaning that it was powered to detect a difference between the two arms in either direction. In contrast, a one-sided analysis, which ignores the possibility that the control could actually perform better than the experimental drug, needs to hit a stricter cutoff of $P<.025$ to achieve the same level of statistical significance. That's why eagle-eyed observers cried foul in 2018 when resTORbio hailed a "significant" reduction in respiratory tract infections in patients treated with RTB101 in its Phase 2b trial, based on a *P* value of .026 that a footnote disclosed was actually one-sided.[73] After the follow-up Phase 3 PROTECTOR 1 trial failed the following year,[74] the company halted development of the drug in this indication.

---

[1] Pocock SJ, Stone GW. The primary outcome is positive—is that good enough? N Engl J Med. 2016 Sep 8;375(10):971–979. doi: 10.1056/NEJMra1601511. PMID: 27602669.

[2] Colquhoun D. The false positive risk: A proposal concerning what to do about p-values. American Statistician. 2019;73(suppl 1):192–201. doi: 10.1080/00031305.2018.1529622.

[3] Grainger D. Why too many clinical trials fail—and a simple solution that could increase returns on pharma R&D. Forbes.com. January 29, 2016. https://www.forbes.com/sites /davidgrainger/2015/01/29/why-too-many-clinical-trials-fail-and-a-simple-solution-that -could-increase-returns-on-pharma-rd/. Accessed October 15, 2021.

[4] Benjamini Y, Hochberg Y. Controlling the false discovery rate: A practical and powerful approach to multiple testing. J Royal Stat Soc: Series B (Methodological). 1995;57(1):289–300. doi: 10.1111/j.2517-6161.1995.tb02031.x.

[5] Walsh M, Srinathan SK, McAuley DF, Mrkobrada M, Levine O, Ribic C, Molnar AO, Dattani ND, Burke A, Guyatt G, Thabane L, Walter SD, Pogue J, Devereaux PJ. The statistical significance of randomized controlled trial results is frequently fragile: A case for a Fragility Index. J Clin Epidemiol. 2014 Jun;67(6):622–628. doi: 10.1016 /j.jclinepi.2013.10.019. Epub 2014 Feb 5. PMID: 24508144.

[6] Fragility index calculator. ClinCalc.com. https://clincalc.com/Stats/FragilityIndex.aspx. Accessed October 15, 2021. Permalink: https://perma.cc/LLQ6-AM3M.

[7] Del Paggio JC, Tannock IF. The fragility of Phase 3 trials supporting FDA-approved anticancer medicines: A retrospective analysis. Lancet Oncol. 2019 Aug;20(8):1065–1069. doi: 10.1016/S1470-2045(19)30338-9. Epub 2019 Jul 8. PMID: 31296490.

[8] Moreau P, Masszi T, Grzasko N, Bahlis NJ, Hansson M, Pour L, Sandhu I, Ganly P, Baker BW, Jackson SR, Stoppa AM, Simpson DR, Gimsing P, Palumbo A, Garderet L, Cavo M, Kumar S, Touzeau C, Buadi FK, Laubach JP, Berg DT, Lin J, Di Bacco A, Hui AM, van de Velde H, Richardson PG; TOURMALINE-MM1 Study Group. Oral ixazomib, lenalidomide, and dexamethasone for multiple myeloma. N Engl J Med. 2016 Apr 28;374(17):1621–1634. doi: 10.1056/NEJMoa1516282. PMID: 27119237.

[9] Cohen AT, Harrington RA, Goldhaber SZ, Hull RD, Wiens BL, Gold A, Hernandez AF, Gibson CM; APEX Investigators. Extended thromboprophylaxis with betrixaban in acutely ill medical patients. N Engl J Med. 2016 Aug 11;375(6):534–544. doi: 10.1056/NEJMoa1601747. Epub 2016 May 27. PMID: 27232649.

[10] Hattersley G, Harris AG, Simon JA, Constantine GD. Clinical investigation of RAD1901, a novel estrogen receptor ligand, for the treatment of postmenopausal vasomotor symptoms: A Phase 2 randomized, placebo-controlled, double-blind, dose-ranging, proof-of-concept trial. Menopause. 2017 Jan;24(1):92–99. doi: 10.1097/GME.0000000000000726. PMID: 27575546.

[11] Wardell SE, Nelson ER, Chao CA, Alley HM, McDonnell DP. Evaluation of the pharmacological activities of RAD1901, a selective estrogen receptor degrader. Endocr Relat Cancer. 2015 Oct;22(5):713–724. doi: 10.1530/ERC-15-0287. Epub 2015 Jul 10. PMID: 26162914; PMCID: PMC4545300.

[12] Chen P, Nirula A, Heller B, Gottlieb RL, Boscia J, Morris J, Huhn G, Cardona J, Mocherla B, Stosor V, Shawa I, Adams AC, Van Naarden J, Custer KL, Shen L, Durante M, Oakley G, Schade AE, Sabo J, Patel DR, Klekotka P, Skovronsky DM; BLAZE-1 Investigators. SARS-CoV-2 neutralizing antibody LY-CoV555 in outpatients with Covid-19. N Engl J Med. 2021 Jan 21;384(3):229–237. doi: 10.1056/NEJMoa2029849. Epub 2020 Oct 28. PMID: 33113295; PMCID: PMC7646625.

[13] Garon EB, Ciuleanu TE, Arrieta O, Prabhash K, Syrigos KN, Goksel T, Park K, Gorbunova V, Kowalyszyn RD, Pikiel J, Czyzewicz G, Orlov SV, Lewanski CR, Thomas M, Bidoli P, Dakhil S, Gans S, Kim JH, Grigorescu A, Karaseva N, Reck M, Cappuzzo F, Alexandris E, Sashegyi A, Yurasov S, Pérol M. Ramucirumab plus docetaxel versus placebo plus docetaxel for second-line treatment of stage IV non-small-cell lung cancer after disease progression on platinum-based therapy (REVEL): A multicentre, double-blind,

randomised Phase 3 trial. Lancet. 2014 Aug 23;384(9944):665–673. doi: 10.1016/S0140-6736(14)60845-X. Epub 2014 Jun 2. PMID: 24933332.

[14] FDA expands approved use of Cyramza to treat aggressive non-small cell lung cancer. U.S. FDA press release. December 12, 2014. https://www.drugs.com/newdrugs/fda-expands-approved-cyramza-aggressive-non-small-cell-lung-cancer-4120.html. Accessed October 15, 2021. Permalink: https://perma.cc/R5DU-TH45.

[15] Hilal T, Sonbol MB, Prasad V. Analysis of control arm quality in randomized clinical trials leading to anticancer drug approval by the U.S. Food and Drug Administration. JAMA Oncol. 2019 Jun 1;5(6):887–892. doi: 10.1001/jamaoncol.2019.0167. Erratum in: JAMA Oncol. 2019 Jun 20; PMID: 31046071; PMCID: PMC6499129.

[16] Kemp R, Prasad V. Surrogate endpoints in oncology: When are they acceptable for regulatory and clinical decisions, and are they currently overused? BMC Med. 2017 Jul 21;15(1):134. doi: 10.1186/s12916-017-0902-9. PMID: 28728605; PMCID: PMC5520356.

[17] Khanna A, English SW, Wang XS, Ham K, Tumlin J, Szerlip H, Busse LW, Altaweel L, Albertson TE, Mackey C, McCurdy MT, Boldt DW, Chock S, Young PJ, Krell K, Wunderink RG, Ostermann M, Murugan R, Gong MN, Panwar R, Hästbacka J, Favory R, Venkatesh B, Thompson BT, Bellomo R, Jensen J, Kroll S, Chawla LS, Tidmarsh GF, Deane AM; ATHOS-3 Investigators. Angiotensin II for the treatment of vasodilatory shock. N Engl J Med. 2017 Aug 3;377(5):419–430. doi: 10.1056/NEJMoa1704154. Epub 2017 May 21. PMID: 28528561.

[18] Farina N, Bixby A, Alaniz C. Angiotensin II brings more questions than answers. P T. 2018 Nov;43(11):685–687. PMID: 30410284; PMCID: PMC6205124.

[19] Cummings SR, McClung M, Reginster JY, Cox D, Mitlak B, Stock J, Amewou-Atisso M, Powles T, Miller P, Zanchetta J, Christiansen C. Arzoxifene for prevention of fractures and invasive breast cancer in postmenopausal women. J Bone Miner Res. 2011 Feb;26(2):397–404. doi: 10.1002/jbmr.191. Epub 2010 Jul 23. PMID: 20658564.

[20] Lilly reports on outcome of Phase III study of arzoxifene. Eli Lilly press release. August 18, 2009. https://investor.lilly.com/news-releases/news-release-details/lilly-reports-outcome-phase-iii-study-arzoxifene. Accessed October 15, 2021. Permalink: https://perma.cc/S7L3-6255.

[21] Taylor P. CETP inhibitor class finally dies as Merck abandons anacetrapib. PMLiVE. October 13, 2017. http://www.pmlive.com/pharma_news/cetp_inhibitor_class_finally_dies_as_merck_abandons_anacetrapib_1208239. Accessed October 15, 2021.

[22] Giapreza [package insert]. La Jolla Pharmaceutical. 2020. https://firebasestorage.googleapis.com/v0/b/giapreza-db.appspot.com/o/prescribing%2FGIAPREZA.pdf?alt=media. Permalink: https://perma.cc/QQU6-87JY.

[23] Pocock SJ, Stone GW. The primary outcome fails—what next? N Engl J Med. 2016 Sep 1;375(9):861-870. doi: 10.1056/NEJMra1510064. PMID: 27579636.

[24] Hackshaw A, Kirkwood A. Interpreting and reporting clinical trials with results of borderline significance. BMJ. 2011 Jul 4;343:d3340. doi: 10.1136/bmj.d3340. PMID: 21727163.

[25] Paulussen M, Craft AW, Lewis I, Hackshaw A, Douglas C, Dunst J, Schuck A, Winkelmann W, Köhler G, Poremba C, Zoubek A, Ladenstein R, van den Berg H, Hunold A, Cassoni A, Spooner D, Grimer R, Whelan J, McTiernan A, Jürgens H; European Intergroup Cooperative Ewing's Sarcoma Study-92. Results of the EICESS-92 study: Two randomized trials of Ewing's sarcoma treatment—cyclophosphamide compared with ifosfamide in standard-risk patients and assessment of benefit of etoposide added to standard treatment in high-risk patients. J Clin Oncol. 2008 Sep 20;26(27):4385–4393. doi: 10.1200/JCO.2008.16.5720. PMID: 18802150.

[26] Natale RB, Thongprasert S, Greco FA, Thomas M, Tsai CM, Sunpaweravong P, Ferry D, Mulatero C, Whorf R, Thompson J, Barlesi F, Langmuir P, Gogov S, Rowbottom JA, Goss GD. Phase III trial of vandetanib compared with erlotinib in patients with previously treated advanced non-small-cell lung cancer. J Clin Oncol. 2011 Mar 10;29(8):1059–1066. doi: 10.1200/JCO.2010.28.5981. Epub 2011 Jan 31. PMID: 21282542.

[27] Cox GF. The art and science of choosing efficacy endpoints for rare disease clinical trials. Am J Med Genet A. 2018 Apr;176(4):759–772. doi: 10.1002/ajmg.a.38629. Epub 2018 Feb 9. PMID: 29423972.

[28] Elvidge S. Mallinckrodt's rare disease drug set back by confusing trial result. BioPharma Dive. November 8, 2018. https://www.biopharmadive.com/news/mallinckrodts-rare-disease-drug-set-back-by-confusing-trial-result/541733/. Accessed October 15, 2021.

[29] VanMeter S. Clinical update on intrathecal VTS-270 for the treatment of Niemann-Pick disease. Mallinckrodt Pharmaceuticals (investor presentation). June 3, 2019. https://mallinckrodt.gcs-web.com/static-files/e0712994-a013-4658-b8be-0a3bc4da0c5b. Accessed October 15, 2021. Permalink: https://perma.cc/NQP6-63DF.

[30] Adams B. Dermira posts broadly positive results for excessive sweat drug. FierceBiotech. June 2, 2016. https://www.fiercebiotech.com/biotech/dermira-posts-broadly-positive-results-for-excessive-sweat-drug. Accessed October 15, 2021.

[31] Dermira announces positive topline results from two pivotal Phase 3 clinical trials for DRM04 in patients with primary axillary hyperhidrosis. Dermira press release. June 1, 2016. https://investor.dermira.com/news-releases/press-release-details/2016/Dermira-Announces-Positive-Topline-Results-from-Two-Pivotal-Phase-3-Clinical-Trials-for-DRM04-in-Patients-with-Primary-Axillary-Hyperhidrosis/default.aspx. Accessed October 15, 2021. Permalink: https://perma.cc/U4MC-JKXE.

[32] Dermira receives FDA approval for Qbrexza (glycopyrronium) cloth to treat primary axillary hyperhidrosis. Dermira press release. June 29, 2018. https://investor.dermira.com/news-releases/press-release-details/2018/Dermira-Receives-FDA-Approval-for-Qbrexza-glycopyrronium-Cloth-to-Treat-Primary-Axillary-Hyperhidrosis/default.aspx. Accessed October 15, 2021. Permalink: https://perma.cc/ER8P-HW8C.

[33] Hill MD, Goyal M, Menon BK, Nogueira RG, McTaggart RA, Demchuk AM, Poppe AY, Buck BH, Field TS, Dowlatshahi D, van Adel BA, Swartz RH, Shah RA, Sauvageau E, Zerna C, Ospel JM, Joshi M, Almekhlafi MA, Ryckborst KJ, Lowerison MW, Heard K, Garman D, Haussen D, Cutting SM, Coutts SB, Roy D, Rempel JL, Rohr AC, Iancu D, Sahlas DJ, Yu AYX, Devlin TG, Hanel RA, Puetz V, Silver FL, Campbell BCV, Chapot R, Teitelbaum J, Mandzia JL, Kleinig TJ, Turkel-Parrella D, Heck D, Kelly ME, Bharatha A, Bang OY, Jadhav A, Gupta R, Frei DF, Tarpley JW, McDougall CG, Holmin S, Rha JH, Puri AS, Camden MC, Thomalla G, Choe H, Phillips SJ, Schindler JL, Thornton J, Nagel S, Heo JH, Sohn SI, Psychogios MN, Budzik RF, Starkman S, Martin CO, Burns PA, Murphy S, Lopez GA, English J, Tymianski M; ESCAPE-NA1 Investigators. Efficacy and safety of nerinetide for the treatment of acute ischaemic stroke (ESCAPE-NA1): A multicentre, double-blind, randomised controlled trial. Lancet. 2020 Mar 14;395(10227):878–887. doi: 10.1016/S0140-6736(20)30258-0. Epub 2020 Feb 20. PMID: 32087818.

[34] Efficacy and safety of nerinetide in participants with acute ischemic stroke undergoing endovascular thrombectomy excluding thrombolysis (ESCAPE-NEXT). ClinicalTrials.gov identifier: NCT04462536. Updated December 17, 2020. Accessed October 15, 2021.

[35] Belluck P, Kaplan S, Robbins R. How an unproven Alzheimer's drug got approved. New York Times. July 19, 2021. https://www.nytimes.com/2021/07/19/health/alzheimers-drug-aduhelm-fda.html. Accessed November 23, 2021.

[36] FDA grants accelerated approval for Alzheimer's drug. FDA press release. June 7, 2021. https://www.fda.gov/news-events/press-announcements/fda-grants-accelerated-approval-alzheimers-drug. Accessed November 23, 2021. Permalink: https://perma.cc/6CWZ-PYFM.

[37] Multiple endpoints in clinical trials: Guidance for industry (draft guidance). U.S. Food and Drug Administration. January 2017.

[38] Butler J, Packer M, Greene SJ, Fiuzat M, Anker SD, Anstrom KJ, Carson PE, Cooper LB, Fonarow GC, Hernandez AF, Januzzi JL Jr, Jessup M, Kalyani RR, Kaul S, Kosiborod M, Lindenfeld J, McGuire DK, Sabatine MS, Solomon SD, Teerlink JR, Vaduganathan M, Yancy CW, Stockbridge N, O'Connor CM. Heart failure end points in cardiovascular outcome trials of sodium glucose cotransporter 2 inhibitors in patients with type 2 diabetes mellitus: A critical evaluation of clinical and regulatory issues. Circulation. 2019 Dec 17;140(25):2108–2118. doi: 10.1161/CIRCULATIONAHA.119.042155. Epub 2019 Dec 16. PMID: 31841369; PMCID: PMC7027964.

[39] Clayton GL, Schachter AD, Magnusson B, Li Y, Colin L. How often do safety signals occur by chance in first-in-human trials? Clin Transl Sci. 2018 Sep;11(5):471–476. doi: 10.1111/cts.12558. Epub 2018 Apr 27. PMID: 29702733; PMCID: PMC6132364.

[40] David FS, Robey S, Matthews A. *The Pharmagellan Guide to Biotech Forecasting and Valuation*. 1st ed. Pharmagellan; 2016.

[41] Pfeiffer T, Bertram L, Ioannidis JP. Quantifying selective reporting and the Proteus phenomenon for multiple datasets with similar bias. PLoS One. 2011 Mar 29;6(3):e18362. doi: 10.1371/journal.pone.0018362. PMID: 21479240; PMCID: PMC3066227.

[42] Cook D, Brown D, Alexander R, March R, Morgan P, Satterthwaite G, Pangalos MN. Lessons learned from the fate of AstraZeneca's drug pipeline: A five-dimensional framework. Nat Rev Drug Discov. 2014 Jun;13(6):419–431. doi: 10.1038/nrd4309. Epub 2014 May 16. PMID: 24833294.

[43] Morgan P, Brown DG, Lennard S, Anderton MJ, Barrett JC, Eriksson U, Fidock M, Hamrén B, Johnson A, March RE, Matcham J, Mettetal J, Nicholls DJ, Platz S, Rees S, Snowden MA, Pangalos MN. Impact of a five-dimensional framework on R&D productivity at AstraZeneca. Nat Rev Drug Discov. 2018 Mar;17(3):167–181. doi: 10.1038/nrd.2017.244. Epub 2018 Jan 19. PMID: 29348681.

[44] Morgan P, Van Der Graaf PH, Arrowsmith J, Feltner DE, Drummond KS, Wegner CD, Street SD. Can the flow of medicines be improved? Fundamental pharmacokinetic and pharmacological principles toward improving Phase II survival. Drug Discov Today. 2012 May;17(9-10):419–424. doi: 10.1016/j.drudis.2011.12.020. Epub 2011 Dec 29. PMID: 22227532.

[45] Parasrampuria DA, Benet LZ, Sharma A. Why drugs fail in late stages of development: Case study analyses from the last decade and recommendations. AAPS J. 2018 Mar 13;20(3):46. doi: 10.1208/s12248-018-0204-y. PMID: 29536211.

[46] Sun A, Benet LZ. Late-stage failures of monoclonal antibody drugs: A retrospective case study analysis. Pharmacology. 2020;105(3-4):145–163. doi: 10.1159/000505379. Epub 2020 Jan 7. PMID: 31910414.

[47] 22 case studies where Phase 2 and Phase 3 trials had divergent results. U.S. Food and Drug Administration. January 2017.

[48] Yaspan BL, Williams DF, Holz FG, Regillo CD, Li Z, Dressen A, van Lookeren Campagne M, Le KN, Graham RR, Beres T, Bhangale TR, Honigberg LA, Smith A, Henry EC, Ho C, Strauss EC; MAHALO Study Investigators. Targeting factor D of the alternative complement pathway reduces geographic atrophy progression secondary to age-related macular degeneration. Sci Transl Med. 2017 Jun 21;9(395):eaaf1443. doi: 10.1126/scitranslmed.aaf1443. PMID: 28637922.

[49] Holz FG, Sadda SR, Busbee B, Chew EY, Mitchell P, Tufail A, Brittain C, Ferrara D, Gray S, Honigberg L, Martin J, Tong B, Ehrlich JS, Bressler NM; Chroma and Spectri Study Investigators. Efficacy and safety of lampalizumab for geographic atrophy due to age-related macular degeneration: Chroma and Spectri Phase 3 randomized clinical trials. JAMA Ophthalmol. 2018 Jun 1;136(6):666–677. doi: 10.1001/jamaophthalmol.2018.1544. PMID: 29801123; PMCID: PMC6145777.

[50] Jardim DL, Groves ES, Breitfeld PP, Kurzrock R. Factors associated with failure of oncology drugs in late-stage clinical development: A systematic review. Cancer Treat Rev. 2017 Jan;52:12–21. doi: 10.1016/j.ctrv.2016.10.009. Epub 2016 Nov 4. PMID: 27883925.

[51] Witcher J, Fleischmann R, Chindalore VL, Hansen RJ, Hu L, Radtke D, Voelker J, Gomez E, McColm J. Pharmacokinetics and safety of single doses of tabalumab in subjects with rheumatoid arthritis or systemic lupus erythematosus. Br J Clin Pharmacol. 2016 May;81(5):908–917. doi: 10.1111/bcp.12860. Epub 2016 Feb 25. PMID: 26648084; PMCID: PMC4834597.

[52] Genovese MC, Lee E, Satterwhite J, Veenhuizen M, Disch D, Berclaz PY, Myers S, Sides G, Benichou O. A Phase 2 dose-ranging study of subcutaneous tabalumab for the treatment of patients with active rheumatoid arthritis and an inadequate response to methotrexate. Ann Rheum Dis. 2013 Sep 1;72(9):1453–1460. doi: 10.1136/annrheumdis-2012-202864. Epub 2013 Apr 18. PMID: 23599435.

[53] Greenwald M, Szczepanski L, Kennedy A, Veenhuizen M, Komocsar WJ, Polasek E, Guerrettaz K, Berclaz PY, Lee C. A 52-week, open-label study evaluating the safety and efficacy of tabalumab, an anti-B-cell-activating factor monoclonal antibody, for rheumatoid arthritis. Arthritis Res Ther. 2014 Aug 29;16(4):415. doi: 10.1186/s13075-014-0415-2. PMID: 25168268; PMCID: PMC4177512.

[54] Isenberg DA, Petri M, Kalunian K, Tanaka Y, Urowitz MB, Hoffman RW, Morgan-Cox M, Iikuni N, Silk M, Wallace DJ. Efficacy and safety of subcutaneous tabalumab in patients with systemic lupus erythematosus: Results from ILLUMINATE-1, a 52-week, Phase III, multicentre, randomised, double-blind, placebo-controlled study. Ann Rheum Dis. 2016 Feb;75(2):323–331. doi: 10.1136/annrheumdis-2015-207653. Epub 2015 Sep 3. PMID: 26338095.

[55] Merrill JT, van Vollenhoven RF, Buyon JP, Furie RA, Stohl W, Morgan-Cox M, Dickson C, Anderson PW, Lee C, Berclaz PY, Dörner T. Efficacy and safety of subcutaneous tabalumab, a monoclonal antibody to B-cell activating factor, in patients with systemic lupus erythematosus: Results from ILLUMINATE-2, a 52-week, Phase III, multicentre, randomised, double-blind, placebo-controlled study. Ann Rheum Dis. 2016 Feb;75(2):332–340. doi: 10.1136/annrheumdis-2015-207654. Epub 2015 Aug 20. PMID: 26293163.

[56] Plieth J. Restorbio clutches at straws, and investors say that's fine. Evaluate Vantage. July 25, 2018. https://www.evaluate.com/vantage/articles/news/trial-results/restorbio-clutches-straws-and-investors-say-thats-fine. Accessed October 15, 2021.

[57] reSTORbio announces that the Phase 3 PROTECTOR 1 trial of RTB101 in clinically symptomatic respiratory illness did not meet the primary endpoint. resTORbio press release. November 15, 2019. https://www.globenewswire.com/news-release/2019/11/15/1947932/0/en/resTORbio-Announces-That-the-Phase-3-PROTECTOR-1-Trial-of-RTB101-in-Clinically-Symptomatic-Respiratory-Illness-Did-Not-Meet-the-Primary-Endpoint.html. Accessed October 15, 2021. Permalink: https://perma.cc/U242-TU55.

[58] Serruys PW, García-García HM, Buszman P, Erne P, Verheye S, Aschermann M, Duckers H, Bleie O, Dudek D, Bøtker HE, von Birgelen C, D'Amico D, Hutchinson T, Zambanini A, Mastik F, van Es GA, van der Steen AF, Vince DG, Ganz P, Hamm CW, Wijns W, Zalewski A; Integrated Biomarker and Imaging Study-2 Investigators. Effects of the direct lipoprotein-associated phospholipase A(2) inhibitor darapladib on human coronary atherosclerotic plaque. Circulation. 2008 Sep 9;118(11):1172–1182. doi: 10.1161/CIRCULATIONAHA.108.771899. Epub 2008 Sep 1. PMID: 18765397.

[59] White HD, Held C, Stewart R, Tarka E, Brown R, Davies RY, Budaj A, Harrington RA, Steg PG, Ardissino D, Armstrong PW, Avezum A, Aylward PE, Bryce A, Chen H, Chen MF, Corbalan R, Dalby AJ, Danchin N, De Winter RJ, Denchev S, Diaz R, Elisaf M, Flather MD, Goudev AR, Granger CB, Grinfeld L, Hochman JS, Husted S, Kim HS, Koenig W, Linhart A, Lonn E, López-Sendón J, Manolis AJ, Mohler ER 3rd, Nicolau JC, Pais P, Parkhomenko A, Pedersen TR, Pella D, Ramos-Corrales MA, Ruda M, Sereg M, Siddique S, Sinnaeve P, Smith P, Sritara P, Swart HP, Sy RG, Teramoto T, Tse HF, Watson D, Weaver WD, Weiss R, Viigimaa M, Vinereanu D, Zhu J, Cannon CP, Wallentin L;

STABILITY Investigators. Darapladib for preventing ischemic events in stable coronary heart disease. N Engl J Med. 2014 May 1;370(18):1702–1711. doi: 10.1056/NEJMoa1315878. Epub 2014 Mar 30. PMID: 24678955.

[60] O'Donoghue ML, Braunwald E, White HD, Steen DL, Lukas MA, Tarka E, Steg PG, Hochman JS, Bode C, Maggioni AP, Im K, Shannon JB, Davies RY, Murphy SA, Crugnale SE, Wiviott SD, Bonaca MP, Watson DF, Weaver WD, Serruys PW, Cannon CP; SOLID-TIMI 52 Investigators. Effect of darapladib on major coronary events after an acute coronary syndrome: The SOLID-TIMI 52 randomized clinical trial. JAMA. 2014 Sep 10;312(10):1006–1015. doi: 10.1001/jama.2014.11061. Erratum in: JAMA. 2014 Oct 8;312(14):1473. Dylan P. Steen[corrected to Dylan L. Steen]. PMID: 25173516.

[61] Scagliotti GV, Vynnychenko I, Park K, Ichinose Y, Kubota K, Blackhall F, Pirker R, Galiulin R, Ciuleanu TE, Sydorenko O, Dediu M, Papai-Szekely Z, Banaclocha NM, McCoy S, Yao B, Hei YJ, Galimi F, Spigel DR. International, randomized, placebo-controlled, double-blind Phase III study of motesanib plus carboplatin/paclitaxel in patients with advanced nonsquamous non-small-cell lung cancer: MONET1. J Clin Oncol. 2012 Aug 10;30(23):2829–2836. doi: 10.1200/JCO.2011.41.4987. Epub 2012 Jul 2. PMID: 22753922.

[62] Kubota K, Ichinose Y, Scagliotti G, Spigel D, Kim JH, Shinkai T, Takeda K, Kim SW, Hsia TC, Li RK, Tiangco BJ, Yau S, Lim WT, Yao B, Hei YJ, Park K. Phase III study (MONET1) of motesanib plus carboplatin/paclitaxel in patients with advanced nonsquamous nonsmall-cell lung cancer (NSCLC): Asian subgroup analysis. Ann Oncol. 2014 Feb;25(2):529–536. doi: 10.1093/annonc/mdt552. Epub 2014 Jan 13. PMID: 24419239.

[63] Kubota K, Yoshioka H, Oshita F, Hida T, Yoh K, Hayashi H, Kato T, Kaneda H, Yamada K, Tanaka H, Ichinose Y, Park K, Cho EK, Lee KH, Lin CB, Yang JC, Hara K, Asato T, Nakagawa K. Phase III, randomized, placebo-controlled, double-blind trial of motesanib (AMG-706) in combination with paclitaxel and carboplatin in East Asian patients with advanced nonsquamous non-small-cell lung cancer. J Clin Oncol. 2017 Nov 10;35(32):3662–3670. doi: 10.1200/JCO.2017.72.7297. Epub 2017 Sep 13. PMID: 28902534.

[64] Monteleone G, Neurath MF, Ardizzone S, Di Sabatino A, Fantini MC, Castiglione F, Scribano ML, Armuzzi A, Caprioli F, Sturniolo GC, Rogai F, Vecchi M, Atreya R, Bossa F, Onali S, Fichera M, Corazza GR, Biancone L, Savarino V, Pica R, Orlando A, Pallone F. Mongersen, an oral SMAD7 antisense oligonucleotide, and Crohn's disease. N Engl J Med. 2015 Mar 19;372(12):1104–1113. doi: 10.1056/NEJMoa1407250. PMID: 25785968.

[65] Sands BE, Feagan BG, Sandborn WJ, Schreiber S, Peyrin-Biroulet L, Frédéric Colombel J, Rossiter G, Usiskin K, Ather S, Zhan X, D'Haens G. Mongersen (GED-0301) for active Crohn's disease: Results of a Phase 3 study. Am J Gastroenterol. 2020 May;115(5):738–745. doi: 10.14309/ajg.0000000000000493. PMID: 31850931.

[66] Bewtra M, Lichtenstein GR. Mongersen and SMAD-7 inhibition, not a lucky 7 for patients with IBD: When trial design is as important as disease therapy. Am J Gastroenterol. 2020 May;115(5):687–688. doi: 10.14309/ajg.0000000000000564. PMID: 32195732.

[67] Topline results of Lupuzor pivotal Phase III trial. Immupharma press release. April 17, 2018. https://www.immupharma.co.uk/top-line-results-lupuzor-pivotal-phase-iii-trial/. Accessed October 15, 2021. Permalink: https://perma.cc/9JFF-84XP.

[68] Raptor announces clinical results with RP103 in Huntington's disease Phase 2/3 trial. Raptor Pharmaceutical press release. February 20, 2014. https://www.globenewswire.com/news-release/2014/02/20/611824/12430/en/Raptor-Announces-Clinical-Results-With-RP103-in-Huntington-s-Disease-Phase-2-3-Trial.html. Accessed October 15, 2021. Permalink: https://perma.cc/LGZ6-FVUA.

[69] Mesoblast provides topline results from Phase 3 trial of rexlemestrocel-L for advanced chronic heart failure. Mesoblast press release. December 14, 2020. http://investorsmedia.mesoblast.com/static-files/162dd76a-6deb-47e9-b950-3497dfce1fbc. Accessed October 15, 2021. Permalink: https://perma.cc/7B7W-VWEH.

[70] Herper M. Were researchers wrong to move the goalposts on remdesivir? In the end, it may not have mattered. STAT. May 5, 2020. https://www.statnews.com/2020/05/05/were-researchers-wrong-to-move-the-goalposts-on-remdesivir-in-the-end-it-may-not-have-mattered/. Accessed October 15, 2021.

[71] CytoDyn's Phase 3 trial demonstrates safety, a 24% reduction in mortality and faster hospital discharge for mechanically ventilated critically ill COVID-19 patients treated with leronlimab. CytoDyn press release. March 5, 2021. https://www.cytodyn.com/newsroom/press-releases/detail/501/cytodyns-phase-3-trial-demonstrates-safety-a-24. Accessed October 15, 2021. Permalink: https://perma.cc/ENJ3-EVE2.

[72] Adams B. CytoDyn's chief scientific officer Rahman quietly exits amid leronlimab limbo. FierceBiotech. April 8, 2021. https://www.fiercebiotech.com/biotech/cytodyn-s-chief-scientific-officer-rahman-quietly-exits-amid-leronlimab-limbo. Accessed October 15, 2021.

[73] Bell J. ResTORbio rockets up on questionable data. BioPharma Dive. July 25, 2018. https://www.biopharmadive.com/news/restorbio-rockets-up-on-questionable-data/528592/. Accessed October 15, 2021.

[74] reSTORbio announces that the Phase 3 PROTECTOR 1 trial of RTB101 in clinically symptomatic respiratory illness did not meet the primary endpoint. resTORbio press release. November 15, 2019. https://www.globenewswire.com/news-release/2019/11/15/1947932/0/en/resTORbio-Announces-That-the-Phase-3-PROTECTOR-1-Trial-of-RTB101-in-Clinically-Symptomatic-Respiratory-Illness-Did-Not-Meet-the-Primary-Endpoint.html. Accessed October 15, 2021. Permalink: https://perma.cc/U242-TU55.

9.

RESULTS—SAFETY

ONE OF THE MOST COMMON and misused claims in biotech press releases is that a drug is "safe and well tolerated." There is no agreement about what this phrase means, and it lacks important details about how patients reacted to an experimental therapy.

In general, readers of clinical trial reports on development-stage agents need to answer two main questions about the drug's safety profile. First, does the drug increase the odds a patient will experience a particular kind of adverse event? And if so, how significant is this finding to the drug's ability to be approved or its commercial prospects?

Unfortunately, both these questions are difficult to answer. Randomized controlled trials (RCTs) of new drugs are powered to detect differences in efficacy, not uncommon safety signals, so it is impossible to perform standard statistical tests to compare the incidence of safety events, even when they are relatively common. For most drugs, the true tests of safety and tolerability occur only when a drug has been used on the market by a much larger number of people. This can make it challenging to predict from clinical trials how a drug's safety profile will affect its perception among regulators, physicians, and patients.

Notwithstanding these challenges, in this chapter we highlight some key considerations in evaluating safety results presented in reports from efficacy trials as well as some guidance on interpreting companies' disclosures of events during ongoing studies. Our focus here is on safety results from middle- and late-stage studies (Phase 2a and later) because those are the ones that are most

---

commonly released to the public. Although many points are applicable to interpreting results from first-in-human studies, readers specifically interested in Phase 1 trials may want to consult resources that focus specifically on clinical pharmacology and early clinical development.[1,2,3,4]

Key definitions in drug safety

Grading of drug safety signals

First developed in cancer, the Common Terminology Criteria for Adverse Events (CTCAE)[5] classifies **adverse events (AEs)** into clinical categories and defines grades from 1 (mild) to 5 (death) within each of them. The grades are defined based on a mix of objective criteria like laboratory findings, subjective clinical criteria, and treatments. Not all categories employ all five grades. For example, within nausea AEs, the CTCAE defines grade 1 as loss of appetite without alteration in eating habits, grade 2 as decreased oral intake without significant weight loss, dehydration, or malnutrition, and grade 3 as inadequate oral intake that requires tube feeding, total parenteral nutrition, or hospitalization.

The U.S. Food and Drug Administration (FDA) specifically defines **serious adverse events (SAEs)** as those that result in death, persistent or significant disability, a congenital anomaly or birth defect, hospitalization or prolongation of existing hospitalization, or a life-threatening adverse experience.[6] In some situations, a less clinically impactful event may be classified as an SAE if it required medical or surgical intervention to prevent an SAE, such as allergic bronchospasm that requires intensive therapy to prevent a life-threatening respiratory emergency.[7] Note that the correlation between SAEs and the 5-point AE grading scheme is imperfect because the interpretation of "life threatening" and criteria for hospitalization can vary between studies, study sites, or investigators.[8] In other words, an AE might be graded as "severe" based on CTCAE criteria but not meet the FDA's strict definition of an SAE.

An important but blurry distinction in clinical trials is between safety and **tolerability**. Although press releases commonly refer to drugs as being "well tolerated," there is no agreed-upon definition of the term. Portola reported in 2017 that its Syk/Jak inhibitor cerdulatinib for lymphoma was "generally well tolerated" in an interim look at data from a single-arm Phase 2a study, even though two patients died from infections.[9] And even when a drug doesn't cause SAEs,

lower-severity AEs can be uncomfortable or persistent enough to cause patients to cease treatment or seek alternatives before even beginning therapy.

Cause and timing of safety signals

Many adverse effects in clinical trials are unrelated to the study drug. Side effects like nausea, drowsiness, headache, and minor itching are common in all drug trials, even on placebo. One analysis found that as many as 26% of non-drug-treated patients in statin trials discontinued therapy during the study.[10] **Treatment-emergent AEs (TEAEs)** are defined strictly on the basis of their timing: they were either not present before initiation of the treatments and manifested on therapy, or they were already present but worsened in intensity or frequency after drug exposure. No causality is implied.

In contrast, **adverse drug reactions (ADRs)**, which are sometimes called **drug-related AEs**, are defined as AEs that have "at least a reasonable possibility" to have been caused by a drug, based on so-called ICH guidelines from the International Council for Harmonisation of Technical Requirements for Pharmaceuticals for Human Use.[11] During a trial, determining whether a safety event is an ADR can be complicated because not every AE that befalls a patient in a trial is necessarily due to the study drug. Patients with life-threatening, progressive diseases like cancer can die or become seriously ill for reasons unrelated to a study. And even in trials in less severe indications, patients' underlying chronic diseases like asthma, hypertension, or diabetes may progress or cause serious health events for reasons unrelated to the study drug.

For ongoing studies, the FDA requires that sponsors report all SAEs with a "reasonable possibility" of having been caused by the study drug within 15 days,[12] and these reports are often made public. However, there is typically a lag after reporting while study physicians dig into the clinical details to assess the timing of onset, the patient's prior clinical history, and other factors to determine the likelihood that the event was attributable to the drug. Investors drove the stock of Ziopharm down 22% after news broke in 2016 that a patient enrolled in the company's Phase 1 study of a gene therapy, Ad-RTS-hIL-12, in glioblastoma multiforme died of an intracranial hemorrhage.[13] But four days later, the study's safety review committee concluded that the death was unrelated to the study drug.[14] The trial continued, and the stock regained almost all its losses within a few weeks.

Factors to consider when assessing safety results

Safety and tolerability results are extremely challenging to interpret, requiring both quantitative and qualitative assessments. Determining the implications of apparent AEs for the possible R&D, regulatory, or commercial fate of a drug development program typically involves assessing the "preponderance of the evidence" in light of the context around the drug and the clinical indication. Key factors to consider include:

- **Absolute and relative numbers of events:** The absolute incidence of safety events in a trial is highly dependent on the number of treated patients. Many SAEs are thankfully extremely rare and thus almost impossible to observe in small and medium-sized trials. For this reason, absence of evidence of clinically significant side effects is not necessarily evidence of absence, and negative or extremely weak signals should always be viewed in the context of the trial size. At the same time, an apparent safety signal in a small, early-stage study may have arisen spuriously and may not accurately reflect the drug's clinical profile.[15] We discuss how to calculate a range of uncertainty in these sorts of scenarios in Chapter 12 on *P* values and confidence intervals.

  For studies that compare a drug against a control arm, one should note numerical imbalances in AEs overall, by grade, and by specific classes or types. Such imbalances could be random noise, but even in small studies, they may carry more weight if there is evidence of dose dependency or the findings reinforce prior evidence or expectations, as discussed below.

  Obviously, the magnitude and type of risk are extremely context-dependent. For example, a 0.4% absolute increase in the odds of stroke might be deemed a tolerable risk for patients with a debilitating, progressive disease in exchange for a reasonable level of efficacy. But when Merck found such a safety signal in 2016 in an osteoporosis Phase 3 RCT of its cathepsin K inhibitor odanacatib,[16] the company scrapped further development. It did so even in the context of a substantial decrease in fracture risk, presumably due to skepticism that a drug with that profile would be approved for a primary care indication.[17]

  Importantly, although *P* values are commonly reported in safety tables, formal tests of statistical significance within or between studies are not valid for safety data.[18] This is because even the largest Phase 3 RCTs are designed to quantify efficacy and are not big enough to evaluate different incidences of rare safety events. (Chapter 13 is devoted to discussing the relationship between study size and statistical power.) In this context, a *P* value above .05 is highly likely to be a false negative, due to the insufficient powering of the study, and a "significant" *P* value is likely to be a false positive due to multiple hypothesis testing.

- **Fit with prior knowledge and data:** Many drugs enter clinical testing with some pre-existing evidence of a possible safety liability from preclinical studies or results from clinical trials of other agents in the same class. When these "expected" AEs are observed, even in small studies, it is appropriate to view them with heightened attention and concern. Drugs targeting nerve growth factor (NGF) have been known to increase the risk of serious joint-related AEs since 2010, when reports from ongoing and completed studies of tanezumab (Pfizer/Lilly) led the FDA to temporarily halt development until the agency studied the issue and defined more-stringent monitoring of joint safety.[19] In that context, it was not surprising when the FDA issued a clinical hold on another anti-NGF drug, fasinumab (Regeneron/Teva), in 2016 after a single patient in a Phase 2b study in low back pain developed advanced joint disease.[20] Similarly, interim results from a first-in-human study reported in 2019 of the antibody-drug conjugate GSK2857916 (Blenrep; GlaxoSmithKline), also called belantamab mafodotin-blmf, in multiple myeloma showed that over half of enrolled patients developed corneal toxicity as detected by formal ophthalmologic testing.[21] Regular eye exams are not standard in drug trials, but they were incorporated into the trial protocol because the chemotherapeutic conjugate was already known to have ocular toxicity. As expected, the corneal findings persisted throughout drug development, and when the therapy was approved in 2020 an explicit warning was incorporated into the drug's label.[22]
- **Emergence of "surprising" AEs:** As mentioned, side effects like nausea, drowsiness, headache, and minor itching are common in all drug trials, even on placebo and at levels high enough that patients withdraw from control arms.[23] But the emergence of less common side effects, even at low severity, often merits close attention. In two separate Phase

1 studies, AstraZeneca's JAK2 inhibitor AZD1480 induced a substantial number of low-grade adverse neuropsychiatric effects, including ataxia, aphasia, confusion, and dizziness.[24,25] These were unexpected and unexplainable by the drug's mechanism of action and most likely contributed to the sponsor's decision in 2012 to discontinue the program.[26]

- **Clinical context:** An excessive risk of death or other SAEs is almost always a cause for concern for a new drug, but even low-grade, "manageable" tolerability signals can make a drug candidate commercially non-viable in certain target indications. AstraZeneca formulated its TLR7 agonist AZD8848 for local delivery in an attempt to minimize the incidence of systemic immune responses, which were well known and expected from this class. But an inhaled form of the agent at a dose that induced an efficacy biomarker led four out of six healthy volunteers to experience flu-like symptoms on repeat treatment,[27] and in an RCT in mild asthma, an intranasal form induced flu-like symptoms in more than half of drug-treated patients at a dose that failed on the primary efficacy endpoint.[28] The side effects in both trials were mild to moderate and resolved rapidly. But the sponsor determined that the tolerability profile was incompatible with clinical uptake and commercial success in the mild respiratory illnesses being addressed and discontinued development in 2014.[29,30]

  Even in oncology, where the threshold for halting development based on AEs is typically higher than in other clinical areas, it is important to consider the safety profile in context. Many reports of cancer drug trials use general language like "generally well tolerated" or "manageable toxicities" to describe safety findings even when the incidence or severity of events is potentially highly significant to patients.[31] Of note, many reports from oncology drug studies lump together all AEs of grade 3 or higher in the text of papers or press releases, even though significant imbalances in SAEs might be evident from more detailed tables.
- **Withdrawals:** A detailed accounting of the number of patients who leave a trial due to adverse events can often yield crucial insights about the "tolerability" of low-grade AEs. Phase 3 studies of Merck's first-in-class P2X3 receptor antagonist gefapixant for chronic cough demonstrated efficacy in 2020, but about 60% of patients experienced taste disturbances, and 15%–20% quit the study as a result.[32] If the drug is approved, it may

nonetheless leave the door open for future competitors if they can show equivalent efficacy and a lower incidence of taste disturbances.

- **Impact of the study protocol on safety results:** Detection and reporting of low-severity AEs are highly dependent on the level of stringency the protocol mandates for each study visit. In the run-up to pivotal testing of its apo B antisense drug mipomersen (Kynamro) in familial hypercholesterolemia, Ionis accidentally disclosed in 2013 that it intended to reduce the frequency of laboratory testing and avoid actively asking patients about flu-like symptoms or injection site reactions, presumably to skew the safety results more favorably.[33]

Regulatory implications of unfavorable safety results

When regulators evaluate a new drug's application for marketing approval, they balance efficacy and safety findings to determine whether there is a net benefit. This is an extremely subjective determination, and regulators have wide latitude for how to handle safety findings during drug approval:

- **Warnings in product insert:** The agency can decide to simply grant full approval, in which case the safety data are typically included in the package insert as a summary of "warnings and precautions" on the first page, with more detailed data later in the multi-page document.
- **Black box warning:** Regulators can mandate a "black box warning," the most stringent safety notice the agency applies to drug labels. Such warnings more prominently highlight particular safety concerns in boldface type at the top of the first page of the package insert. The example in Figure 9-1 is from the U.S. product insert for fluoxetine (Prozac; Pfizer).[34] In addition to making the safety issues more prominent, these warnings sometimes strongly recommend additional testing or monitoring that could make therapy significantly more burdensome. This is the case for the belantamab mafodotin-blmf example discussed earlier, where the recommended ophthalmologic exams in the label are not part of standard oncology care and generate additional hassle for patients and physicians.
- **Requirement for additional studies:** Regulators can require additional safety studies either as a requirement for approval or as a post-marketing commitment.[35] For example, when the FDA granted accelerated approval to carfilzomib (Kyprolis; Onyx/Amgen) in 2012, the

agency required the sponsor to conduct additional sub-studies within an ongoing RCT to specifically characterize cardiac and pulmonary toxicities, the safety of different dosing regimens, and safety and pharmacokinetics in patients with reduced liver or renal function.[36]

- **Mandated risk mitigation program:** Regulatory authorities may require the sponsor to institute a Risk Evaluation and Mitigation Strategy (REMS) to reduce the frequency or severity of a specific type of adverse event.[37] REMS programs are negotiated on a case-by-case basis between regulators and the company and can include features like certifications or other limitations on prescribers or dispensers, restrictions on the setting in which the drug can be provided, requirements for lab tests before dispensing, patient monitoring, and patient registries.
- **Rejection:** And of course, regulators can decide to reject a drug outright if the agency determines that the safety/efficacy balance is unfavorable.

FIGURE 9-1: Example of drug label with black box warning.

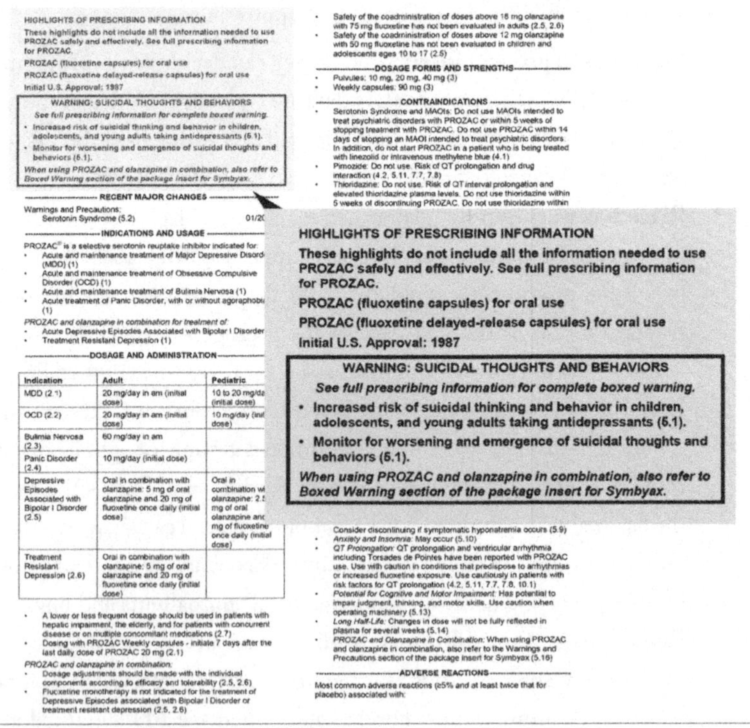

HIGHLIGHTS OF PRESCRIBING INFORMATION
These highlights do not include all the information needed to use PROZAC safely and effectively. See full prescribing information for PROZAC.
PROZAC (fluoxetine capsules) for oral use
PROZAC (fluoxetine delayed-release capsules) for oral use
Initial U.S. Approval: 1987

WARNING: SUICIDAL THOUGHTS AND BEHAVIORS
See full prescribing information for complete boxed warning.
- Increased risk of suicidal thinking and behavior in children, adolescents, and young adults taking antidepressants (5.1).
- Monitor for worsening and emergence of suicidal thoughts and behaviors (5.1).

When using PROZAC and olanzapine in combination, also refer to Boxed Warning section of the package insert for Symbyax.

RECENT MAJOR CHANGES
Warnings and Precautions:
Serotonin Syndrome (5.2) 01/20

INDICATIONS AND USAGE
PROZAC® is a selective serotonin reuptake inhibitor indicated for:
- Acute and maintenance treatment of Major Depressive Disord (MDD) (1)
- Acute and maintenance treatment of Obsessive Compulsive Disorder (OCD) (1)
- Acute and maintenance treatment of Bulimia Nervosa (1)
- Acute treatment of Panic Disorder, with or without agoraphobi (1)

PROZAC and olanzapine in combination for treatment of:
- Acute Depressive Episodes Associated with Bipolar I Disorder
- Treatment Resistant Depression (1)

DOSAGE AND ADMINISTRATION

Indication	Adult	Pediatric
MDD (2.1)	20 mg/day in am (initial dose)	10 to 20 mg/da (initial dose)
OCD (2.2)	20 mg/day in am (initial dose)	10 mg/day (init dose)
Bulimia Nervosa (2.3)	60 mg/day in am	
Panic Disorder (2.4)	10 mg/day (initial dose)	
Depressive Episodes Associated with Bipolar I Disorder (2.5)	Oral in combination with olanzapine: 5 mg of oral olanzapine and 20 mg of fluoxetine once daily (initial dose)	Oral in combination wi olanzapine: 2.5 mg of oral olanzapine anc mg of fluoxetine once daily (initial dose)
Treatment Resistant Depression (2.6)	Oral in combination with olanzapine: 5 mg of oral olanzapine and 20 mg of fluoxetine once daily (initial dose)	

- A lower or less frequent dosage should be used in patients with hepatic impairment, the elderly, and for patients with concurrent disease or on multiple concomitant medications (2.7)
- Dosing with PROZAC Weekly capsules - initiate 7 days after the last daily dose of PROZAC 20 mg (2.1)

PROZAC and olanzapine in combination:
- Dosage adjustments should be made with the individual components according to efficacy and tolerability (2.5, 2.6)
- Fluoxetine monotherapy is not indicated for the treatment of Depressive Episodes associated with Bipolar I Disorder or treatment resistant depression (2.5, 2.6)
- Safety of the coadministration of doses above 18 mg olanzapine with 75 mg fluoxetine has not been evaluated in adults (2.5, 2.6)
- Safety of the coadministration of doses above 12 mg olanzapine with 50 mg fluoxetine has not been evaluated in children and adolescents ages 10 to 17 (2.5)

DOSAGE FORMS AND STRENGTHS
- Pulvules: 10 mg, 20 mg, 40 mg (3)
- Weekly capsules: 90 mg (3)

CONTRAINDICATIONS
- Serotonin Syndrome and MAOIs: Do not use MAOIs intended to treat psychiatric disorders with PROZAC or within 5 weeks of stopping treatment with PROZAC. Do not use PROZAC within 14 days of stopping an MAOI intended to treat psychiatric disorders. In addition, do not start PROZAC in a patient who is being treated with linezolid or intravenous methylene blue (4.1)
- Pimozide: Do not use. Risk of QT prolongation and drug interaction (4.2, 5.11, 7.7, 7.8)
- Thioridazine: Do not use. Risk of QT interval prolongation and elevated thioridazine plasma levels. Do not use thioridazine within 5 weeks of discontinuing PROZAC. Do not use thioridazine within

HIGHLIGHTS OF PRESCRIBING INFORMATION
These highlights do not include all the information needed to use PROZAC safely and effectively. See full prescribing information for PROZAC.
PROZAC (fluoxetine capsules) for oral use
PROZAC (fluoxetine delayed-release capsules) for oral use
Initial U.S. Approval: 1987
WARNING: SUICIDAL THOUGHTS AND BEHAVIORS
See full prescribing information for complete boxed warning.
• Increased risk of suicidal thinking and behavior in children, adolescents, and young adults taking antidepressants (5.1).
• Monitor for worsening and emergence of suicidal thoughts and behaviors (5.1).
When using PROZAC and olanzapine in combination, also refer to Boxed Warning section of the package insert for Symbyax.

Consider discontinuing if symptomatic hyponatremia occurs (5.9)
- *Anxiety and Insomnia:* May occur (5.10)
- *QT Prolongation:* QT prolongation and ventricular arrhythmia including Torsades de Pointes have been reported with PROZAC use. Use with caution in conditions that predispose to arrhythmias or increased fluoxetine exposure. Use cautiously in patients with risk factors for QT prolongation (4.2, 5.11, 7.7, 7.8, 10.1)
- *Potential for Cognitive and Motor Impairment:* Has potential to impair judgment, thinking, and motor skills. Use caution when operating machinery (5.13)
- *Long Half-Life:* Changes in dose will not be fully reflected in plasma for several weeks (5.14)
- *PROZAC and Olanzapine in Combination:* When using PROZAC and olanzapine in combination, also refer to the Warnings and Precautions section of the package insert for Symbyax (5.16)

ADVERSE REACTIONS
Most common adverse reactions (≥5% and at least twice that for placebo) associated with:

Figure note: First page of package insert with black box warning at top left and enlarged in inset. See text for details.

Regulators use all these approaches, and as an outside observer, it is hard to predict how they will handle different types and quantities of safety findings from clinical trials. For example, in a Phase 3 RCT in familial chylomicronemia syndrome published in 2019, a third of patients treated with the ApoC-III antisense agent volanesorsen (Waylivra; Ionis) developed thrombocytopenia, or low blood platelet count, with two severe, grade 4 events of less than 25,000 platelets per microliter.[38] After those two events, the investigators amped up the trial's platelet monitoring program with more frequent testing and more stringent requirements for reducing or pausing dosing, after which no more declines below 50,000 platelets per microliter were observed. The European Medicines Agency (EMA) approved the drug with post-marketing requirements for a safety-focused educational program and a registry-based thrombocytopenia study.[39] However, the FDA rejected it outright.[40]

It is important to note that regulators can and do look at the totality of safety data across multiple studies when making their assessments. In a Phase 3 study of the CB1 cannabinoid receptor antagonist rimonabant for treating obesity (Acomplia; Sanofi), the fraction of trial dropouts was roughly equivalent between placebo and the 5 mg arm (7.0% and 8.4%), and higher in the 20 mg arm (15.0%).[41] But closer examination revealed that withdrawals from both experimental arms were much more likely to be attributed to "depression," "major depression," or "depressed mood": two of 24 withdrawals on placebo, compared with eight of 29 on low-dose therapy and 14 of 52 on the higher dose. Similar results were obtained in several other large Phase 3 studies.[42,43] European regulators approved the drug in 2006 but yanked it from the market two years later after meta-analyses of both published and unpublished data confirmed the increased risk of depression and suicidal ideations. The FDA never granted approval.[44] In retrospect, regulators were probably swayed by several factors, including the apparent severity of the psychiatric symptoms that led patients to withdraw from the study; the reproducibility across trials of the numerical imbalance in AEs; and the fact that the drug had been suggested to induce anxiety-like responses in preclinical testing.[45]

Another case where regulators took into account safety data across multiple studies is Janssen's IL-6 antagonist sirukumab. The drug yielded positive findings in three Phase 3 trials in rheumatoid arthritis, each of which individually showed minimal safety signals.[46] However, in 2017 an FDA advisory committee found in a pooled analysis that 34 of the 35 deaths across all three studies occurred in sirukumab-treated patients and did not recommend the drug for approval.[47]

Even when a new drug's safety profile in clinical trials is clean, regulators often incorporate safety warnings into the label based on "class effects" seen in closely related therapies.[48] For example, in 2008 the FDA updated the safety information for antimicrobial drugs in the fluoroquinolone class to move the risk of tendinitis and tendon rupture from the main text of the product insert into a black box warning.[49] Regulators made this update based on their study of events reported in the agency's MedWatch adverse event reporting system for several marketed drugs in the class. Since then, labels for all newly approved fluoroquinolones, such as delafloxacin (Baxdela; Melinta), which was approved in 2017, have had this black box warning even when they didn't exhibit any such events in clinical trials.[50]

Notably, although a 2011 study found significant differences between black box warnings among drugs in the same mechanistic class,[51] closer analysis reveals that these differences appeared only when drugs were in different chemical families that would be unlikely to share the same clinical risks. For example, lamotrigine (Lamictal; GlaxoSmithKline) and oxcarbazepine (Trileptal; Novartis) are both sodium channel blockers indicated for the treatment of partial-onset seizures. Clinical trials of lamotrigine, a member of the triazine chemical family, showed an increased incidence of severe rash[52] that the FDA incorporated into a black box warning upon approval in 1994.[53] But oxcarbazepine, which as a dibenzazepine is chemically distinct from lamotrigine, has been on the market in the U.S. since 2000 with no such warning.[54]

Specific safety issues with small molecules and biologics

For small molecules, particularly common causes of clinical failure, regulatory failure, and post-marketing withdrawal are cardiac rhythm toxicities, which typically manifest as prolongation or shortening of the QT interval on electrocardiographic measurements,[55,56] and drug-induced liver injury (DILI), which often first appears as so-called Hy's law cases with unexplained liver enzyme elevations.[57,58,59]

Companies and regulators are on high alert for evidence of adverse cardiac or hepatic effects during preclinical or clinical development of small molecule drugs, although the decision by sponsors to halt a program based on such findings is often complex. Development of the GPR40 agonist fasiglifam (TAK-875; Takeda) in type 2 diabetes was halted during Phase 3 in 2013 as a result of liver toxicity.[60] About five years later, the sponsor disclosed that the drug had been known before entering human testing to cause hepatotoxicity in dogs, but the company elected to move forward with a liver safety monitoring plan rather than kill the program before clinical trials.[61] It does not appear that there were any publicly available data before 2013 that could have enabled outside observers to predict the drug's adverse effect.

For biologic therapies, a specific pharmacologic issue that can impair both tolerability and efficacy is the formation of anti-drug antibodies (ADAs) due to an immunologic reaction against a therapeutic protein or monoclonal antibody.[62] ADAs can have highly idiosyncratic effects on the pharmacokinetics of these therapies, leading to either increased or decreased drug exposure at a given dose and also to infusion-site reactions. Like hepatotoxicity from small molecules, the true incidence and effect of ADAs may be evident only in large, late-stage trials. The PCSK9 inhibitor bococizumab (Pfizer), intended to reduce LDL levels and improve cardiovascular outcomes, produced detectable ADAs in 7% of the 354 patients in a Phase 2 study published in 2015. The authors noted that this was in line with results from other PCSK9 inhibitors and did not lead to significant infusion-site reactions.[63] But in two of the main Phase 3 studies, involving 27,438 patients, almost half of those who received bococizumab developed ADAs, which most likely contributed to the high 10% rate of treatment-related infusion-site reactions and the drug's lack of clinical efficacy.[64] From an external perspective, it is not clear what Pfizer did (or could have done) after reviewing the Phase 2 data to predict or mitigate the risk of ADAs in the pivotal study.

---

[1] Piazzi G, Mari E, Reeve R, Smith B. Oncology Phase 1 trials: A scientific and operational review. IQVIA; 2017. Available at https://www.iqvia.com/library/white-papers/oncology-phase-1-trials. Accessed October 15, 2021.

[2] Association of the British Pharmaceutical Industry. Guidelines for Phase I clinical trials, 2018 edition. 2018. Available at https://www.abpi.org.uk/publications/guidelines-for-phase-i-clinical-trials-2018-edition/. Accessed October 15, 2021. Permalink: https://perma.cc/3S3S-S7LK.

[3] Shen J, Swift B, Mamelok R, Pine S, Sinclair J, Attar M. Design and conduct considerations for first-in-human trials. Clin Transl Sci. 2019 Jan;12(1):6–19. doi: 10.1111/cts.12582. Epub 2018 Aug 24. PMID: 30048046; PMCID: PMC6342261.

[4] Le Tourneau C, Lee JJ, Siu LL. Dose escalation methods in Phase I cancer clinical trials. J Natl Cancer Inst. 2009 May 20;101(10):708–720. doi: 10.1093/jnci/djp079. Epub 2009 May 12. PMID: 19436029; PMCID: PMC2684552.

[5] Common terminology criteria for adverse events (CTCAE). U.S. National Cancer Institute. https://ctep.cancer.gov/protocoldevelopment/electronic_applications/ctc.htm. Updated September 21, 2020. Accessed October 15, 2021. Permalink: https://perma.cc/2KPE-W4Y6.

[6] What is a serious adverse event? U.S. Food and Drug Administration. https://www.fda.gov/safety/reporting-serious-problems-fda/what-serious-adverse-event. Updated February 1, 2016. Accessed October 15, 2021. Permalink: https://perma.cc/2RYZ-3M9Z.

[7] Reviewer guidance: Conducting a clinical safety review of a new product application and preparing a report on the review. U.S. Food and Drug Administration. February 2005.

[8] Smit MD, Casak SJ, Lemergy S, Keegan P, McKee AE. FDA analysis of grade 3–4 safety events. J Clin Oncol. 2017 May 20. 35(15 suppl):2544. doi: 10.1200/JCO.2017.35.15_suppl.2544.

[9] Portola Pharmaceuticals presents interim Phase 2a safety and efficacy data for cerdulatinib at International Congress of Malignant Lymphoma. Portola Pharmaceuticals press release. June 15, 2017. https://investors.portola.com/Portola-Pharmaceuticals-Presents-Interim-Phase-2a-Safety-and-Efficacy-Data-for-Cerdulatinib-at-the-International-Congress-of-Malignant-Lymphoma. Accessed October 15, 2021. Permalink: https://perma.cc/34HU-Z7X6.

[10] Rief W, Avorn J, Barsky AJ. Medication-attributed adverse effects in placebo groups: Implications for assessment of adverse effects. Arch Intern Med. 2006 Jan 23;166(2):155–160. doi: 10.1001/archinte.166.2.155. PMID: 16432082.

[11] International Conference on Harmonisation of Technical Requirements for Registration of Pharmaceuticals for Human Use. Clinical Safety Data Management: Definitions and Standards for Expedited Reporting E2A. March 1995. https://www.fda.gov/media/71188/download. Accessed October 15, 2021.

[12] Sherman RB, Woodcock J, Norden J, Grandinetti C, Temple RJ. New FDA regulation to improve safety reporting in clinical trials. N Engl J Med. 2011 Jul 7;365(1):3–5. doi: 10.1056/NEJMp1103464. Epub 2011 Jun 8. PMID: 21651388.

[13] Arif A. Ziopharma craters on report of patient death in gene therapy study. Endpoints News. July 15, 2016. https://endpts.com/ziopharm-craters-on-report-of-patient-death-in-gene-therapy-study/. Accessed October 15, 2021.

[14] Ziopharm provides update regarding Phase 1 study of gene therapy candidate Ad-RTS-hIL-12 in brain cancer. Ziopharm Oncology press release. July 19, 2016. https://ir.ziopharm.com/news-releases/news-release-details/ziopharm-provides-update-regarding-phase-i-study-gene-therapy. Accessed October 15, 2021. Permalink: https://perma.cc/T9TG-ECQJ.

[15] Mehrotra DV, Heyse JF. Use of the false discovery rate for evaluating clinical safety data. Stat Methods Med Res. 2004 Jun; 13(3):227–238. doi: 10.1191/0962280204sm363ra. PMID: 15198488.

[16] McClung MR, O'Donoghue ML, Papapoulos SE, Bone H, Langdahl B, Saag KG, Reid IR, Kiel DP, Cavallari I, Bonaca MP, Wiviott SD, de Villiers T, Ling X, Lippuner K, Nakamura T, Reginster JY, Rodriguez-Portales JA, Roux C, Zanchetta J, Zerbini CAF, Park JG, Im K, Cange A, Grip LT, Heyden N, DaSilva C, Cohn D, Massaad R, Scott BB, Verbruggen N, Gurner D, Miller DL, Blair ML, Polis AB, Stoch SA, Santora A, Lombardi A, Leung AT, Kaufman KD, Sabatine MS; LOFT Investigators. Odanacatib for the treatment of postmenopausal osteoporosis: Results of the LOFT multicentre, randomised, double-blind, placebo-controlled trial and LOFT Extension study. Lancet Diabetes Endocrinol. 2019 Dec;7(12):899–911. doi: 10.1016/S2213-8587(19)30346-8. Epub 2019 Oct 31. PMID: 31676222.

[17] Carroll J. Stroke risk forces Merck to scrap its long-neglected PhIII osteoporosis drug odanacatib. Endpoints News. September 2, 2016. https://endpts.com/merck-scraps-its-long-neglected-phiii-osteoporosis-drug-odanacatib/. Accessed October 15, 2021.

[18] Phillips R, Hazell L, Sauzet O, Cornelius V. Analysis and reporting of adverse events in randomised controlled trials: A review. BMJ Open. 2019 Mar 1;9(2):e024537. doi: 10.1136/bmjopen-2018-024537. PMID: 30826796; PMCID: PMC6398660.

[19] BLA 761130 (tanezumab): Joint meeting of Arthritis Advisory Committee and Drug Safety and Risk Management Advisory Committee. U.S. Food and Drug Administration. March 24–25, 2021. https://www.fda.gov/media/146867/download. Accessed October 15, 2021. Permalink: https://perma.cc/KTF8-DX2S.

[20] Carroll J. Safety threat forces FDA to put a hold on Regeneron, Teva's big NGF pain drug fasinumab. Endpoints News. October 17, 2016. https://endpts.com/fda-slaps-a-hold-on-regeneron-tevas-big-ngf-pain-drug-fasinumab/. Accessed October 15, 2021.

[21] Trudel S, Lendvai N, Popat R, Voorhees PM, Reeves B, Libby EN, Richardson PG, Anderson LD Jr, Sutherland HJ, Yong K, Hoos A, Gorczyca MM, Lahiri S, He Z, Austin DJ, Opalinska JB, Cohen AD. Targeting B-cell maturation antigen with GSK2857916 antibody-drug conjugate in relapsed or refractory multiple myeloma (BMA117159): A dose escalation and expansion Phase 1 trial. Lancet Oncol. 2018 Dec;19(12):1641–1653. doi: 10.1016/S1470-2045(18)30576-X. Epub 2018 Nov 12. PMID: 30442502; PMCID: PMC6328058.

[22] FDA granted accelerated approval to belantamab mafodotin-blmf for multiple myeloma. FDA press release. August 6, 2020. https://www.fda.gov/drugs/resources-information-approved-drugs/fda-granted-accelerated-approval-belantamab-mafodotin-blmf-multiple-myeloma. Accessed October 15, 2021. Permalink: https://perma.cc/5VGB-NE62.

[23] Rief W, Avorn J, Barsky AJ. Medication-attributed adverse effects in placebo groups: Implications for assessment of adverse effects. Arch Intern Med. 2006 Jan 23;166(2):155–160. doi: 10.1001/archinte.166.2.155. PMID: 16432082.

[24] Plimack ER, Lorusso PM, McCoon P, Tang W, Krebs AD, Curt G, Eckhardt SG. AZD1480: A Phase I study of a novel JAK2 inhibitor in solid tumors. Oncologist. 2013;18(7):819–820. doi: 10.1634/theoncologist.2013-0198. Epub 2013 Jul 11. PMID: 23847256; PMCID: PMC3720635.

[25] Verstovsek S, Hoffman R, Mascarenhas J, Soria JC, Bahleda R, McCoon P, Tang W, Cortes J, Kantarjian H, Ribrag V. A Phase I, open-label, multi-center study of the JAK2 inhibitor AZD1480 in patients with myelofibrosis. Leuk Res. 2015 Feb;39(2):157–163. doi: 10.1016/j.leukres.2014.11.018. Epub 2014 Nov 29. PMID: 25530567.

[26] Development pipeline as at 31 December 2012. AstraZeneca. https://www.astrazeneca.com/content/dam/az/our-company/our-company-052017/investor-relations/presentations-and-webcast/2013/Download-RampD-Pipeline-Summary.pdf. Accessed October 15, 2021. Permalink: https://perma.cc/FKU5-H2LE.

[27] Delaney S, Biffen M, Maltby J, Bell J, Asimus S, Aggarwal A, Kraan M, Keeling D. Tolerability in man following inhalation dosing of the selective TLR7 agonist, AZD8848. BMJ Open Respir Res. 2016 Feb 23;3(1):e000113. doi: 10.1136/bmjresp-2015-000113. PMID: 26933507; PMCID: PMC4769423.

[28] Leaker BR, Singh D, Lindgren S, Almqvist G, Eriksson L, Young B, O'Connor B. Effects of the Toll-like receptor 7 (TLR7) agonist, AZD8848, on allergen-induced responses in patients with mild asthma: A double-blind, randomised, parallel-group study. Respir Res. 2019 Dec 19;20(1):288. doi: 10.1186/s12931-019-1252-2. PMID: 31856838; PMCID: PMC6924002.

[29] Morgan P, Brown DG, Lennard S, Anderton MJ, Barrett JC, Eriksson U, Fidock M, Hamrén B, Johnson A, March RE, Matcham J, Mettetal J, Nicholls DJ, Platz S, Rees S, Snowden MA, Pangalos MN. Impact of a five-dimensional framework on R&D productivity at AstraZeneca. Nat Rev Drug Discov. 2018 Mar;17(3):167–181. doi: 10.1038/nrd.2017.244. Epub 2018 Jan 19. PMID: 29348681.

[30] AstraZeneca development pipeline, 30 September 2014. AstraZeneca. https://www.astrazeneca.com/content/dam/az/our-company/our-company-052017/investor-relations/presentations-and-webcast/2014/Development-pipeline-table.pdf. Accessed October 15, 2021. Permalink: https://perma.cc/GN7W-VB2Z.

[31] Gyawali B, Shimokata T, Honda K, Ando Y. Reporting harms more transparently in trials of cancer drugs. BMJ. 2018 Nov 1;363:k4383. doi: 10.1136/bmj.k4383. Erratum in: BMJ. 2018 Nov 22;363:k4930. PMID: 30385466.

[32] Feuerstein A. Merck chronic cough drug shows mixed results in late-stage clinical trials, raising questions about its future. STAT. September 8, 2020. https://www.statnews.com/2020/09/08/merck-chronic-cough-drug-shows-mixed-results-in-late-stage-clinical-trials-raising-questions-about-its-future/. Accessed October 15, 2021.

[33] Feuerstein A. Biotech stock mailbag: Ionis, trust issues and "Oops! Don't look at that slide deck." TheStreet. August 5, 2016. https://www.thestreet.com/investing/stocks/biotech-stock-mailbag-ionis-trust-issues-and-oops-don-t-look-at-that-slide-deck-13665173. Accessed October 15, 2021.

[34] Prozac [package insert]. Pfizer. January 2017. https://www.accessdata.fda.gov/drugsatfda_docs/label/2017/018936s108lbl.pdf. Accessed October 15, 2021. Permalink: https://perma.cc/4CZF-B8HJ.

[35] Postmarketing requirements and commitments: Introduction. U.S. Food and Drug Administration. https://www.fda.gov/drugs/guidance-compliance-regulatory-information/postmarket-requirements-and-commitments. Updated January 12, 2016. Accessed October 15, 2021. Permalink: https://perma.cc/B4Y8-SWQA.

[36] Approval package for Kyprolis (carfilzomib). U.S. Food and Drug Administration. July 20, 2012. https://www.accessdata.fda.gov/drugsatfda_docs/nda/2012/202714Orig1s000Approv.pdf. Permalink: https://perma.cc/NH3J-798K.

[37] Risk evaluation and mitigation strategies | REMS. U.S. Food and Drug Administration. https://www.fda.gov/drugs/drug-safety-and-availability/risk-evaluation-and-mitigation-strategies-rems. Updated August 8, 2019. Accessed October 15, 2021. Permalink: https://perma.cc/3YSK-UDV4.

[38] Witztum JL, Gaudet D, Freedman SD, Alexander VJ, Digenio A, Williams KR, Yang Q, Hughes SG, Geary RS, Arca M, Stroes ESG, Bergeron J, Soran H, Civeira F, Hemphill L, Tsimikas S, Blom DJ, O'Dea L, Bruckert E. Volanesorsen and triglyceride levels in familial chylomicronemia syndrome. N Engl J Med. 2019 Aug 8;381(6):531–542. doi: 10.1056/NEJMoa1715944. PMID: 31390500.

[39] Assessment report for Waylivra (volanesoren). European Medicines Agency. February 28, 2019. Available at https://www.ema.europa.eu/en/medicines/human/EPAR/waylivra. Accessed October 15, 2021. Permalink: https://perma.cc/4FR7-GFBU.

[40] Brown A, Gardner J. Ionis feels the pain as the U.S. FDA finally bares its teeth. Evaluate Vantage. August 28, 2018. https://www.evaluate.com/vantage/articles/news/policy-and-regulation/ionis-feels-pain-us-fda-finally-bares-its-teeth. Accessed October 15, 2021.

[41] Després JP, Golay A, Sjöström L; Rimonabant in Obesity-Lipids Study Group. Effects of rimonabant on metabolic risk factors in overweight patients with dyslipidemia. N Engl J Med. 2005 Nov 17;353(20):2121–2134. doi: 10.1056/NEJMoa044537. PMID: 16291982.

[42] Scheen AJ, Finer N, Hollander P, Jensen MD, Van Gaal LF; RIO-Diabetes Study Group. Efficacy and tolerability of rimonabant in overweight or obese patients with type 2 diabetes: A randomised controlled study. Lancet. 2006 Nov 11;368(9548):1660–72. doi: 10.1016/S0140-6736(06)69571-8. Erratum in: Lancet. 2006 Nov 11;368(9548):1650. PMID: 17098084.

[43] Van Gaal LF, Rissanen AM, Scheen AJ, Ziegler O, Rössner S; RIO-Europe Study Group. Effects of the cannabinoid-1 receptor blocker rimonabant on weight reduction and cardiovascular risk factors in overweight patients: 1-year experience from the RIO-Europe study. Lancet. 2005 Apr 16–22;365(9468):1389-97. doi: 10.1016/S0140-6736(05)66374-X. Erratum in: Lancet. 2005 Jul 30–Aug 5;366(9483):370. PMID: 15836887.

[44] Sam AH, Salem V, Ghatei MA. Rimonabant: From RIO to ban. J Obes. 2011;2011:432607. doi: 10.1155/2011/432607. Epub 2011 Jul 6. PMID: 21773005; PMCID: PMC3136184.

[45] Navarro M, Hernández E, Muñoz RM, del Arco I, Villanúa MA, Carrera MR, Rodríguez de Fonseca F. Acute administration of the CB1 cannabinoid receptor antagonist SR 141716A induces anxiety-like responses in the rat. Neuroreport. 1997 Jan 20;8(2):491–496. doi: 10.1097/00001756-199701200-00023. PMID: 9080435.

[46] Sun A, Benet LZ. Late-stage failures of monoclonal antibody drugs: A retrospective case study analysis. Pharmacology. 2020;105(3-4):145–163. doi: 10.1159/000505379. Epub 2020 Jan 7. PMID: 31910414.

[47] BLA 761057 (sirukumab; Janssen): Arthritis Advisory Committee Meeting (briefing document). U.S. Food and Drug Administration. August 2, 2017. https://www.fda.gov/media/106325/download. Accessed October 15, 2021. Permalink: https://perma.cc/U4X6-NGAV.

[48] Panagiotou OA, Contopoulos-Ioannidis DG, Papanikolaou PN, Ntzani EE, Ioannidis JP. Different black box warning labeling for same-class drugs. J Gen Intern Med. 2011 Jun;26(6):603–610. doi: 10.1007/s11606-011-1633-9. Epub 2011 Feb 1. PMID: 21286838; PMCID: PMC3101972.

[49] Information for healthcare professionals: Fluoroquinolone antimicrobial drug [ciprofloxacin (marketed as Cipro and generic ciprofloxacin), ciprofloxacin extended-release (marketed as Cipro XR and Proquin XR), gemifloxacin (marketed as Factive), levofloxacin (marketed as Levaquin), moxifloxacin (marketed as Avelox), norfloxacin (marketed as Avelox), norfloxacin (marketed as Noroxin), and ofloxacin (marketed as Floxin)]. U.S. Food and Drug Administration press release. July 8, 2006. Permalink: http://wayback.archive-it.org/7993/20170112032310/http://www.fda.gov/Drugs/DrugSafety/PostmarketDrugSafetyInformationforPatientsandProviders/ucm126085.htm.

[50] Baxdela [package insert]. Melinta Therapeutics. October 2019. https://www.accessdata.fda.gov/drugsatfda_docs/label/2019/208610s007,208611s006lbl.pdf. Accessed October 15, 2021. Permalink: https://perma.cc/PYC5-97GK.

[51] Panagiotou OA, Contopoulos-Ioannidis DG, Papanikolaou PN, Ntzani EE, Ioannidis JP. Different black box warning labeling for same-class drugs. J Gen Intern Med. 2011 Jun;26(6):603–610. doi: 10.1007/s11606-011-1633-9. Epub 2011 Feb 1. PMID: 21286838; PMCID: PMC3101972.

[52] Betts T, Goodwin G, Withers RM, Yuen AW. Human safety of lamotrigine. Epilepsia. 1991;32(suppl 2):S17–21. doi: 10.1111/j.1528-1157.1991.tb05881.x. PMID: 1837776.

[53] Lamictal [package insert]. GlaxoSmithKline. March 2015. https://www.accessdata.fda.gov/drugsatfda_docs/label/2015/020241s045s051lbl.pdf. Accessed October 15, 2021. Permalink: https://perma.cc/JZP3-NVU5.

[54] Trileptal [package insert]. Novartis. June 2014. https://www.accessdata.fda.gov/drugsatfda_docs/label/2014/021014s033,021285s027lbl.pdf. Accessed October 15, 2021. Permalink: https://perma.cc/644K-9ZX9.

[55] Lester RM, Paglialunga S, Johnson IA. QT assessment in early drug development: The long and the short of it. Int J Mol Sci. 2019 Mar 15;20(6):1324. doi: 10.3390/ijms20061324. PMID: 30884748; PMCID: PMC6471571.

[56] Guidance for industry: E14 clinical evaluation of QT/QTc interval prolongation and proarrhythmic potential for non-antiarrhythmic drugs. U.S. Food and Drug Administration. October 2005.

[57] Kaplowitz N. Idiosyncratic drug hepatotoxicity. Nat Rev Drug Discov. 2005 Jun;4(6):489–499. doi: 10.1038/nrd1750. PMID: 15931258.

[58] Navarro VJ, Senior JR. Drug-related hepatotoxicity. N Engl J Med. 2006 Feb 16;354(7):731–739. doi: 10.1056/NEJMra052270. PMID: 16481640.

[59] Guidance for industry: Drug-induced liver injury: Premarketing clinical evaluation. U.S. Food and Drug Administration. July 2009.

[60] Takeda announces termination of fasiglifam (TAK-875) development. Takeda press release. December 25, 2013. https://www.takeda.com/en-us/newsroom/news-releases/2013/takeda-announces-termination-of-fasiglifam-tak-875-development/. Accessed October 15, 2021. Permalink: https://perma.cc/JH5U-YZ5Y.

[61] Marcinak JF, Munsaka MS, Watkins PB, Ohira T, Smith N. Liver safety of fasiglifam (TAK-875) in patients with type 2 diabetes: Review of the global clinical trial experience. Drug Saf. 2018 Jun;41(6):625–640. doi: 10.1007/s40264-018-0642-6. Erratum in: Drug Saf. 2018 Dec;41(12):1431-1437. PMID: 29492878.

[62] Sailstad JM, Amaravadi L, Clements-Egan A, Gorovits B, Myler HA, Pillutla RC, Pursuhothama S, Putman M, Rose MK, Sonehara K, Tang L, Wustner JT; Global Bioanalysis Consortium. A white paper—consensus and recommendations of a global harmonization team on assessing the impact of immunogenicity on pharmacokinetic measurements. AAPS J. 2014 May;16(3):488–498. doi: 10.1208/s12248-014-9582-y. Epub 2014 Mar 29. PMID: 24682765; PMCID: PMC4012055.

[63] Ballantyne CM, Neutel J, Cropp A, Duggan W, Wang EQ, Plowchalk D, Sweeney K, Kaila N, Vincent J, Bays H. Results of bococizumab, a monoclonal antibody against proprotein convertase subtilisin/kexin type 9, from a randomized, placebo-controlled, dose-ranging study in statin-treated subjects with hypercholesterolemia. Am J Cardiol. 2015 May 1;115(9):1212–1221. doi: 10.1016/j.amjcard.2015.02.006. Epub 2015 Feb 12. PMID: 25784512.

[64] Ridker PM, Revkin J, Amarenco P, Brunell R, Curto M, Civeira F, Flather M, Glynn RJ, Gregoire J, Jukema JW, Karpov Y, Kastelein JJP, Koenig W, Lorenzatti A, Manga P, Masiukiewicz U, Miller M, Mosterd A, Murin J, Nicolau JC, Nissen S, Ponikowski P, Santos RD, Schwartz PF, Soran H, White H, Wright RS, Vrablik M, Yunis C, Shear CL, Tardif JC; SPIRE Cardiovascular Outcome Investigators. Cardiovascular efficacy and safety of bococizumab in high-risk patients. N Engl J Med. 2017 Apr 20;376(16):1527–1539. doi: 10.1056/NEJMoa1701488. Epub 2017 Mar 17. PMID: 28304242.

PART 2:

SPECIAL TOPICS

10.

FIGURES

FIGURES ARE OFTEN A KEY ELEMENT of presentations at scientific meetings and investor updates. In these settings, figures may provide a crucial first look at results before more details about methods and findings are disclosed in full journal articles.

In this chapter, we review several types of figures that commonly appear in reports of clinical trials, including some particular nuances and red flags that are important to note. We exclude from this chapter time-to-event studies, Kaplan-Meier curves, and event curves, which are more complicated and are the topics of Chapter 11.

Plots comparing a single parameter between groups

One of the simplest and most common types of figures in reports of clinical trial data is a direct comparison of a single parameter between two or more groups, at least one being the control and at least one drug-treated. They can take several forms, including bar, box, and dot plots; the examples in Figures 10-1a and 10-1b are adapted from a clinical study of reproxalap AC (Aldeyra) for seasonal allergy reported in 2018[1] and a trial of Moderna's COVID-19 mRNA vaccine that was reported in 2020,[2] respectively.

The Pharmagellan Guide to Analyzing Biotech Clinical Trials, by Frank S. David.

FIGURE 10-1a: Example of a single-parameter (bar) plot.

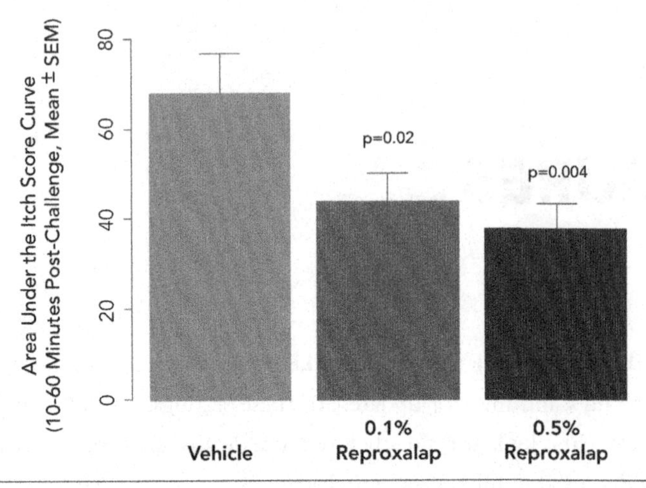

Figure note: Adapted from the original; see text for source information.

FIGURE 10-1b: Example of a single-parameter (box) plot.

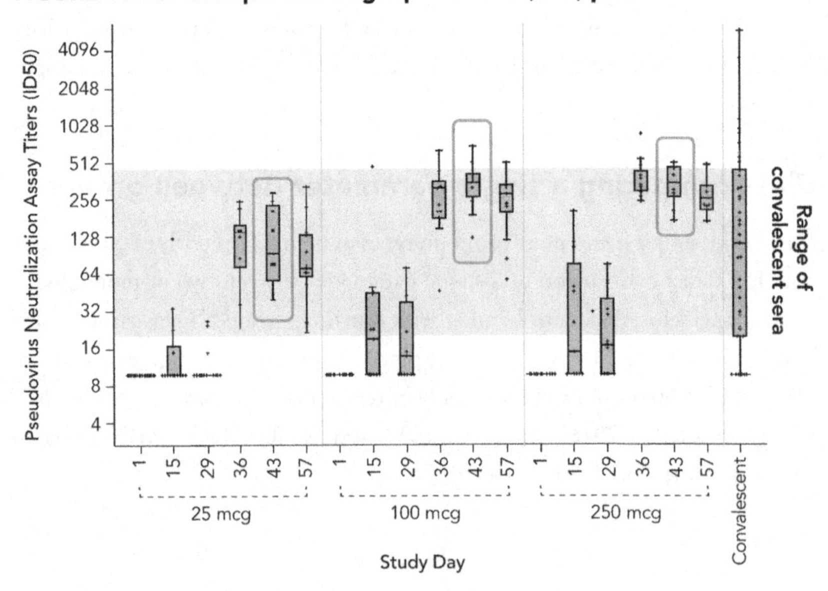

Figure note: Adapted from the original; see text for source information.

In these single-parameter graphs, the y-axis reflects the variable of interest, and each group is in its own column along the x-axis. They display some of the following types of information:

- **Mean or median:** The summary value is indicated by the height of the bar or a horizontal hash mark. The title or y-axis label usually indicates whether the measurement is a mean or a median.
- **Numerical data:** The number of subjects per group is typically indicated under or over each column, and *P* values are often given for various pairwise comparisons. When a study makes multiple statistical comparisons, it is important to verify in the figure or accompanying text/methods whether adjustments were made for multiple hypothesis testing.
- **Distribution of data:** Many graphs also include boxes or T-shaped "plungers" that indicate some aspect of the distribution (standard error of the mean [SEM], 95% confidence interval [CI], interquartile range [IQR], etc.). The legend or methods section should but does not always indicate which metric is shown. Box plots typically present the median value as a horizontal hash mark, the IQR within the box, and the minimum and maximum values as the ends of the "whiskers." Extreme outliers, typically defined as values greater than the third quartile plus 1.5 times the interquartile range, or less than the first quartile minus 1.5 times the interquartile range, are sometimes but not always shown as dots past the ends of the whiskers. Even when outliers are not shown in a bar-and-whiskers plot, however, they are included in statistical analyses.

These figures also often provide *P* values to indicate the statistical significance of specific comparisons. Importantly, the degree to which the boxes or plungers around data points overlap with one another does not necessarily indicate whether the differences are statistically significant. Specifically, nonoverlapping 95% CIs do indeed correspond to statistical significance, but in contrast, 95% CIs can overlap somewhat even when the *P* value of the comparison is less than .05. This topic is discussed in more detail in Chapter 12 on *P* values.

Plots of repeated measures over time

Plots of repeated measures over time show how a continuous outcome changes at various time points after patients initiate treatment. In drug trials, they typically compare patients receiving a placebo or control with those taking one or more experimental treatments, or different doses of the same therapy.

A typical example is shown in Figure 10-2, adapted from a graph in a study reported in 2021 of an anti-beta-amyloid monoclonal antibody, donanemab (Eli Lilly), for Alzheimer's disease.[3] The x-axis is time, with the zero point indicating a baseline pre-treatment measurement. The y-axis can be an absolute measurement of a parameter or, as shown here, the change from baseline, starting from zero and expressed as either a numerical value as in this case or a percentage. Each arm of the study is represented by a set of points—means or medians—connected by line segments. This plot also shows error bars (standard error in this case, although they could also be SEM or 95% CI) for each point and select *P* values for comparisons across the two arms, although as discussed shortly, these aspects are extremely problematic.

FIGURE 10-2: Example of a plot of repeated measures over time.

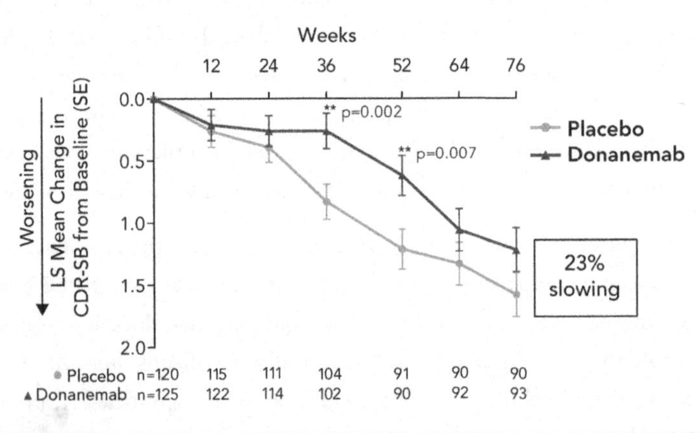

Figure note: Adapted from the original; see text for source information. CDR-SB, clinical dementia rating scale.

The sample figure illustrates several red flags and challenges with analyzing repeated measure plots that are extremely common. The investigators reported the statistical significance of the difference between the two arms at each time point and highlighted the ones that were "significant." However, this type of analysis is conceptually flawed. Because successive observations for individual patients are likely to be highly correlated, this approach raises the odds of spuriously detecting a false positive result unless appropriate analytic methods are used.[4,5] Furthermore, the *P* values presented in these sorts of analyses are almost never corrected for multiplicity, further increasing the chance that one will see a spuriously significant result, particularly as the number of measurements increases. Most concerningly in the example is that the only statistically significant comparisons were at a handful of intermediate time points, even though the overall trend would suggest that the difference should either grow or remain consistent over time. This raises further concerns that any nominally "positive" findings are a red herring absent any plausible biological explanation to the contrary.

In practice, the most appropriate way to evaluate plots of repeated measures is to perform and report the results from a single statistical test that compares the two arms on a single summary parameter. The most common pattern for a plot of repeated measures in clinical trials, illustrated in the figure, is when a clinical outcome grows or declines steadily over time, with the last value reflecting the maximum or minimum value. This is most often and appropriately analyzed by evaluating the final (maximum or minimum) value or the difference between the starting and ending measurements, although in theory one could assess the slope or the amount of time to reach a particular value. A less common situation is a "peak and decay" pattern that might arise in response to a single dose of therapy and could be quantified via the overall mean value, area under the curve, or maximum or minimum value across the entire time period. Before diving into the quantitative details of a repeat measure plot, it is always worth considering what sort of pattern one would expect and what single parameter might best express its behavior, based on known aspects of the biology being studied.

Additional details about appropriate methods for analyzing responses over time are discussed in Chapter 14 on statistical tests.

Forest plots

Forest plots are most commonly seen in meta-analyses to compare results across multiple studies. In reports of individual clinical trials, they are used to display estimates of treatment effects across different subgroups of patients. Figure 10-3 shows a post hoc analysis of a failed Phase 2 trial of a troponin activator, reldesemtiv (CK-601; Cytokinetics) in amyotrophic lateral sclerosis[6]:

FIGURE 10-3: Example of a forest plot.

Percent Predicted SVC

	No. of Patients (*pbo/reldesemtiv*)	LSM Difference (95% CI)	Estimate	*P* value
Percent predicted SVC at baseline				
<80	38/102		1.037	0.5935
≥80	52/187		2.135	0.0834
ALSFRS-R total score at baseline				
<Median (38.0)	43/118		2.886	0.1.41
≥Median (38.0)	47/171		0.451	0.7146
ALSAQ-5 total score at baseline				
<150	49/159		0.568	0.6689
≥150	41/130		3.489	0.0287
Anatomic site of disease onset				
Limb	73/234		2.309	0.0448
Bulbar	17/55		-0.027	0.9923
Time since ALS symptom onset				
<2 Years	50/188		0.530	0.7211
≥2 Years	40/101		3.640	0.0094
Time since ALS diagnosis				
<1 Year	65/210		0.819	0.5263
≥1 Year	25/79		4.237	0.0172
<6 Months	39/130		1.230	0.4538
≥6 Months	51/159		2.285	0.1024
Pre-study rate of disease progression				
(ALSFRS-R total score reduction per month)				
1st tertile ≤(0.3667)	29/107		0.663	0.6361
2nd tertile >(0.3667)=(0.6673)	35/94		2.960	0.0976
3rd tertile ≤(0.6673)	26/88		1.620	0.4597

-15 -10 -5 0 5 10 15

Favors Placebo ← → Favors Treatment

Figure note: Adapted from the original; see text for source information. SVC, slow vital capacity. LSM, least squares mean.

In biotech clinical trial reports, forest plots are typically displayed in one of two scenarios:

- **Positive overall study (significant treatment effect in the entire population):** Here, the forest plot shows whether the effect is accentuated or eliminated in particular subgroups.
- **Negative overall study (no significant treatment effect in the entire population):** In this case, as in the example above, the forest plot is intended to show whether a particular subgroup exhibited a positive or more promising response, notwithstanding the overall negative result.

In both situations, the forest plots share common characteristics. The x-axis is a relative measure of treatment effect—relative risk, odds ratio, or hazard ratio. Typically, 1.0 for no effect is at the midpoint, and the two sides of the forest plot indicate superiority of the experimental therapy or the control. Each row corresponds to a subset of the population, and a "dot and whiskers" plot indicates the estimated relative effect for that subgroup with its 95% CI. In particularly large studies, the area of the dot may be proportional to the number of patients in the subgroup.

A vertical line in a forest plot usually indicates the 1.0 level, signifying equivalent response across the two arms, and labels indicate which side of the line shows responses favoring the experimental drug versus the control. In an overall positive study, a second vertical line typically shows the overall treatment effect for the entire population. The whiskers (95% CI) of each subgroup indicate whether it is meaningfully different from the equivalence level of 1.0 or the result in the bulk population.

Interpreting forest plots requires an understanding of subgroup analyses and relative measures of treatment effects, which are covered in Chapter 7 on analysis and Chapter 14 on statistical tests, respectively. In terms of the figure, several features are worth noting:

- **X-axis scale:** Depending on the context, the x-axis may be in linear or log scale. Either is acceptable, but it is important to carefully examine the figure before jumping to conclusions based on visual appearance.
- **Subgroup sizes and confidence intervals:** CIs will necessarily become wider as subgroups become smaller. Thus, results in a forest plot from the largest subgroups should generally be considered with more confidence. Most forest plots will provide the absolute number of patients and events for each subgroup as well as the numerical values for the relative effect and 95% CI.
- **"Positive" subgroup results in negative trials:** As discussed in a separate section, false positives are common in subgroup analyses due to multiple hypothesis testing, and it is extremely unusual for the appropriate corrections to be incorporated into these sorts of fishing expeditions unless the subgroup analysis was limited to a small number of predefined subsets with obvious clinical importance. Key information is usually found in the methods, not in the forest plot itself.
- **"Negative" subgroup results in positive trials:** When an overall trial result is positive, the goal of the forest plot is to visually assess whether this effect appears in only some patient subgroups. If the 95% CIs for

the subgroup and the entire population overlap, this indicates that the effect in the subgroup is concordant with that in the bulk population—irrespective of whether the subgroup's 95% CI crosses 1.0.[7]

Plots of single patient responses

Several types of figures are used to display the responses of individual patients. Because of their visual density, they are most compatible with small studies of roughly 40 patients or fewer. Although they can be used in various clinical settings, they are particularly common in early-stage, single-arm trials, especially in oncology. They are largely descriptive and rarely raise any significant methodologic red flags.

Spider/spaghetti plots

These figures illustrate the responses of individual patients over time. The x-axis is time on study for each patient, and the y-axis is a relative value or change from baseline for a variable of interest. Each patient is plotted as a set of points connected by line segments, starting at a value of zero at the point when the baseline measurement was taken, typically to the left of zero on the x-axis. Figure 10-4 is adapted from a 2018 presentation of responses to CX-072 (CytomX), an anti-PD-L1 antibody-based therapy, in the Phase 1 Proclaim study of patients with multiple tumor types who received different doses of the experimental drug[8]:

FIGURE 10-4: Example of a spider plot.

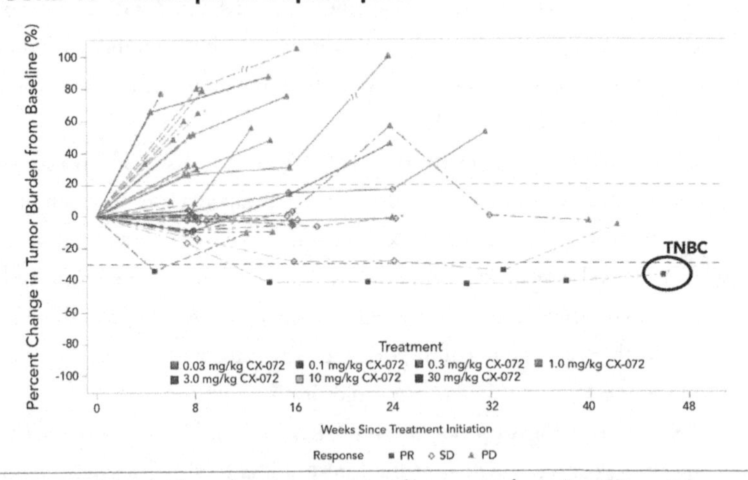

Figure note: Adapted from the original; see text for source information. PR, partial response. SD, stable disease. PD, progressive disease. TNBC, triple-negative breast cancer.

The figure is typical for cancer studies in that the y-axis measures "tumor burden" as the change from baseline in the sum of diameters of the target lesions (SLD), and y-axis thresholds of –30% and +20% are indicated with horizontal lines. These levels are significant in oncology because they distinguish between partial response, stable disease, and progressive disease according to RECIST criteria.[9] In the figure, the investigators highlighted a patient with triple-negative breast cancer (TNBC) who achieved a sustained partial response to therapy.

Outside of oncology, one challenge of spider plots is that it may be difficult to interpret the clinical significance of various relative levels of change in the y-axis measurement. For example, a study of the PD-L1 inhibitor avelumab (Bavencio; Pfizer) in patients with recurrent respiratory papillomatosis[10] showed a spider plot measuring the change in patients' Derkay score, an anatomic rating system specific to this indication.[11] Although all patients exhibited a relative decrease after initiating therapy, more diligence would be required to determine the level of improvement that is clinically significant in this setting.

In addition to providing information about each patient's final measured response, spider plots also show how quickly individual patients manifested responses to therapy and the durability of their responses. For this reason, they have become common in immuno-oncology in particular, where although only a minority of patients may respond to a therapy, their responses may be long-lived.[12]

Despite their widespread use, spider plots are extremely challenging to interpret as they selectively draw the viewer's attention toward longer-duration patients. Because patients all start at x=0 when they enter the study but continue for different lengths of time, spider plots can look like "hairballs" from which a small number of lines emerge. In the figure above, note the density of lines before 16 weeks compared with the sparseness after week 32. This makes it likely that one will pay outsized attention to results from those patients who were in the study the longest, even though they may not be representative of the larger group. This phenomenon is even more problematic when the number of patients expands, further increasing the density of the "hairball" at early time points. For this reason, spider plots are best evaluated in conjunction with other tables and figures to obtain a full picture of patients' responses to therapy over time.

Waterfall plots

Such figures display how individual patients' "best responses" are distributed in the study population. Each patient is represented as a bar along the x-axis, typically organized from least to greatest response from left to right. The y-axis reflects each individual patient's response compared with his or her baseline. Thus, a value of 0% indicates that the patient experienced no change over the study period. Figure 10-5 is adapted from a 2018 press release of Phase 1b data of a combination of the anti-galectin-3 agent GR-MD-02 (Galectin Therapeutics) and pembrolizumab (Keytruda; Merck) in metastatic melanoma[13]:

FIGURE 10-5: Example of a waterfall plot.

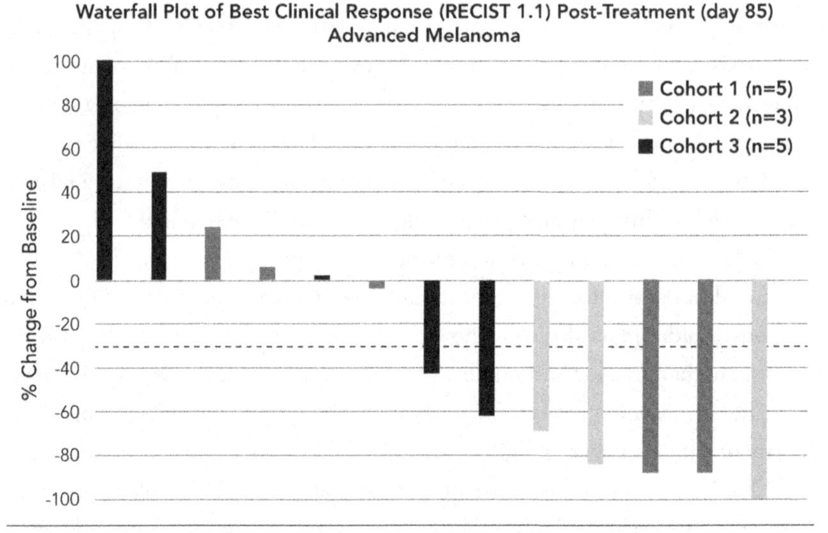

Figure note: Adapted from the original; see text for source information.

Compared with spider plots, waterfall plots can make it easier to see how various patient subgroups responded differently to therapy, especially if the plot uses different colors to reflect different dose levels. In the example above, the press release indicated that patients in cohort 1 received the lowest dose of therapy and those in cohort 3 got the highest dose, so the lack of a clear dose-response relationship is obvious. A weakness of waterfall plots versus spider plots is that because they show the best response for each patient, they provide no information about the speed of achieving that response or whether it is durable for a long period.

Swimmer plots

Like spider plots, swimmer plots are mainly used in oncology to describe how individual patients' responses evolve over time. Each "swim lane" is a horizontal bar representing an individual patient with time on the x-axis. Typically, different symbols are used to denote the points at which a patient's response to therapy began, ended, or transitioned among complete response, partial response, and progression. Compared with spider plots, these figures make it easier to assess the responses of patients who were treated for shorter durations. They also clearly note which patients are still enrolled in the study, typically with arrowheads. Figure 10-6 shows interim data as of early 2017 on responses to trilaciclib (Cosela; G1 Therapeutics), a CDK4/6 inhibitor, in a Phase 1b study in small cell lung cancer[14]:

FIGURE 10-6: Example of a swimmer plot.

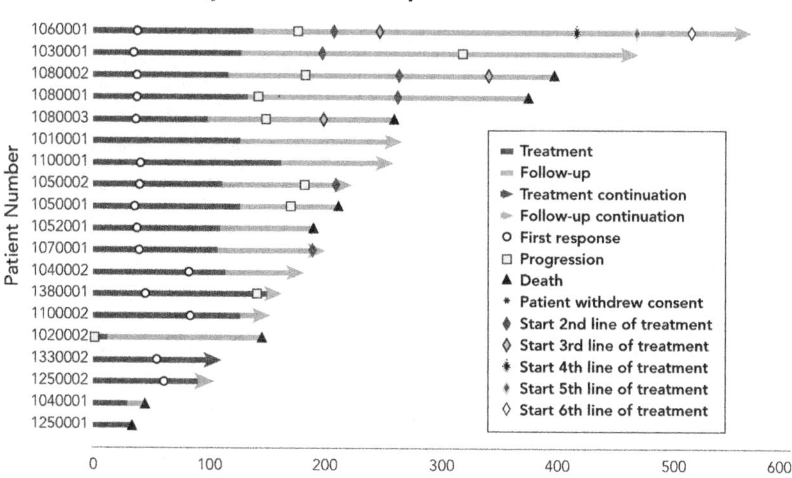

Figure note: Adapted from the original; see text for source information.

---

[1] Aldeyra Therapeutics (ALDX). Form 10-K for fiscal year ended December 31, 2018. https://www.sec.gov/Archives/edgar/data/1341235/000156459019006997/aldx-10k_20181231.htm.

[2] Miller JM. mRNA-1273 Clinical Development Program; Presentation at Centers for Disease Control and Prevention's Advisory Committee on Immunization Practices (ACIP) Meeting. August 26, 2020. https://investors.modernatx.com/static-files/34f97bb2-d89a-45e4-a770-cae0591fa807. Accessed October 15, 2021. Permalink: https://perma.cc/G8D6-S978.

[3] Eli Lilly. Donanemab update (investor presentation). March 15, 2021. https://investor.lilly.com/static-files/8238c02c-6a84-4c8d-be02-bd12218e9d6b. Accessed October 15, 2021. Permalink: https://perma.cc/EC8C-7KQL.

[4] Schober P, Vetter TR. Repeated measures designs and analysis of longitudinal data: If at first you do not succeed—try, try again. Anesth Analg. 2018 Aug;127(2):569–575. doi: 10.1213/ANE.0000000000003511. PMID: 29905618; PMCID: PMC6072386.

[5] Matthews JN, Altman DG, Campbell MJ, Royston P. Analysis of serial measurements in medical research. BMJ. 1990 Jan 27;300(6719):230–235. doi: 10.1136/bmj.300.6719.230. PMID: 2106931; PMCID: PMC1662068.

[6] Cytokinetics. Corporate presentation. September 20, 2021. https://ir.cytokinetics.com/static-files/d97eea18-cd38-49c1-9fa7-b32ac3940e76. Accessed October 15, 2021. Permalink: https://perma.cc/L9U4-DYVV.

[7] Cuzick J. Forest plots and the interpretation of subgroups. Lancet. 2005 Apr 9–15;365(9467):1308. doi: 10.1016/S0140-6736(05)61026-4. PMID: 15823379.

[8] CytomX Therapeutics. Proclaim CX-072: ESMO 2018 clinical presentations (investor presentation). October 22, 2018. Available at https://www.sec.gov/Archives/edgar/data/0001501989/000156459018024564/0001564590-18-024564-index.html. Accessed October 15, 2021.

[9] RECIST Working Group (home page). https://recist.eortc.org/. Accessed October 15, 2021. Permalink: https://perma.cc/ZMD8-4RX5.

[10] Allen CT, Lee S, Norberg SM, Kovalovsky D, Ye H, Clavijo PE, Hu-Lieskovan S, Schlegel R, Schlom J, Strauss J, Gulley JL, Trepel J, Hinrichs CS. Safety and clinical activity of PD-L1 blockade in patients with aggressive recurrent respiratory papillomatosis. J Immunother Cancer. 2019 May 3;7(1):119. doi: 10.1186/s40425-019-0603-3. PMID: 31053174; PMCID: PMC6500000.

[11] Hester RP, Derkay CS, Burke BL, Lawson ML. Reliability of a staging assessment system for recurrent respiratory papillomatosis. Int J Pediatr Otorhinolaryngol. 2003 May;67(5):505–509. doi: 10.1016/s0165-5876(03)00007-7. PMID: 12697352.

[12] Tsimberidou AM, Levit LA, Schilsky RL, Averbuch SD, Chen D, Kirkwood JM, McShane LM, Sharon E, Mileham KF, Postow MA. Trial Reporting in Immuno-Oncology (TRIO): An American society of clinical oncology-society for immunotherapy of cancer statement. J Immunother Cancer. 2018 Oct 19;6(1):108. doi: 10.1186/s40425-018-0426-7. PMID: 30340549; PMCID: PMC6195705.

[13] Galectin Therapeutics, Inc. announces positive preliminary results from Phase 1b clinical trial of GR-MD-02 and Keytruda in advanced melanoma and expansion of the trial. Galectin Therapeutics press release. September 20, 2018. https://investor.galectintherapeutics.com/news-releases/news-release-details/galectin-therapeutics-inc-announces-positive-preliminary-results. Accessed October 15, 2021. Permalink: https://perma.cc/GTW6-DK9P.

[14] G1 Therapeutics (GTHX). Form S-1. February 7, 2017. https://www.sec.gov/Archives/edgar/data/1560241/000095012317001279/filename1.htm. Accessed October 15, 2021.

11.

TIME-TO-EVENT STUDIES, KAPLAN-MEIER CURVES, AND EVENT CURVES

TIME-TO-EVENT (TTE) STUDIES are among the most prevalent yet most poorly understood analyses in modern drug development. They give rise to the classic "staircase" Kaplan-Meier curves and event curves that are a staple of conferences and investor presentations, particularly in oncology and cardiology. Understanding them is critical for professionals who work in and around drug development. But interpreting these curves is complicated. Unlike most biopharma analyses, which are based solely on observed data, TTE analyses also incorporate an approximation of what *would* have happened to patients who did not experience an event during the trial.

In this chapter, we first explain the methods of TTE studies, which are critical to understand in order to interpret the resultant figures, as well as several red flags in studies that use these analyses. We then discuss how to visually assess key aspects of Kaplan-Meier curves and event curves.

Basic principles of time-to-event analyses

TTE studies estimate the fraction of patients that will experience an event as a function of time in situations where at the end of the observation period many patients still have not experienced events. For example, in a cancer study with

---

survival as an endpoint, some patients are typically still alive at the end of the trial. And even in multi-year cardiovascular trials that measure death from heart attack or stroke, only a small fraction of patients will have had such events by the time the study ends.

If patients don't experience an event during an observation period, we can't know exactly what they might experience in the future. All we know is the amount of time during which they did *not* have events. In a TTE study, these patients are "censored" and excluded from both the numerator and the denominator of the analysis going forward. Thus, the resultant curves and statistics do not solely reflect actual events. Instead, TTE studies use observed data to approximate the cumulative incidence over time for the entire study population, including patients who did not experience events during the trial. More details on how raw data are handled in TTE analyses using simplified examples are provided elsewhere.[1,2,3,4]

There are several reasons why censoring might occur. If the patient was still event-free at the end of the study, she or he will be **administratively censored**. If a cancer trial has a minimum 24-month follow-up period but takes 18 months to fully enroll, then patients' actual on-study durations will range from 24 to 42 months. At the end of the study, the last patients enrolled will be administratively censored at or shortly after the 24-month time point if they are still in the trial and haven't had events by that time. Patients can also be censored prematurely if they have **competing events** that preclude ever experiencing the endpoint of interest. For example, death from a non-cardiac cause is a competing event in a trial that measures cardiac-specific deaths because a patient who dies from cancer cannot subsequently die from a heart attack or a stroke. Finally, patients may be censored without experiencing events if they **withdraw** from the study or are **lost to follow-up**.

For trials of new therapies, an important assumption underlying TTE analyses is that of **uninformative censoring**. This means that at any time, patients who are censored without having had an event must have the same odds of experiencing a future event as those who continue to be followed in the study. Returning to the oncology example, a TTE analysis would assume that all patients who made it to 24 months had the same future probability of experiencing an event, regardless of how much longer they actually remained in the study.

A second key assumption in TTE studies is that **proportional hazards** are maintained. This means the relative risk between the arms of the trial must remain constant over time. But several clinical trial scenarios may violate this assumption. For example, in a study comparing surgical stent placement versus medical management for cardiovascular disease, patients in the surgery arm may have a slightly greater risk of dying early than those in the medical arm due to intraoperative and postoperative complications, but the risks may flip in favor of the surgical arm after the acute post-surgical period. Similarly, immune checkpoint inhibitors tend to have a delayed effect on tumors compared with chemotherapy or tyrosine kinase inhibitors, so in a head-to-head study, the risk of death or progression in the arm receiving the checkpoint inhibitors may be higher at early time points, before the immune therapy has kicked in, but the profiles may be reversed later. This can lead the curves in a Kaplan-Meier figure to cross, as discussed later in this chapter. Another example is if prolonged exposure to an anti-cancer therapy leads to the emergence of resistance, so patients alive at later time points are at higher risk than they were at the outset of the trial. Finally, in long TTE studies the case mix or clinical care standard could evolve over the course of the trial and change the risk profile for patients who enrolled earlier versus later.

Quantitative outputs from time-to-event studies

The main statistical output that sponsors typically report for TTE studies is the **hazard ratio (HR)**, which measures the ratio of the risk of experiencing events in the experimental arm to that in the control arm.[5,6] Each component of the ratio is referred to as that arm's hazard rate. Although the hazard rate in each arm changes over the course of the trial, the ratio between them (the HR) remains constant under the assumption of proportional hazards. An HR of 1 indicates the two therapies are equivalent, and values below 1 favor the experimental therapy. In addition to the HR, TTE studies typically also report the *P* value or 95% confidence interval (CI) as a measure of statistical significance.

Consider a hypothetical randomized controlled trial of a drug intended to prevent heart attacks and strokes. An HR of 0.75 would mean that the risk of cardiovascular events in patients on the study drug was 75% of the risk for those on placebo. One can also re-express the HR as a relative improvement in duration; the HR of 0.75 means that patients treated with the experimental therapy experienced on average a 33% increase (because 1 ÷ 0.75 = 1.33) in the amount of time before they experienced a cardiovascular event compared with the control arm. These approaches are similar to how one would interpret relative risk values, which are discussed in Chapter 14 on statistical tests.

Because the HR reflects a relative improvement due to the drug, it needs to be assessed in the context of the absolute event rates in the two arms. In our cardiovascular example, the HR of 0.75 is equivalent to a 25% reduction in relative risk at any point in time. Time-to-event studies also often present the amount of absolute risk reduction (ARR) between the two arms. If this study showed an ARR of 5% between the two arms, for example, it would mean that the absolute difference in risk between the two arms, 5%, was equivalent to the 25% relative reduction from the value in the control arm. This would correspond to an absolute risk of 20% for patients in the control group versus 15% for those treated with the drug.

As with all discussions of risk, a full interpretation of the results from a TTE study requires looking at not just the HR but also the absolute risk reduction and other parameters that are relevant to patient care. In cancer studies, most readers look toward the median overall survival (OS) as a more appropriate measure of clinical benefit than the HR. This is particularly relevant in rapidly progressing cancers, where a sizable HR could be associated with a minimal absolute increase in life span.

Finally, note that some studies report both an "unadjusted" HR and an "adjusted" one. The adjusted rate is typically more relevant to readers as it reflects the output from a multivariate analysis that controls for differences in important prognostic factors between patients in the two arms.

Red flags in the design and execution of time-to-event analyses

Several potential scenarios in TTE analyses should be noted because they may require the use of specialized methods or cause one to reconsider the strength of the results. The most common issues that arise in drug trials are:

- **Informative censoring:** As noted above, a key assumption underlying TTE analyses is that all censoring is uninformative. If this assumption does not completely hold, it could partially or completely invalidate the analysis.

  One common cause of potentially informative censoring arises due to competing events in studies that assess an endpoint other than all-cause mortality. For example, many cardiovascular studies use cardiac-specific death or morbidity as a primary endpoint and censor patients who die from other causes such as cancer. However, patients with advanced malignancies are often prone to blood clots and thus may be at greater risk of cardiovascular death than patients without cancer. That means that a conventional TTE analysis would underestimate the future risk of cardiac death for a patient who died of breast cancer because the fact that her *specific* cause of non-cardiac death was cancer told us that her risk of a future event was different from her risk if she died at the same time of another cause, like uncontrolled asthma or a car accident. Special analytic methods may be required in this situation.[7]
- **Non-competing but related events:** In some cases, patients may experience events that don't directly compete with the event of interest but still affect the future probability of experiencing it. For example, in a cancer prevention trial with the primary endpoint of ovarian cancer incidence, a patient diagnosed with breast cancer during the study might have her ovaries removed prophylactically, which would significantly reduce her subsequent risk of developing ovarian cancer and distort the results.
- **Imprecise time assignment:** If an endpoint requires a physician visit, like progression-free survival in cancer, it is impossible to pinpoint the timing more accurately than to say it occurred between one visit and the next. This can be particularly challenging if the visits occur at irregular intervals.
- **Violations of proportional hazards:** As noted earlier, standard TTE analyses assume that the relative event-free probability for all patients in each arm must be constant over time. If this is not the case, however, standard methods for analyzing TTE may not be appropriate. Alternative

analytical approaches beyond our scope, like the Max-Combo test, can be employed in some of these scenarios.[8]

- **Recurrent events:** Some TTE studies measure endpoints that could occur repeatedly, such as hospitalizations, disease exacerbations, or other non-fatal events.[9,10] These trials are extremely complicated to analyze and require specialized statistical tools that are beyond our scope to address.

For most readers of TTE study reports, the only feasible course of action is to identify the potential for these problems to arise, get additional details from investigators or sponsors when possible, and keep them in mind when evaluating the strength of the findings. These red flags are rarely explicitly addressed in reports of biopharma clinical trial results, even in full journal articles and especially in press releases and investor presentations. In addition, it is impossible for a reader to vet most of these issues in detail without access to the primary data. And finally, although TTE studies with these issues can still be conducted if the correct methods are employed, the choice and application of the proper statistical methods are extremely complex and almost impossible to vet even when fully described without access to the underlying patient-level data.

Main features of Kaplan-Meier curves and event curves

TTE analysis plots can take two forms, depending on whether one displays the probability of experiencing or avoiding the event in question. Both types of curves use the same underlying analytic methods:

- **Event curve:** In preventive care indications, therapies are typically intended to reduce the incidence of relatively rare negative events, like death or stroke. The y-axis measures *occurrence* of the event, starting at 0% at the beginning of the study. As time advances along the x-axis, the staircases for the control and experimental therapies rise as patients experience events. An effective drug will yield a less steep (more horizontal) staircase than the control, indicating that at any given time, fewer patients experienced events.

- **Kaplan-Meier (KM) curve:** In oncology, the outcome of interest is *avoidance* of a bad event such as death or tumor progression. So in this format, both curves start at 100% on the y-axis because at the outset of the study all patients are alive, or no one has progressed. The two staircases descend over the course of the study. An effective drug will have a smaller rate of decline than the control because fewer patients die or progress at any given time.

Examples of each plot are shown below. Figure 11-1a is adapted from an event curve of results published in 2018 from the REDUCE-IT study of icosapent ethyl (Vascepa; Amarin) to reduce the incidence of cardiovascular events in high-risk patients.[11] Figure 11-b is adapted from a Kaplan-Meier curve presented in 2017 of a Phase 2b study of L-asparaginase encapsulated within erythrocytes (eryaspase; Erytech) in second-line pancreatic cancer.[12]

FIGURE 11-1a: Example of an event curve.

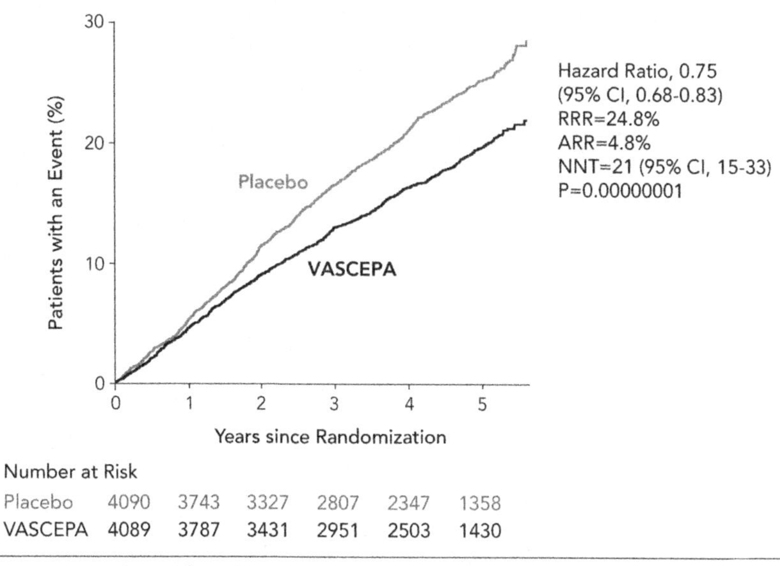

Figure note: Adapted from the original; see text for source information. CI, confidence interval. RRR, relative risk reduction. ARR, absolute risk reduction. NNT, number needed to treat.

FIGURE 11-1b: Example of a Kaplan-Meier curve.

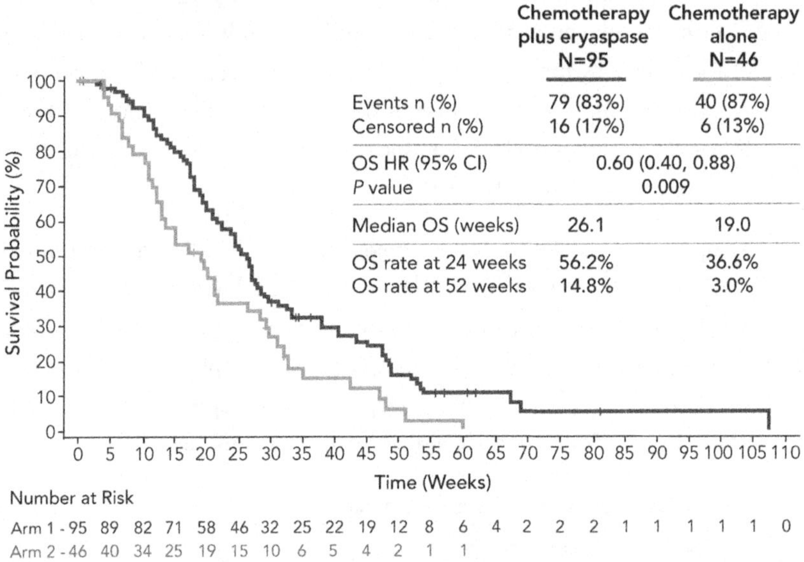

	Chemotherapy plus eryaspase N=95	Chemotherapy alone N=46
Events n (%)	79 (83%)	40 (87%)
Censored n (%)	16 (17%)	6 (13%)
OS HR (95% CI)	0.60 (0.40, 0.88)	
P value	0.009	
Median OS (weeks)	26.1	19.0
OS rate at 24 weeks	56.2%	36.6%
OS rate at 52 weeks	14.8%	3.0%

Survival Probability (%)

Time (Weeks)

Number at Risk

Time (Weeks)	0	5	10	15	20	25	30	35	40	45	50	55	60	65	70	75	80	85	90	95	100	105	110
Arm 1	95	89	82	71	58	46	32	25	22	19	12	8	6	4	2	2	2	1	1	1	1	1	0
Arm 2	46	40	34	25	19	15	10	6	5	4	2	1	1										

Figure note: Adapted from the original; see text for source information. OS, overall survival.

Although virtually all TTE analyses are accompanied by results from statistical analyses, the graphs themselves often provide additional important information. Three aspects of Kaplan-Meier and event curves are particularly important to assess:

1. **Balance and distribution of censoring:** A key assumption underlying TTE studies is that the censoring was uninformative. Although this is virtually impossible to comprehensively assess without patient-level data, many TTE graphs provide some useful information by indicating censored patients with hash marks or other symbols. Figure 11-2 is adapted from interim results published in 2017 of KEYNOTE-045, a study of pembrolizumab (Keytruda; Merck) versus chemotherapy in recurrent/ progressive metastatic or locally advanced urothelial carcinoma.[13] It is typical in that the censoring mostly occurs toward later time points, after the minimum duration of follow-up of 9.9 months, suggesting it was due to dropouts or other administrative causes.

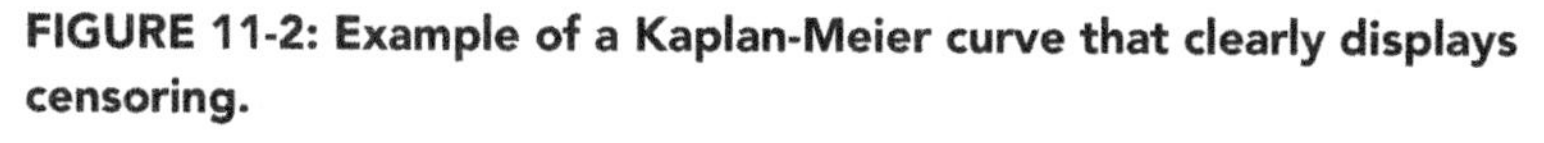

FIGURE 11-2: Example of a Kaplan-Meier curve that clearly displays censoring.

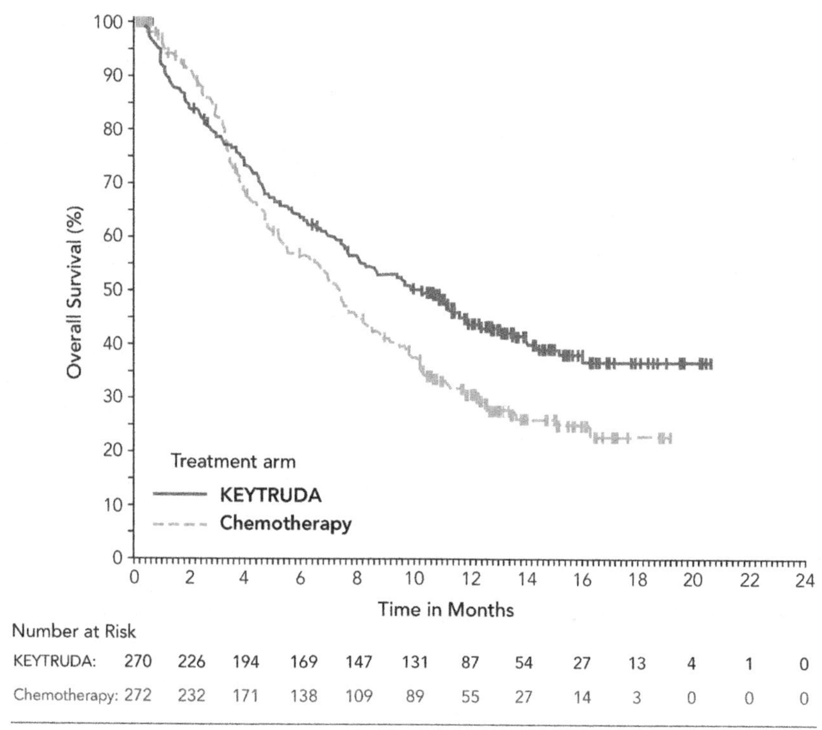

Figure note: Adapted from the original; see text for source information.

An important thing to visually assess is whether there is an obvious imbalance in censoring between the two trial arms. Apparent censoring imbalances at later time points as in the figure above are relatively common and typically assumed to be uninformative. However, from public information it is impossible to exclude the possibility that some of these could reflect potentially informative withdrawals or competing events.

Censoring imbalances at early time points are more worrisome and are not easily explained. If patients were randomly assigned, one would normally expect roughly the same number of patients in each arm to withdraw or be lost to follow-up at these early points. But a large absolute and relative number of censored events at early points could imply informative censoring.

An example of potentially informative early censoring is shown in Figure 11-3, adapted from an academic study reported in 2020 of gastric cancer patients treated with S-1 plus either oxaliplatin or cisplatin.[14] Why were so many more patients censored at early time points in the oxaliplatin arm? One possibility is that these events reflect withdrawals due to side effects; elsewhere in the paper, the authors report that oxaliplatin-treated patients had substantially higher rates of low-grade hematologic side effects, and almost all of them required treatment with the blood cell growth factor G-CSF to raise neutrophil counts and prevent infections. Thus, the early censoring events could reflect voluntary withdrawals due to poor tolerability, and in theory these could be informative if the patients who withdrew were more likely to die more quickly, leaving behind in the oxaliplatin-treated arm only those patients with higher odds of longer-term survival. Importantly, the imbalance in early censoring events is not itself evidence that the study is invalid, but it does raise additional questions about the analysis and interpretation of the trial data that should be explored.

FIGURE 11-3: Example of a Kaplan-Meier curve with early censoring.

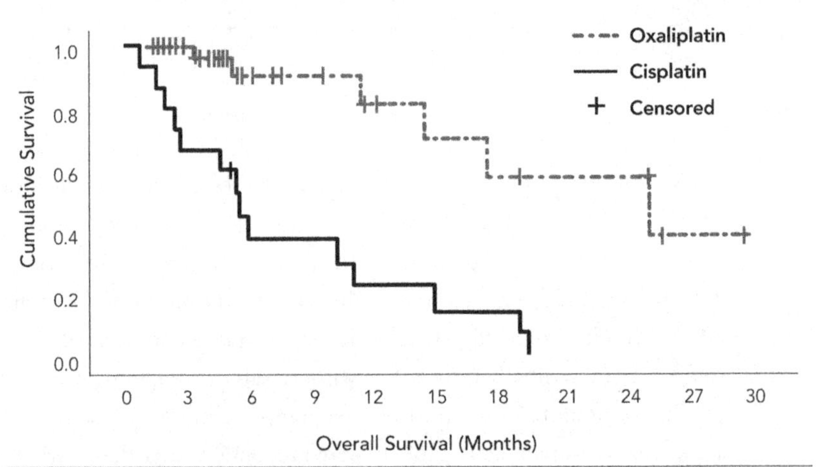

Figure note: Adapted from the original; see text for source information.

2. **Timing of curve divergence:** Under the proportional hazards assumption, the difference between the two arms in a positive TTE study should increase steadily over time, indicated by a gradually widening

gap between the curves. But this is not always the case. Figure 11-4 is adapted from results disclosed in 2019 of the OS in the ITT population for neratinib (Nerlynx; Puma) plus capecitabine versus lapatinib plus capecitabine in HER2-positive breast cancer[15]:

FIGURE 11-4: Example of a Kaplan-Meier curve with late divergence.

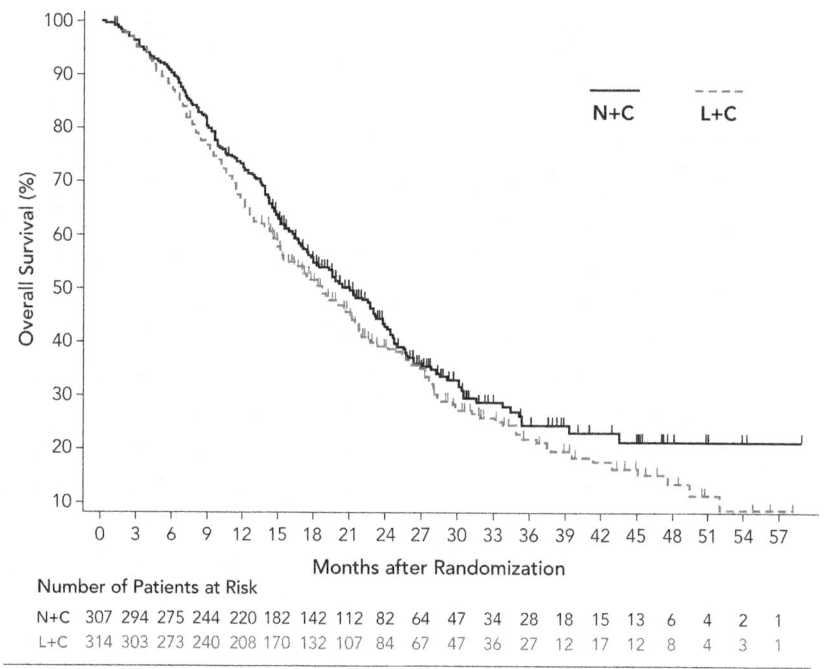

N+C	307	294	275	244	220	182	142	112	82	64	47	34	28	18	15	13	6	4	2	1
L+C	314	303	273	240	208	170	132	107	84	67	47	36	27	12	17	12	8	4	3	1

Figure note: Adapted from the original; see text for source information. N+C, neratinib plus capecitabine. L+C, lapatinib plus capecitabine.

When TTE curves diverge at later time points, one's eye is naturally drawn to the large difference on the far right-hand side, but this is commonly an over-representation of the true difference. Although late divergence could indicate that the proportional hazards assumption has been violated, which would be worthy of investigation, it more frequently reflects the high uncertainty associated with later points that are derived from analyzing smaller numbers of patients.[16]

In the absence of standard error bars, which are rarely provided in these sorts of figures, it is often helpful to check how many patients contributed to the results when the curves started to diverge. A good rule of thumb is to put less stock in results at time points when fewer than 20% of patients who entered the trial remained at risk. In the neratinib example above, most of the divergence occurred after 36 weeks, at which point the table under the x-axis reveals that fewer than 10% of the patients (28 of 307 in the experimental arm and 27 of 314 in the control arm) were still included in the analysis. At the latest point at which 20% of patients remained at risk (27–30 weeks), the curves were essentially overlapping, which calls the magnitude of benefit from neratinib into question.

3. **Crossing curves:** When the two curves in a KM or survival plot cross, this typically indicates that the relative risk of experiencing an event between the treatment arms changes over the course of the study. This is technically a violation of the proportional hazards assumption that the relative risk in each arm must remain constant over time.

   Violations of the proportional hazards assumption are plausible and expected in some clinical scenarios. As noted earlier, immune modulators are known to exert their effects more slowly than other anti-cancer therapies, and therefore commonly exhibit crossing Kaplan-Meier curves as in Figure 11-2. Even in these expected situations, however, it may be worthwhile to seek expert statistical input to confirm that the appropriate methods were used to account for the proportional hazards violation.

   Even if there is no obvious rationale, curve crossings toward the right side of a TTE graph are generally less concerning than those toward the left. As discussed in the context of curve divergence, later data points are associated with a larger amount of uncertainty, so apparent violations of the proportional hazards assumption at these times, especially if fewer than 20% of patients remain at risk, are probably not worrisome.

---

[1] Young KD, Menegazzi JJ, Lewis RJ. Statistical methodology: IX. survival analysis. Acad Emerg Med. 1999 Mar;6(3):244–249. doi: 10.1111/j.1553-2712.1999.tb00165.x. PMID: 10192678.

[2] Stel VS, Dekker FW, Tripepi G, Zoccali C, Jager KJ. Survival analysis I: The Kaplan-Meier method. Nephron Clin Pract. 2011;119(1):c83–88. doi: 10.1159/000324758. Epub 2011 Jun 15. PMID: 21677442.

[3] Rich JT, Neely JG, Paniello RC, Voelker CC, Nussenbaum B, Wang EW. A practical guide to understanding Kaplan-Meier curves. Otolaryngol Head Neck Surg. 2010 Sep;143(3):331–336. doi: 10.1016/j.otohns.2010.05.007. PMID: 20723767; PMCID: PMC3932959.

[4] Clark TG, Bradburn MJ, Love SB, Altman DG. Survival analysis part I: Basic concepts and first analyses. Br J Cancer. 2003 Jul 21;89(2):232–238. doi: 10.1038/sj.bjc.6601118. PMID: 12865907; PMCID: PMC2394262.

[5] Barraclough H, Simms L, Govindan R. Biostatistics primer: What a clinician ought to know: Hazard ratios. J Thorac Oncol. 2011 Jun;6(6):978–982. doi: 10.1097/JTO.0b013e31821b10ab. Erratum in: J Thorac Oncol. 2011 Aug;6(8):1454. PMID: 21623277.

[6] Clark TG, Bradburn MJ, Love SB, Altman DG. Survival analysis part I: Basic concepts and first analyses. Br J Cancer. 2003 Jul 21;89(2):232–238. doi: 10.1038/sj.bjc.6601118. PMID: 12865907; PMCID: PMC2394262.

[7] Austin PC, Lee DS, Fine JP. Introduction to the analysis of survival data in the presence of competing risks. Circulation. 2016 Feb 9;133(6):601–609. doi: 10.1161/CIRCULATIONAHA.115.017719. PMID: 26858290; PMCID: PMC4741409.

[8] Duke-Margolis Center for Health Policy. Public Workshop: Oncology Clinical Trials in the Presence of Non-Proportional Hazards (meeting summary). National Press Club, February 5, 2018. https://healthpolicy.duke.edu/sites/default/files/2020-03/oncology_trials_workshop_meeting_summary_0.pdf. Accessed October 15, 2021. Permalink: https://perma.cc/N6GK-WAKM.

[9] Rogers JK, McMurray JJ, Pocock SJ, Zannad F, Krum H, van Veldhuisen DJ, Swedberg K, Shi H, Vincent J, Pitt B. Eplerenone in patients with systolic heart failure and mild symptoms: Analysis of repeat hospitalizations. Circulation. 2012 Nov 6;126(19):2317–2323. doi: 10.1161/CIRCULATIONAHA.112.110536. Epub 2012 Oct 5. PMID: 23042980.

[10] Solomon SD, Rizkala AR, Gong J, Wang W, Anand IS, Ge J, Lam CSP, Maggioni AP, Martinez F, Packer M, Pfeffer MA, Pieske B, Redfield MM, Rouleau JL, Van Veldhuisen DJ, Zannad F, Zile MR, Desai AS, Shi VC, Lefkowitz MP, McMurray JJV. Angiotensin receptor neprilysin inhibition in heart failure with preserved ejection fraction: Rationale and design of the PARAGON-HF trial. JACC Heart Fail. 2017 Jul;5(7):471–482. doi: 10.1016/j.jchf.2017.04.013. Epub 2017 Jun 26. PMID: 28662936.

[11] Amarin. Results from the Vascepta (icosapent ethyl) CV outcomes trial (REDUCE-IT). https://investor.amarincorp.com/static-files/7eed9f2b-3f7a-493f-9113-99d981a198b1. Accessed October 15, 2021. Permalink: https://perma.cc/NJF9-9772.

[12] Erytech Pharma (ERYP). Form F-1. October 6, 2017. https://www.sec.gov/Archives/edgar/data/1624422/000119312517306022/d373760df1.htm. Accessed October 15, 2021.

[13] Keytruda [package insert]. Merck. March 2021. https://www.accessdata.fda.gov/drugsatfda_docs/label/2021/125514s096lbl.pdf. Accessed October 15, 2021. Permalink: https://perma.cc/RL4G-8Y5V.

[14] Koumarianou A, Ntavatzikos A, Vallilas C, Kampoli K, Kakoseou Z, Karamouzis MV. Survival outcomes following combination of first-line platinum-based chemotherapy with S-1 in patients with advanced gastric cancer. Cancers (Basel). 2020 Dec 15;12(12):3780. doi: 10.3390/cancers12123780. PMID: 33333977; PMCID: PMC7765389.

[15] Nerlynx [package insert]. Puma Biotechnology. February 2020. https://www.accessdata.fda.gov/drugsatfda_docs/label/2020/208051s005s006lbl.pdf. Accessed October 15, 2021. Permalink: https://perma.cc/LH64-39RM.

[16] Pocock SJ, Clayton TC, Altman DG. Survival plots of time-to-event outcomes in clinical trials: Good practice and pitfalls. Lancet. 2002 May 11;359(9318):1686–1689. doi: 10.1016/S0140-6736(02)08594-X. PMID: 12020548.

12.

P VALUES AND CONFIDENCE INTERVALS

LOVE THEM OR LOATHE THEM, *P* values are a key element in assessing and communicating the significance of drug trial results. They are the cornerstone of scientific abstracts and papers, and many readers of press releases and investor presentations base their impressions of a study on whether it hit the "$P<.05$" threshold. In the regulatory sphere, *P* values have endured as a make-or-break metric in regulators' drug approval criteria and are likely to remain so.

P values are one of the most misinterpreted "basic" concepts in statistics, and most professionals who read trial results every day—including physicians, investors, and journalists—do not properly understand them. In this chapter, we summarize the basics of what *P* values do and do not say about the significance of a study, as well as the relationship between *P* values and confidence intervals. Common examples of statistical manipulations known as "*P*-hacking" are covered in Chapter 8 on efficacy results.

Definition of *P* values

The clearest definition of a *P* value for most readers of the biomedical research literature is that "the *P* value represents the probability that the data would be at least as extreme as those observed, if the null hypothesis were true."[1] For randomized controlled trials, this means that the *P* value is the chance of obtaining results as good as or better than what the study showed, if the experimental treatment didn't actually work any better than the comparator.

Consider a simple example of a clinical trial of a cardiovascular drug versus placebo, testing whether the new therapy reduces systolic blood pressure (SBP). The null hypothesis is that there is no difference between them and the drug doesn't work. So if the study shows that the drug confers a 20-point decrease in SBP compared with placebo with two-sided $P = .05$, then *even if the drug and the placebo were actually no different*, there would have been only a 5% chance in this trial that we would have seen at least a 20-point difference in SBP between the two arms in one direction or the other.

There are several important points to remember about *P* values:

1. **The *P* value measures probability, not "truth."** As with all probabilities, a *P* value does not prove or disprove any hypothesis. It merely measures the likelihood that in this particular study, designed in this particular way, there would have been a difference of a given magnitude or greater if the true effects of the two therapies were, in fact, the same.
2. **The *P* value is highly dependent on study design.** A large *P* value ($> .05$) in a drug trial does not mean that a therapy does not have any effect. More precisely, it means that *this particular study* was unable to reject with more than 95% confidence the possibility that the control arm could have created an effect at least as large as found with the drug. Another trial, designed differently, could have yielded a result with a smaller *P* value.
3. **The *P* value is not the "false positive rate."** Many readers assume that if a study yields $P < .05$, then there is less than a 5% chance the results are false, but that's not quite accurate. A study testing homeopathic doses of orange juice versus water in colon cancer might detect a survival advantage from Tropicana with $P < .05$. But all that would mean is that *this particular study* rejected the null hypothesis with more than 95% certainty, even though the likelihood on basic scientific grounds that this is a false positive finding is astronomically high. This concept is discussed in more detail in the context of the false discovery rate in Chapter 8 on efficacy results.

4. ***P* values say nothing about the *clinical* significance of a finding.** It is possible to obtain results from a study that yield a low *P* value but are not meaningful to patient care because the amount of benefit from the new therapy is so minuscule. Sanofi's ziv-afilbercept (Zaltrap) was approved in 2012 for patients with metastatic colorectal cancer based on a highly significant study (P=.0032) that showed a median survival gain of only 42 days.[2] After the drug's $11,000-a-month price was announced, Memorial Sloan Kettering Cancer Center refused to offer the therapy.[3] This topic is explored in more depth in Chapter 8 on efficacy results.

One- and two-sided *P* values

Most drug trials calculate and report two-sided *P* values, sometimes called two-tailed *P* values. This refers to whether the comparison is designed to test for statistical significance in both directions from the comparator or only in one direction. Consider the hypertension example. If a new drug yields a systolic blood pressure of 110 mm Hg compared with 130 mm Hg in the control group with a two-sided *P* value of .05, it means there was a 5% chance of observing a 20-point difference between the experimental therapy and the comparator in either direction, even if there was no actual difference. In other words, in that experiment there was a 5% chance that the experimental drug would have yielded a result of *either* ≤110 mm Hg *or* ≥150 mm Hg, even if the null hypothesis were true and its effect was the same as that of the control. Each of these possibilities would have equal odds of 2.5%.

In principle, it is logical to argue that a one-sided test for significance is appropriate in most studies of new experimental therapies. After all, we mainly care about whether the new drug is superior to the control, not whether it's superior *or* inferior. That is true, but only if we were to give up the sanctity of the P=.05 threshold. In other words, the convention of the classic 5% threshold, which we will discuss more later, is based on the assumption that we are talking about a two-sided test. For one-sided comparisons, the *P* value cutoff should generally be halved to .025.[4] The CoreValve trial as reported in 2014, which compared mortality with transcatheter aortic valve replacement versus surgery, was designed with a one-tailed threshold of .05 for both non-inferiority (the primary endpoint) and superiority (a secondary endpoint).[5] The one-tailed *P* values for the two analyses were <.001 and .04, respectively, and the study claimed success on both counts. However, the one-tailed *P* value for superiority of .04 would have been called a failure in a typical Phase 3 biopharma study.

Finally, although two-tailed *P* values are the norm in clinical trials, reporting can be ambiguous in press releases and even in some high-profile journal articles. A 2018 paper reporting results from a Phase 3 study of brentuximab vedotin (Adcetris; Seattle Genetics) in Hodgkin's lymphoma was unnecessarily confusing when it said it was designed "at a one-sided significance level of 0.025," but then reported an improvement in progression-free survival (PFS) with *P*=.04 that was presumably two-sided but not defined.[6] It would have been clearer for the authors to either stipulate to a two-sided cutoff of .05 or to explicitly report the one-sided *P* value for their analysis.

Factors that affect the *P* value

In general, the *P* value *decreases* as any of these things happens:

- The **observed difference** between the two arms *increases.*
- The **standard deviation** of the measurement within each arm *decreases.*
- The **number of samples** in each arm *increases.*

Returning to the hypertension example—imagine that another hypertension study found that a different drug was superior to the same comparator with a *P* value of .005, or one-tenth what was seen in the first study.

One possible explanation for the smaller *P* value in the second study is that the second drug is actually more likely to be effective than the first in reducing blood pressure, but there are several other possible explanations. For example:

- **Bigger trial:** The second study may have been much larger than the first.
- **Better testing device:** The outcomes in the second study may have been less variable because the device for measuring blood pressure yielded more consistent or more accurate results.
- **Different testing method:** The second study may have had less variability in its outcomes because it used a different method for measuring blood pressure that had less variability.
- **More homogeneous population:** The outcomes in the second study may have been less variable because the patient population was more homogeneous. For example, a trial conducted in a small number of sites

or countries might yield a smaller *P* value than an identically designed study with more diverse participating centers and patients.

In any of these scenarios, the second trial would be likely to yield a smaller *P* value than the first, even if the two anti-hypertensive drugs were equally effective. Thus, comparing the *P* values from separate studies tells one nothing about the relative efficacies of two active agents. The relationships between the *P* value and the observed difference, standard deviation, and sample size are discussed in more detail in Chapter 13 on statistical power.

Regulatory significance of *P*<.05

Since the mid-20th century, a two-sided *P* value less than a significance cutoff (α) of .05 has been the generally accepted threshold for declaring that trial results are significant[7]—but in fact, this threshold is arbitrary. There is no inherent reason why one should view a *P* value of 5% as substantially more impactful than one of 6% and less so than one of 4%.

In the context of studies intended for regulatory submission, however, this value has outsized significance because since 1998 the U.S. Food and Drug Administration (FDA) has explicitly defined $P<.05$ as the general standard for drug approval. The 5% threshold has taken on such importance in clinical development that some industry analysts, and even some sponsors, report results as "$P<.05$" or "$P>.05$" and don't even provide the specific values, even though most top-tier medical journals frown on this practice.[8]

In general, the FDA has held firm on the $P<.05$ standard for full, unconditional drug approval. For example, although one of the initial Phase 3 trials of sipuleucel-T (Provenge; Dendreon) for prostate cancer yielded $P<.05$ on the primary endpoint of time to progression, another reported a *P* value of .052. Agency reviewers rejected the company's case for declaring efficacy based on a post hoc analysis of the second study but subsequently approved the drug after a new Phase 3 trial published in 2011 reported results with $P<.05$.[9]

In rare cases, the FDA has relaxed the $P<.05$ standard for new drugs but only when a secondary analysis that met the 5% threshold was deemed compelling enough to justify approval. The first instance of this was carvedilol (Coreg; SmithKline Beecham) for congestive heart failure in 1995.[10] More recently, the Phase 3 study of betrixaban (Bevyxxa; Portola) to prevent thromboembolic events in hospitalized patients yielded a non-significant result (*P*=.054) using a pre-specified analysis focusing on a high-risk subset with elevated baseline D-dimer.[11] However, the drug was granted approval in 2017 based on a revised analysis of the full population, which achieved *P*=.006.[12,13]

Most cases where the FDA relaxes the *P*<.05 standard are conditional on performing additional confirmatory studies. Two trials of treprostinil (Remodulin; United Therapeutics) for pulmonary arterial hypertension narrowly missed the 5% threshold. Although the FDA's statistical reviewers recommended that the drug be rejected, the agency granted approval in 2002 based on the results of a surrogate endpoint analysis that was statistically significant, with a requirement to conduct a confirmatory post-marketing study with "endpoints that are clearly clinically relevant."[14] Another example is the Phase 2 study of olaratumab (Lartruvo; Lilly) in soft tissue sarcoma, which was designed to detect an improvement in PFS with a two-sided *P* value of .2. The results showed longer PFS with the experimental drug (*P*=.0615), as well as an improvement in overall survival (OS), a secondary endpoint (*P*=.003).[15] Based on these data, the FDA granted accelerated approval in 2016 for treating soft tissue sarcoma, conditional on obtaining positive results from another study.[16] Notably, the subsequent Phase 3 trial did not demonstrate improved OS, and in 2019 Lilly announced it was withdrawing the drug from the market.[17]

There are two main situations in which the FDA imposes an even more demanding requirement than *P*<.05 to grant approval of a new drug:

- **Approvals based on a single study:** When sponsors request approval based on a single trial instead of the typical standard of two well-controlled experiments, the agency requires that the single trial show a "statistically very persuasive finding."[18] Although "very persuasive" is not explicitly defined, in several instances over the years the FDA has suggested that a significance level of .0010 to .00125 is appropriate in this scenario,[19] in line with statistical arguments to this effect.[20,21] Indeed, an analysis of 20 cancer drug approvals from 2000 to 2016 that were granted based on a single randomized, controlled trial revealed that 12 met the *P*<.00125 threshold.[22]
- **Approvals based on multiple hypothesis testing:** Assessing a drug's effect on multiple possible endpoints increases the odds that one of the comparisons will yield a significant *P* value, discussed in more detail in

Chapter 7 on analysis. A similar problem can arise in other multiplicity scenarios, such as tests of different time periods or drug doses. FDA guidance clearly indicates the need to account for multiple hypothesis testing and provides various methodologic options.[23] All these methods have the net effect of reducing the effective *P* value threshold. The most stringent one, the well-known Bonferroni method, yields an effective *P* value cutoff of .05 divided by the number of analyses being conducted.

Interpretation of very small *P* values

It is common for cursory readers of clinical trial results to conclude that a result with a very small *P* value (say, *P*=.001) is extremely reliable and important. However, regardless of the degree of statistical significance of the results, it is important to closely examine the effect size and the study size:

- **Results that are statistically significant but clinically insignificant:** The magnitude of the *P* value says nothing about the importance of the absolute difference between the experimental arm and the comparator. Regardless of the results of the statistical test, it is possible—some would even say common—for a study to yield findings that are statistically significant but clinically insignificant. An oft-cited example is the finding published in 2007 that erlotinib plus gemcitabine confers a 10-day improvement in OS in pancreatic cancer over gemcitabine alone, with a *P* value of .038.[24] Regardless of the statistical significance of the result, its magnitude is unimpressive.
- **Large study size that "bought" statistical power:** As noted above, for any given level of treatment effect, it is possible to "buy" statistical power and thus a smaller *P* value by increasing the study size or making other changes to the trial design. This concept is discussed in more detail in Chapter 13 on statistical power.

It is technically true that if one is comparing two positive trials that were designed and executed *in exactly the same way,* a smaller *P* value would increase one's confidence that the difference would not have been observed if the drug and the control were, in fact, the same. But in practice, there are almost always subtle and substantive differences between trials that preclude a direct comparison.

Interpretation of borderline *P* values

In practice, "barely significant" *P* values such as .049 in drug trials should usually raise extra concerns, particularly if they arise in studies executed by small biotechs to support regulatory filings or corporate financing efforts. In these scenarios, one should be particularly vigilant for the use of inappropriate analytic techniques to get the *P* value below .05, such as multiple hypothesis testing without the appropriate corrections.

In Phase 2 studies, *P* values slightly above the .05 threshold often warrant a closer look for evidence that the drug has a clinically meaningful effect. When these trials are intended to be hypothesis-generating, there is no a priori reason to conclude that the justification for running a confirmatory study is substantially lower if the *P* value is .049 versus .051, .06, or even .10. Depending on the scenario, any of these results may provide essentially equivalent support for exploring the hypothesis in a subsequent trial, appropriately powered to detect a clinically meaningful difference and win regulatory approval.

More generally, borderline *P* values should be viewed in the context of the entire study, including its design, comparator arm, size, and statistical power. This topic is discussed more extensively in Chapter 8 on efficacy results.

Interconverting *P* values and confidence intervals

Many reports of clinical trial results present the 95% confidence interval (CI) alongside or instead of the *P* value. The 95% CI provides complementary information about the magnitude of uncertainty associated with the study results and can be particularly valuable in assessing the clinical implications of the findings. CIs of 95% are also the norm for reporting the results of non-inferiority studies.

Mathematically, the 95% CI is the range encompassing 95% of the results that would have been obtained if one had data from the entire population, instead of the group of patients examined in the trial. If two 95% CIs from independent samples do not overlap, then the two-tailed *P* value is less than .05. However, if the two 95% CIs do overlap, it does not necessarily mean that the two-tailed *P* value exceeds .05. This disconnect arises because the *P* value applies to the difference between the two mean values, whereas the CIs reflect the estimates of each group's mean, not the difference between them. Readers who are interested in more technical details can consult various sources.[25,26,27,28]

The 95% CI can be particularly informative in studies that are classified as negative based on their *P* values. The ORBITA study reported in 2017 compared percutaneous coronary intervention to a sham procedure for stable angina.[29] The primary endpoint was the amount of exercise time. The study found "no significant difference," with a *P* value of .200 for the difference between the two groups. However, the 95% CI of the difference ranged from −8.9 seconds to +42.0 seconds, which says that although there are reasonable odds that a treated patient would experience an increase in exercise capacity, one can be 95% confident that the benefit would be less than 42.0 seconds of additional exercise time. The impact of that information on patients, physicians, or regulators would obviously require additional clinical context.[30]

In many common scenarios, one can interconvert two-sided *P* values and 95% CIs; note that the equations below are not valid in extreme failure scenarios of $P>.50$.[31,32]

Interconverting *P* values and 95% CIs for differences between proportions or means

To derive the 95% CI from a *P* value in this scenario, one first needs to calculate the standard error (SE):

$$SE = \frac{|\Delta|}{z} \qquad \textit{(Eqn. 1)}$$

where Δ is the difference between the two arms, and z is the test statistic for a normal distribution test, derived from the two-sided *P* value. The easiest way to get z from a two-sided *P* value is to use the NORM.S.INV function in Excel, where z = NORM.S.INV(1-*P*/2). Alternatively, you can use the following equation as an approximation:

$$z = -0.862 + \sqrt{0.743 - 2.404 \times \ln(P)} \qquad \textit{(Eqn. 2)}$$

(Per standard terminology, ln is the natural logarithm.) Then:

$$95\%\ \text{CI} = [\Delta - (1.96 \times SE)]\ \text{to}\ [\Delta + (1.96 \times SE)] \qquad \textit{(Eqn. 3)}$$

To perform the reverse calculation and derive the *P* value from the 95% CI, one first determines the SE:

$$SE = \frac{(u - l)}{2 \times 1.96} \qquad (Eqn.\ 4)$$

where u and l are the upper and lower limits of the 95% CI. From the SE, one can calculate z using Eqn. 1. One can then calculate the *P* value using the NORM.S.DIST function in Excel, where the two-sided *P* value equals 2 x NORM.S.DIST(z), or the following approximate equation:

$$P = e^{(-0.717 \times |z| - 0.416 \times z^2)} \qquad (Eqn.\ 5)$$

Note that Eqn. 2 and Eqn. 5 are related via the quadratic equation.[33]

- **Example:** A Phase 3 study reported in 2020 of pimavanserin (Nuplazid; Acadia) for major depression yielded an improvement of 9.0 points on the HAMD-17 score with the drug, compared with an improvement of 8.1 points with placebo,[34] a difference of 0.9 points that did not reach statistical significance (P= .296). Thus, z=1.045 via Excel, SE=0.86 via Eqn. 1, and the 95% CI is (–0.79, +2.59), so the range is from an advantage of 2.57 points in favor of pimavanserin to a deficit of 0.77 points in favor of placebo.

Interconverting *P* values and 95% CIs for ratios

When dealing with odds ratios or hazard ratios (HRs), the approach is virtually identical, except that u and l in Eqn. 3 are replaced with the natural logs of the upper and lower limits of the 95% CI, and Δ in Eqn. 1 is replaced with the natural log of the ratio.

- **Example:** A study of baricitinib (Eli Lilly) plus remdesivir versus remdesivir alone for hospitalized patients with COVID-19 infection reported in 2021 a 30% higher odds of improvement in clinical status on day 15 in the experimental arm—an odds ratio of 1.3—with a 95% CI of 1.0 to 1.6.[35] Thus, u equals ln(1.6)=0.470, l equals ln(1.0)=0, and Δ equals ln(1.3)=0.262. These inputs yield SE=0.12 via Eqn. 4, z=2.18 via Eqn. 1, and two-sided P=.029 via Excel.
- **Example:** The Checkmate-9ER Phase 3 study measured PFS in renal cell carcinoma patients treated with cabozantinib (Cabometyx; Exelixis)

plus nivolumab (Opdivo; Bristol Myers Squibb) versus those treated with sunitinib, and in 2020 investigators reported a top-line HR of 0.51 ($P<.0001$).[36] If we conservatively take the *P* value to be .0001, then z=3.89 via Excel, *SE*=0.173 via Eqn. 1, and the 95% CI in natural log scale is (–1.012,–0.334). Thus, the 95% CI for the HR ranges from $e^{-1.012}$ to $e^{-0.334}$, or 0.36 to 0.72. This is a conservative estimate of the 95% CI, because the actual *P* value was less than .0001.

Confidence intervals and single-armed studies

Event rates from single-armed clinical trials are difficult to interpret, particularly when a study is small. We know intuitively that a 5% response rate based on observing one event in 20 drug-treated subjects is less trustworthy than one that finds five events in 100 patients—but *how much* less trustworthy? And similarly, seeing zero safety events in a 2,000-patient study is more comforting than if one sees no signal out of just 20 patients—but *how much* more comforting?

To put these sorts of results in context, it can sometimes be informative to explicitly quantify the CI around the reported result. An approach that can be applied to even the small, skewed samples commonly encountered in drug trials involves calculating three quantities[37,38]:

$$A = 2r + z^2$$

$$B = z\sqrt{z^2 + 4r(1-p)}$$

$$C = 2(n + z^2)$$

where z=1.96 for a 95% CI, r is the number of observed events among drug-treated patients, n is the number of drug-treated patients, and p is the proportion of drug-treated patients with the observed event (i.e., r/n). (Note that this p is not the same as the *P* value.) Then, the 95% CI is:

$$\frac{A-B}{C} < p < \frac{A+B}{C}$$

For example, if a single response were observed among 20 patients treated with a study drug (i.e., r=1, n=20, yielding p=5%), then one can be 95% confident that the true efficacy rate is between 0.9% and 24%. But if the same proportion were observed in 100 drug-treated patients (r=5, n=100), the range of the 95% CI would shrink to between 2.2% and 11%.

For safety data, this method can also be useful to understand the implications of unobserved events. In this simple case (r=0), the maximum value of the 95% CI simplifies to

$$p < \frac{z^2}{n + z^2}, i.e., p < \frac{3.84}{n + 3.84}$$

So if no cases of grade 4 liver failure were observed among 20 drug-treated patients, then the 95% CI of the true incidence could span up to 16%. But if 100 patients were treated with no cases of this adverse event, then the true incidence is 95% certain to be less than 3.7%.

CIs of 95% are also helpful when comparing the results from a single-armed study with an external standard. A pivotal single-arm trial assessed the ability of a magnetic implantable device (LINX; Torax Medical) to reduce the amount of esophageal acid exposure in patients with gastroesophageal reflux.[39] The primary endpoint was the fraction of patients whose acid exposure either normalized or decreased by at least 50% at one year, with a pre-specified threshold for success of at least 60% of patients achieving the primary outcome. The trial failed to achieve statistical significance; 64% of patients hit the endpoint, with a 95% CI of 54% to 73%, encompassing the 60% threshold. However, FDA reviewers determined that even the non-significant 54% improvement was still clinically meaningful and corresponded to a positive risk/reward profile, and the agency approved the device in 2012.[40]

---

[1] Vickers A. *What is a p-value anyway? 34 Stories to Help You Actually Understand Statistics.* 1st ed. Pearson; 2009.

[2] U.S. FDA approves Zaltrap (ziv-aflibercept) after priority review for previously treated metastatic colorectal cancer. Sanofi press release. August 3, 2012. https://www.news.sanofi.us/2012-08-03-U.S.-FDA-Approves-ZALTRAP-ziv-aflibercept-After-Priority-Review-for-Previously-Treated-Metastatic-Colorectal-Cancer. Accessed October 15, 2021. Permalink: https://perma.cc/LN3E-52CC.

[3] Hall SS. The cost of living. New York Magazine. October 18, 2013. https://nymag.com/news/features/cancer-drugs-2013-10/. Accessed October 15, 2021.

[4] Multiple endpoints in clinical trials: Guidance for industry (draft guidance). U.S. Food and Drug Administration. January 2017.

[5] Adams DH, Popma JJ, Reardon MJ, Yakubov SJ, Coselli JS, Deeb GM, Gleason TG, Buchbinder M, Hermiller J Jr, Kleiman NS, Chetcuti S, Heiser J, Merhi W, Zorn G, Tadros P, Robinson N, Petrossian G, Hughes GC, Harrison JK, Conte J, Maini B, Mumtaz M, Chenoweth S, Oh JK; U.S. CoreValve Clinical Investigators. Transcatheter aortic-valve replacement with a self-expanding prosthesis. N Engl J Med. 2014 May 8;370(19):1790–1798. doi: 10.1056/NEJMoa1400590. Epub 2014 Mar 29. PMID: 24678937.

[6] Connors JM, Jurczak W, Straus DJ, Ansell SM, Kim WS, Gallamini A, Younes A, Alekseev S, Illés Á, Picardi M, Lech-Maranda E, Oki Y, Feldman T, Smolewski P, Savage KJ, Bartlett NL, Walewski J, Chen R, Ramchandren R, Zinzani PL, Cunningham D, Rosta A, Josephson NC, Song E, Sachs J, Liu R, Jolin HA, Huebner D, Radford J; ECHELON-1 Study Group. Brentuximab vedotin with chemotherapy for stage III or IV Hodgkin's lymphoma. N Engl J Med. 2018 Jan 25;378(4):331–344. doi: 10.1056/NEJMoa1708984. Epub 2017 Dec 10. Erratum in: N Engl J Med. 2018 Mar 1;378(9):878. PMID: 29224502; PMCID: PMC5819601.

[7] Kennedy-Shaffer L. When the alpha is the omega: P-values, "substantial evidence," and the 0.05 standard at FDA. Food Drug Law J. 2017;72(4):595–635. PMID: 30294197; PMCID: PMC6169785.

[8] Harrington D, D'Agostino RB Sr, Gatsonis C, Hogan JW, Hunter DJ, Normand ST, Drazen JM, Hamel MB. New guidelines for statistical reporting in the journal. N Engl J Med. 2019 Jul 18;381(3):285–286. doi: 10.1056/NEJMe1906559. PMID: 31314974.

[9] Anassi E, Ndefo UA. Sipuleucel-T (provenge) injection: The first immunotherapy agent (vaccine) for hormone-refractory prostate cancer. P T. 2011 Apr;36(4):197–202. PMID: 21572775; PMCID: PMC3086121.

[10] Fisher LD, Moyé LA. Carvedilol and the Food and Drug Administration approval process: An introduction. Control Clin Trials. 1999 Feb;20(1):1–15. doi: 10.1016/s0197-2456(98)00052-x. PMID: 10027497.

[11] Cohen AT, Harrington RA, Goldhaber SZ, Hull RD, Wiens BL, Gold A, Hernandez AF, Gibson CM; APEX Investigators. Extended thromboprophylaxis with betrixaban in acutely ill medical patients. N Engl J Med. 2016 Aug 11;375(6):534–544. doi: 10.1056/NEJMoa1601747. Epub 2016 May 27. PMID: 27232649.

[12] FDA approved betrixaban (Bevyxxa, Portola) for the prophylaxis of venous thromboembolism (VTE) in adult patients. U.S. FDA press release. June 23, 2017. https://www.fda.gov/drugs/resources-information-approved-drugs/fda-approved-betrixaban-bevyxxa-portola-prophylaxis-venous-thromboembolism-vte-adult-patients. Accessed October 15, 2021. Permalink: https://perma.cc/2B64-F86L.

[13] Grainger D. Portola's APEX trial design was too clever by half. Forbes.com. https://www.forbes.com/sites/davidgrainger/2016/03/31/portolas-lesson-for-innovative-clinical-trial-designers/. Accessed October 15, 2021.

[14] NDA 21-272 (Remodulin; United Therapeutics): Approval letter. U.S. Food and Drug Administration. February 8, 2002. https://www.accessdata.fda.gov/drugsatfda_docs/nda/2002/21-272_Remodulin_Approv.pdf. Accessed October 15, 2021. Permalink: https://perma.cc/AX4W-2AKA.

[15] Tap WD, Jones RL, Van Tine BA, Chmielowski B, Elias AD, Adkins D, Agulnik M, Cooney MM, Livingston MB, Pennock G, Hameed MR, Shah GD, Qin A, Shahir A, Cronier DM, Ilaria R Jr, Conti I, Cosaert J, Schwartz GK. Olaratumab and doxorubicin versus doxorubicin alone for treatment of soft-tissue sarcoma: An open-label Phase 1b and randomised Phase 2 trial. Lancet. 2016 Jul 30;388(10043):488–497. doi: 10.1016/S0140-6736(16)30587-6. Epub 2016 Jun 9. Erratum in: Lancet. 2016 Jul 30;388(10043):464. PMID: 27291997; PMCID: PMC5647653.

[16] BLA 761038 (Lartruvo; Eli Lilly): Approval letter. U.S. Food and Drug Administration. October 19, 2016. https://www.accessdata.fda.gov/drugsatfda_docs/appletter/2016/761038Orig1s000ltr.pdf. Accessed October 15, 2021. Permalink: https://perma.cc/TP95-6EEJ.

[17] Eli Lilly and Co.; Announcement of the revocation of the biologics license for Lartruvo, 85 Fed. Reg. 43587 (July 17, 2020).

[18] Demonstrating substantial evidence of effectiveness for human drug and biological products: Guidance for industry (draft guidance). U.S. Food and Drug Administration. December 2019.

[19] Kennedy-Shaffer L. When the alpha is the omega: P-values, "substantial evidence," and the 0.05 standard at FDA. Food Drug Law J. 2017;72(4):595–635. PMID: 30294197; PMCID: PMC6169785.

[20] Fisher LD. One large, well-designed, multicenter study as an alternative to the usual FDA paradigm. Ther Innov Regul Sci. 1999 Jan;33:265–271. doi: 10.1177/009286159903300130.

[21] NDA 21-272 (Uniprost; United Therapeutics): Statistical review. U.S. Food and Drug Administration. May 7, 2001. https://www.accessdata.fda.gov/drugsatfda_docs/nda/2002/21-272_Remodulin_statr.pdf. Accessed October 15, 2021. Permalink: https://perma.cc/E3PT-4542.

[22] Ladanie A, Speich B, Briel M, Sclafani F, Bucher HC, Agarwal A, Ioannidis JPA, Pereira TV, Kasenda B, Hemkens LG. Single pivotal trials with few corroborating characteristics were used for FDA approval of cancer therapies. J Clin Epidemiol. 2019 Oct;114:49–59. doi: 10.1016/j.jclinepi.2019.05.033. Epub 2019 May 31. PMID: 31158450.

[23] Multiple endpoints in clinical trials: Guidance for industry (draft guidance). U.S. Food and Drug Administration. January 2017.

[24] Moore MJ, Goldstein D, Hamm J, Figer A, Hecht JR, Gallinger S, Au HJ, Murawa P, Walde D, Wolff RA, Campos D, Lim R, Ding K, Clark G, Voskoglou-Nomikos T, Ptasynski M, Parulekar W; National Cancer Institute of Canada Clinical Trials Group. Erlotinib plus gemcitabine compared with gemcitabine alone in patients with advanced pancreatic cancer: A Phase III trial of the National Cancer Institute of Canada Clinical Trials Group. J Clin Oncol. 2007 May 20;25(15):1960–1966. doi: 10.1200/JCO.2006.07.9525. Epub 2007 Apr 23. PMID: 17452677.

[25] Frost J. Using confidence intervals to compare means. Statistics by Jim. https://statisticsbyjim.com/hypothesis-testing/confidence-intervals-compare-means/. Accessed October 15, 2021. Permalink: https://perma.cc/SX6P-7AK5.

[26] Austin PC, Hux JE. A brief note on overlapping confidence intervals. J Vasc Surg. 2002 Jul;36(1):194–195. doi: 10.1067/mva.2002.125015. PMID: 12096281.

[27] Cumming G. Inference by eye: Reading the overlap of independent confidence intervals. Stat Med. 2009 Jan 30;28(2):205–220. doi: 10.1002/sim.3471. PMID: 18991332.

[28] Cumming G, Finch S. Inference by eye: Confidence intervals and how to read pictures of data. Am Psychol. 2005 Feb–Mar;60(2):170–180. doi: 10.1037/0003-066X.60.2.170. PMID: 15740449.

[29] Al-Lamee R, Thompson D, Dehbi HM, Sen S, Tang K, Davies J, Keeble T, Mielewczik M, Kaprielian R, Malik IS, Nijjer SS, Petraco R, Cook C, Ahmad Y, Howard J, Baker C, Sharp A, Gerber R, Talwar S, Assomull R, Mayet J, Wensel R, Collier D, Shun-Shin M, Thom SA, Davies JE, Francis DP; ORBITA investigators. Percutaneous coronary intervention in stable angina (ORBITA): A double-blind, randomised controlled trial. Lancet. 2018 Jan 6;391(10115):31–40. doi: 10.1016/S0140-6736(17)32714-9. Epub 2017 Nov 2. Erratum in: Lancet. 2018 Jan 6;391(10115):30. PMID: 29103656.

[30] Harrell F. Statistical errors in the medical literature. Statistical Thinking. Updated August 2, 2021. https://www.fharrell.com/post/errmed/. Accessed October 15, 2021. Permalink: https://perma.cc/BE2B-UGFR.

[31] Altman DG, Bland JM. How to obtain the P value from a confidence interval. BMJ. 2011;343:d2304. doi: 10.1136/bmj.d2304. PMID: 22803193.

[32] Altman DG, Bland JM. How to obtain the confidence interval from a P value. BMJ. 2011 Aug 8;343:d2090. doi: 10.1136/bmj.d2090. PMID: 21824904.

[33] Lin JT. Approximating the Normal Tail Probability and its inverse for use on a pocket calculator. J Royal Stat Soc: Series C (Applied Statistics). 1989;38(1):69–70. doi: 10.2307/2347681.

[34] Acadia Pharmaceuticals announces top-line results from the Phase 3 CLARITY study evaluating pimavanserin for the adjunctive treatment of major depressive disorder. Acadia Pharmaceuticals press release. July 20, 2020. https://ir.acadia-pharm.com/news-releases/news-release-details/acadia-pharmaceuticals-announces-top-line-results-phase-3-0. Accessed October 15, 2021. Permalink: https://perma.cc/P65E-B442.

[35] Kalil AC, Patterson TF, Mehta AK, Tomashek KM, Wolfe CR, Ghazaryan V, Marconi VC, Ruiz-Palacios GM, Hsieh L, Kline S, Tapson V, Iovine NM, Jain MK, Sweeney DA, El Sahly HM, Branche AR, Regalado Pineda J, Lye DC, Sandkovsky U, Luetkemeyer AF, Cohen SH, Finberg RW, Jackson PEH, Taiwo B, Paules CI, Arguinchona H, Erdmann N, Ahuja N, Frank M, Oh MD, Kim ES, Tan SY, Mularski RA, Nielsen H, Ponce PO, Taylor BS, Larson L, Rouphael NG, Saklawi Y, Cantos VD, Ko ER, Engemann JJ, Amin AN, Watanabe M, Billings J, Elie MC, Davey RT, Burgess TH, Ferreira J, Green M, Makowski M, Cardoso A, de Bono S, Bonnett T, Proschan M, Deye GA, Dempsey W, Nayak SU, Dodd LE, Beigel JH; ACTT-2 Study Group Members. Baricitinib plus remdesivir for hospitalized adults with Covid-19. N Engl J Med. 2021 Mar 4;384(9):795–807. doi: 10.1056/NEJMoa2031994. Epub 2020 Dec 11. PMID: 33306283; PMCID: PMC7745180.

[36] Brown A. Bristol and Exelixis score in kidney cancer, but will it be enough? Evaluate Vantage. April 20, 2020. https://www.evaluate.com/vantage/articles/news/snippets/bristol-and-exelixis-score-kidney-cancer-will-it-be-enough. Accessed October 15, 2021.

[37] Newcombe RG, Altman DG. Proportions and their differences. In Altman D, Machin D, Bryant T, Gardner M, eds. *Statistics with Confidence: Confidence Intervals and Statistical Guidelines*. 2nd ed. Wiley; 2000.

[38] Wilson EB. Probable inference, the law of succession, and statistical inference. J Am Stat Assoc. 1927;22(158): 209–212. doi: 10.1080/01621459.1927.10502953.

[39] Ganz RA, Peters JH, Horgan S, Bemelman WA, Dunst CM, Edmundowicz SA, Lipham JC, Luketich JD, Melvin WS, Oelschlager BK, Schlack-Haerer SC, Smith CD, Smith CC, Dunn D, Taiganides PA. Esophageal sphincter device for gastroesophageal reflux disease. N Engl J Med. 2013 Feb 21;368(8):719–727. doi: 10.1056/NEJMoa1205544. PMID: 23425164.

[40] PMA P100049 (LINX Reflux Management System; Torax Medical): FDA summary of safety and efficacy data. U.S. Food and Drug Administration. March 22, 2012. https://www.accessdata.fda.gov/cdrh_docs/pdf10/P100049b.pdf. Accessed October 15, 2021. Permalink: https://perma.cc/8R3M-2RDE.

13.

STUDY SIZE AND STATISTICAL POWER

ONE OF THE MOST COMMON CLAIMS people make about negative clinical studies is that they were "underpowered"—by which they mean, "If the study had been bigger, it might have yielded a positive result."

That may be true in some cases, but it masks key details that are important for readers of clinical trial results to understand. In most biotech studies, the statistical power is fixed, and the main factor affecting the planned trial size is the minimum effect size the investigators deem important to detect. In other words, if a study is designed appropriately to detect a clinically meaningful improvement, then a negative trial isn't underpowered—it's just negative.

Readers of clinical trial results or protocols typically have two practical questions about the sample size of a study. First, given the size of a trial and reasonable assumptions about variability, what difference was it powered to detect, and is this difference clinically significant? And second, under reasonable assumptions of a trial's variability and the amount of difference it seeks to detect, was it appropriately sized or too small (underpowered)?

In some simple cases it is possible to do some ballpark calculations to answer these questions. In more complex scenarios, however, it is possible only to address them qualitatively. In this chapter, we review the basic concepts underlying sample size, effect size, and statistical power, and provide guidance on how to evaluate the sample size of both planned and completed studies.

Key factors related to study size

When investigators plan clinical trials, they start with key assumptions and inputs about the study and use those factors to calculate the appropriate study size. But readers of clinical trials face the opposite scenario: the study size is known, and the issue is whether it was correctly chosen based on one's external view of the appropriate assumptions and inputs.

To understand how to evaluate the size of a planned or completed trial, it is important to know the factors that go into that determination. What follows is a somewhat simplified view of the major factors, specific to interventional clinical studies:

- **Minimum clinically important difference (MCID):** The MCID is the smallest effect size that would be meaningful to define as a positive result. The choice of MCID is highly subjective and depends on the clinical context. For example, an oncology drug might be deemed successful if it extends life span by at least a few months, but that same amount of difference may not be seen as worthwhile by patients with many chronic diseases. Similarly, reducing the 10-year risk of death in patients with hypertension by 1% could be extremely meaningful from a public health perspective, but in a rapidly progressive disease with 50% annual mortality, such a small reduction in the absolute odds of dying in a year may not have much perceived benefit.

  In most study designs, the size depends on not just the relative effect but also the absolute magnitude of effect in each arm. A stroke trial intended to identify a decrease in death rate from 6% to 5% requires more patients than one designed to see an improvement from 10% to 9% (same absolute difference) or 60% to 50% (same relative difference). The mathematical details are discussed in the section on approximate power and sample size calculations.
- **Variability:** As the name implies, variability indicates the distribution of outcomes; for normally distributed data, it can be expressed with the standard deviation. The variability depends in part on the factor being assessed and the population, but it is also influenced by the precision of the specific assay used to make the measurement. Thus, some aspects

of variability are intrinsic to the study design, but others depend on the mechanics of how the data are collected.

- **Power:** The power of a clinical trial is equal to $1-\beta$, where β is the type II error rate. The type II error rate is essentially the false negative rate of the study: it is the chance of failing to conclude that there is a difference between the two groups when one actually exists. Most interventional clinical trials of new drugs and devices set the power at 80% or 90% (β of .2 or .1, respectively).
- **Significance:** A study's significance level, also called α or the type I error rate, is the chance of detecting a difference at least as extreme as was observed if there is in fact no difference. In almost all Phase 3 drug and device trials, α is set at 5% (.05). This also corresponds to the *P* value threshold for the analysis.

  The study size also depends on whether the statistical analysis is designed to be one- or two-sided. For simplicity in this chapter, all calculations and illustrative examples assume two-sided tests, which are used in the vast majority of biopharma and medical device trials. This topic is discussed in more detail in Chapter 12 on *P* values.

As almost all clinical trials set the significance level at 5%, the important relationships for readers of clinical trials to understand are those between study size, power, MCID, and variability. All else being equal, for trials that do not measure time-to-event endpoints:

- **Detecting a smaller MCID requires a larger study size:** A trial with more patients is powered to detect a smaller difference than a smaller study. In many scenarios, the sample size varies inversely as the square of the MCID. That is, detecting half the absolute difference between the arms requires four times as many patients. As noted earlier, this can sometimes lead to a situation in which a study is overpowered to detect a difference that is statistically significant but clinically unimportant.
- **Higher variability in the outcome requires a larger study size:** A trial that assesses a more heterogeneous patient population or uses a less precise tool to measure the endpoint needs to be larger to detect the same MCID than one with less variability.

- **Higher power requires a larger study size:** The U.S. Food and Drug Administration (FDA) defines the minimum acceptable power for interventional trials at 80%, and this threshold is common in many scenarios. However, it is perfectly acceptable to design a study with even lower odds of obtaining a false negative finding by increasing the power; this requires increasing the study size. In practice, the choice of lower versus higher power reflects a strategic trade-off between managing risk on the one hand and R&D time and cost on the other.

Note that for time-to-event analyses, the same basic principles apply except that it is the number of observed events, not the sample size per se, that drives the study power.

Underpowering in failed trials

A common scenario in biotech is when a trial fails to meet its primary endpoint even though it met its recruitment target. A discussion often ensues about whether the data indicate the therapy does not work, or whether the study was merely too small and thus underpowered to deliver a positive result.

This is not exactly the right way to think about this scenario. If the agent has *any* intrinsic activity at all, then there is *some* trial size that could successfully detect an infinitesimal positive effect. So in that sense, almost every failed study can be considered to have been potentially underpowered, even though the effect size in that alternate scenario might not be clinically meaningful.[1] The more relevant question is not whether the trial was too small but instead whether the sample size was appropriately matched to the target effect size and assumptions about variability.

Commentators sometimes call a failed trial underpowered as shorthand to say that a redo with a larger sample size might have yielded the opposite result. But if the study was designed appropriately, then a failure is just a failure.

Underpowering due to an over-aggressive target effect size

The only situation in which it makes sense to call a failed trial underpowered is when the sponsors decide mainly for financial reasons to make the study too small to show a difference that would be clinically meaningful. For example, consider a scenario in which a 10% improvement in some parameter would be clinically meaningful. If it would take 1,000 patients to detect an improvement of that size, but the company can afford only a 500-patient trial, then the study might be able to detect only a much larger difference. If the drug actually yields an 11% improvement, the smaller study will fail because it was underpowered.

Thus, to call a study "underpowered," one needs to know the minimum effect size that would be clinically meaningful, as well as the effect size the study was designed to detect. The first parameter typically comes from discussions with clinicians and patients. The second is often explicitly stated in a trial's statistical analysis plan, but if it is not explicitly given, one can often estimate it from available information, as discussed in a later section.

Underpowering is quite common in Phase 2 studies, but it can occur in later-stage trials as well. A review of abstracts of Phase 3 randomized controlled trials presented at a large annual oncology meeting found that more than half were powered to detect only a "large" treatment effect and were too small to detect more modest effect sizes that could still have been clinically meaningful.[2]

Accidental underpowering

In some cases, a failed trial wasn't misdesigned per se, but it nonetheless ended up being accidentally underpowered due to issues with recruitment or incorrect event rate estimates, and new information gleaned from it might provide the chance to improve the design of a follow-up study. For example, the CREATE trial reported in 2006 analyzed the ability of epoetin beta (NeoRecormon; Roche) to increase the time to first cardiac event in patients with chronic kidney disease.[3] The study was designed under the assumption that the 600 enrolled patients would experience 200 events during the observation period. The fact that only 105 events occurred may have contributed to the negative result, and a larger study might have succeeded.

In the preceding example, it might have been worth considering a new, larger study powered using an updated assumption of the event rate. But in other cases, determining why a study ended up being underpowered may not necessarily suggest a feasible path forward for a follow-up trial. The CARE study published in 2019 of plazomicin (Zemdri; Achaogen) for bloodstream infections due to carbapenem-resistant Enterobacteriaceae failed to detect a statistically significant improvement in outcomes, but the 37-patient study fell well short of its target enrollment of 358 participants.[4] Although some members of an FDA advisory committee argued that the trend toward statistical significance and high unmet need warranted approval, the majority disagreed,[5] and the drug was subsequently rejected in this indication. The study's lack of power is a question not of trial design but of execution feasibility. Similarly, trials that fail to achieve their primary endpoints due to higher-than-expected placebo response, as seen in many psychiatric indications,[6] or larger-than-expected measurement variability may not be salvageable with larger follow-up studies, unless there is a way to design the subsequent trial to either control for or predict the unexpected factor.

Overpowering in successful trials

Some positive trials detect a therapeutic effect that is statistically significant but clinically meaningless. This indicates that the study was designed with an inappropriately small MCID and that the investigators overpowered the trial by making it large enough to detect an unimportant effect.

A Phase 3 study of vericiguat (Verquvo; Merck) in heart failure was designed with a primary outcome of either death from cardiovascular causes or first hospitalization for heart failure.[7] However, the sample size was chosen to provide 80% power for detecting only the first component—cardiovascular death—and thus had 98% power for the composite primary outcome. The trial did, indeed, report marginally positive results on the overpowered composite outcome (hazard ratio [HR], 0.90, 95% confidence interval [CI], 0.82 to 0.98, *P*=.02), but it failed to detect any reduction in cardiovascular deaths. Subsequently, some investigators questioned in 2020 whether the positive but unimpressive results from the excessively large study were clinically meaningful.[8]

Because one can "buy" statistical power by increasing the study size, it is not uncommon for sponsors of a Phase 3 trial to overpower the study to increase the odds it will yield a positive finding. Thus, it is important to carefully evaluate the actual effect size of any successful trial to determine whether its clinical impact is truly meaningful.

Methods for approximate sample size calculations

Many readers of top-line findings, meeting presentations, and study registrations on clinicaltrials.gov want to determine either the effect that a trial of a given size was or is powered to detect, or the study size that would be needed for a target effect size. However, outside of journal articles reporting Phase 3 trial results, most completed and registered clinical studies do not disclose detailed sample size analyses.

Although sample size calculations generally benefit from rigorous biostatistics input, for some straightforward trial designs, a non-expert with basic math skills can use historical results or information from a completed study, whether failed or successful, to explore the relationship between MCID, variability, and sample size. The simplified analyses described below, adapted from published work of others,[9,10,11] apply to three common two-armed trial scenarios. Sample size analyses for more complicated trial designs, such as studies including multiple endpoints and adaptive sample size re-estimation, are beyond our scope here.

Key parameters

The first two simplified analyses are based on the same basic equation:

$$n = \frac{2}{d^2} \times c_{p,power} \qquad \textit{(Eqn. 1)}$$

where n is the number of subjects *in each arm*, assuming 1:1 randomization, and d is the standardized difference. The standardized difference is a way to normalize the effect size based on the observed variability. As described below, the method for calculating it depends on the specific scenario.

$c_{p,power}$ is a constant that depends on the significance level (α; see Chapter 12 on *P* values) and power (1-β). In the most common scenario in biopharma (80% power, α=.05), $c_{p,power}$ equals 7.9. Values for other situations and more technical details are provided elsewhere.[12]

The third simplified scenario uses a slight variation of Eqn. 1, adapted to apply to survival analyses.

Simplified scenario 1: Difference in proportions between equal-sized arms

When comparing the response rate between two arms of a trial, the standardized difference is calculated as:

$$d = \frac{|(p_1 - p_2)|}{\sqrt{\hat{p}(1-\hat{p})}} \qquad \textit{(Eqn. 2)}$$

where p_1 and p_2 are the proportions in the two arms, and $\hat{p}$ is the mean of the two values $((p_1+p_2)/2)$. So, if the two proportions are 30% and 50%, then d=0.41, which would be incorporated into Eqn. 1, together with an appropriate value of c, to obtain the sample size.

Example: A Phase 3 study of rigerimod (Lupuzor; Immupharma) versus placebo in systemic lupus erythematosus, reported in 2018, was designed to enroll 200 patients.[13]

- **What effect size was the trial powered to detect?** Using n=100 per arm and standard assumptions (α=.05, β=.20) in Eqn. 1 yields a value of d=0.397. To determine p_1, the response rate in the experimental arm, one needs an assumption for p_2, the response with placebo. An earlier Phase 3 study of belimumab (Benlysta; Human Genome Sciences / GlaxoSmithKline) in same disease using the same endpoint showed a response rate of 44% in the control arm.[14] Using trial and error in Eqn. 2 yields a value of p_1=~0.64. In other words, the 200-patient rigerimod study was powered to detect a 20% absolute improvement in response rate under these assumptions. This target is well above the 14% improvement seen in the earlier trial, and not entirely unexpectedly, the rigerimod study failed (53% vs. 45%; P=.2631).
- **At a more appropriate target effect size, how many patients would be required?** If we instead presume that that rigerimod would be comparably effective to high-dose belimumab (i.e., p_1=0.58, p_2=0.44), Eqn. 2 yields a value of d=0.28. Returning to Eqn. 1 and again applying standard assumptions for α and β as above yields n=202. Thus, to detect a 14% improvement in response rate over placebo, on par with what was seen with high-dose belimumab, the rigerimod trial would have needed 202 patients in each arm, or twice as many as were actually enrolled.

Simplified scenario 2: Difference in means between equal-sized arms

For a study comparing two populations in which the endpoint is numerical and normally distributed, the standardized difference is calculated as:

$$d = \frac{Target\ difference}{Standard\ deviation} \qquad \textit{(Eqn. 3)}$$

So, in a study measuring systolic hypertension in which the target difference is 8 mm Hg and the standard deviation (SD) is 10 mm Hg, then d=0.8. As in the prior scenario, this value of d and an appropriate value of c could then be used in Eqn. 1 to obtain n, the number of patients per arm.

Example: The 127-patient Phase 2b T-Force GOLD trial, completed in 2018, assessed the efficacy of valbenazine (Ingrezza; Neurocrine Biosciences) versus placebo in moderate to severe Tourette syndrome as measured by the 25-point Yale Global Tic Severity Scale total tic score (YGTSS-TTS).[15] For comparison, a prior study of clonidine in this indication using the same endpoint in patients unselected for clinical severity showed a high placebo response but a statistically significant effect of the drug.

- **What effect size was the trial powered to detect?** Using n=64 patients per arm and c=7.9 in Eqn. 1 yields a value of d=0.497. To determine the target difference using Eqn. 3, we need a value for the SD based on prior evidence. One reasonable source is a highly comparable study of clonidine versus placebo in this indication.[16] In that trial, the 280-patient clonidine arm yielded a post-treatment mean of 9.87 with standard error of measurement (SEM) 0.43, which corresponds to an SD of 7.20, while the placebo arm (post-treatment mean 11.44, SEM 0.66, n=101) yielded an SD of 6.63. (Note that SEM equals SD divided by the square root of n.) If we use the average of these two SDs, 6.91, as the projected SD for our valbenazine calculations in Eqn. 3, we get a target difference of 3.43. In other words, the T-Force GOLD study appears to have been powered to detect a superiority of at least 3.43 points on the YGTSS-TTS score of valbenazine over placebo. For context, this effect size is more than twice the effect seen with clonidine, and indeed, the T-Force GOLD trial failed to achieve its goal.[17]
- **At a more appropriate target effect size, how many patients would be required?** Using data from the clonidine study for the absolute improvement in post-treatment YGTSS-TTS versus placebo (1.57) and the average SD as above (6.91) in Eqn. 3 yields d=0.23 based on the parameters from the earlier trial. Returning to Eqn. 1 and once again making standard assumptions (α=.05, β=.20) yields n=299 patients per arm, compared with the 64 per arm that were actually studied. Thus, if we believe the difference between treatment and control seen in the clonidine trial is an appropriate threshold for the MCID, then the T-Force

GOLD study appears to have been far too small to detect an equivalent effect of valbenazine.

Simplified scenario 3: Difference in survival rates

For a study comparing two populations via a time-to-event endpoint, the standardized treatment difference is approximated as:

$$d = |\ln(HR)| \qquad \textit{(Eqn. 4)}$$

where ln (*HR*) is the natural log of the assumed hazard ratio between the treatment and control arms. Importantly, this equation is only an approximation and is less valid if the survival curves have irregular shapes or deviate from an exponential distribution.

In most scenarios, it is valid to approximate the HR as the ratio of the median time-to-event durations. So in a hypothetical oncology study, if the median overall survival (OS) is assumed to be 9 months in the control arm and is expected to increase to 12 months with the experimental treatment, the corresponding HR is 12 ÷ 9 = 1.33. Note that because the equation uses absolute value, it doesn't matter which arm is in the numerator versus the denominator; $|\ln(9/12)| = |\ln(12/9)|$.

For survival rate studies, the resulting standardized difference *d* is plugged into a modified version of Eqn. 1 to compute the target number of events, *e*, required *in both arms of the trial combined* (control plus treatment):

$$e = \frac{1}{d^2} \times \frac{1}{P_A \times P_B} \times c_{p,power} \qquad \textit{(Eqn. 5)}$$

where P_A and P_B are the proportion of study subjects in each arm. So, in the simplest case of equal-sized arms, $P_A = P_B = 0.5$, and Eqn. 5 simplifies to:

$$e = \frac{4}{d^2} \times c_{p,power} \qquad \textit{(Eqn. 6)}$$

Converting *e* into the corresponding number of patients requires making additional assumptions related to the event rate, as illustrated in the example below.

Example: A 1,035-patient Phase 3 study published in 2015 assessed the activity of the VEGFR/PDGFR inhibitor linifanib (ABT-869; AbbVie) versus sorafenib in first-line hepatocellular carcinoma patients with good liver function (Child-Pugh class A).[18]

- **What effect size was the trial powered to detect?** The initial step in the analysis is to estimate the number of events that were expected in the 1,035 patients. An earlier study of sorafenib versus placebo expected 148 deaths to occur among 226 sorafenib-treated patients.[19] Using the same ratio as a benchmark, we can estimate that 678 events were expected in the linifanib Phase 3 study, which implies an HR of 1.24 using Eqn. 6 (α=.05, β=.20). In fact, this is almost exactly the same calculation reported when the results were published.

  The next question to ask is whether an HR of 1.24 compared with sorafenib was appropriate. In a prior single-arm Phase 2 study, linifanib demonstrated a median OS of 10.4 months in the Child-Pugh A subset.[20] If one were to expect the same performance of linifanib in the Phase 3 study, then the HR of 1.24 would imply an expected median OS of 8.3 months in the sorafenib arm. But although this is not an unreasonable assumption, sorafenib-treated patients in some earlier studies had much longer median survival times, for example 10.7 months in the SHARP trial, published in 2008.[21,22] If the median OS with sorafenib were even just *one week longer* than expected (8.55 months instead of 8.3 months), this would imply an HR of 1.22, which translates into 824 required events instead of 678, and a total study size of 1,258 patients. Thus, if one would have thought there was a reasonable chance that the predicted outcomes on sorafenib were even slightly lowballed, then one would have concluded that the Phase 3 linifanib study would have been undersized. In fact, the trial failed, and patients on sorafenib had a median OS of 9.8 months.
- **At a more appropriate target effect size, how many patients would be required?** As noted, the Phase 3 linifanib trial was powered to detect an HR of ~1.24 compared with sorafenib, which would correspond to an absolute increase in life span of at least two months. Irrespective of whether this was the appropriate goal to set from the perspective of clinical impact, it may have been the minimum improvement target that was feasible for trial execution. An alternative design, intended to detect a one-month improvement (from ~9.4 months to 10.4 months; HR ~1.1),

would have required ~3,092 events across both arms, corresponding to a ~4.5-fold larger study, or 4,720 total patients.

Caveats to post hoc sample size calculations

These examples illustrate some basic scenarios in which one can determine the rough relationship between sample size, MCID, and other factors in a planned or completed study. However, the simplified and stylized approaches here are mainly intended to provide approximate estimates, and as the design becomes more complex—due to variation in design or analytic methods, multiple endpoints, interim analyses, etc.—input from a biostatistician is almost always needed. For example, in the valbenazine case, we based our analysis on a comparison of the final mean values. However, one could also have designed the trial to assess the average difference in patients' scores from baseline to after therapy. This would have involved a different analytical approach and possibly would have changed the sample size results. And in the linifanib example, our modeling of the shape of the survival curve is oversimplified.

Retrospective sample size analyses are also extremely sensitive to the choice of inputs and comparators. Even in relatively straightforward cases, differences in the population, measurement tools, allocation, intervention, and other factors can render assumptions that are used for such calculations extremely tenuous.

In general, regardless of whether one attempts to do calculations like the ones described here, it is often appropriate for non-experts to look for comparators in the medical literature that used similar populations, endpoints, analytic methods, and effect sizes. Although this approach doesn't yield quantitative results, it can be useful for getting a general sense of whether the size of a study is in the ballpark for its target effect size or is woefully inadequate.

---

[1] Levine M, Ensom MH. Post hoc power analysis: An idea whose time has passed? Pharmacotherapy. 2001 Apr;21(4):405–409. doi: 10.1592/phco.21.5.405.34503. PMID: 11310512.

[2] Bedard PL, Krzyzanowska MK, Pintilie M, Tannock IF. Statistical power of negative randomized controlled trials presented at American Society for Clinical Oncology annual meetings. J Clin Oncol. 2007 Aug 10;25(23):3482–3487. doi: 10.1200/JCO.2007.11.3670. PMID: 17687153.

[3] Drüeke TB, Locatelli F, Clyne N, Eckardt KU, Macdougall IC, Tsakiris D, Burger HU, Scherhag A; CREATE Investigators. Normalization of hemoglobin level in patients with chronic kidney disease and anemia. N Engl J Med. 2006 Nov 16;355(20):2071–2084. doi: 10.1056/NEJMoa062276. PMID: 17108342.

[4] McKinnell JA, Dwyer JP, Talbot GH, Connolly LE, Friedland I, Smith A, Jubb AM, Serio AW, Krause KM, Daikos GL; CARE Study Group. Plazomicin for infections caused by carbapenem-resistant enterobacteriaceae. N Engl J Med. 2019 Feb 21;380(8):791–793. doi: 10.1056/NEJMc1807634. PMID: 30786196.

[5] Tong A. Glass half empty: Achaogen receives split vote from FDA experts on lead antibiotic, shares plunge. Endpoints News. May 3, 2018. https://endpts.com/glass-half-empty-achaogen-receives-split-vote-from-fda-experts-on-lead-antibiotic-shares-plunge/. Accessed October 15, 2021.

[6] Hasnain M, Rudnick A, Bonnell WS, Remington G, Lam RW. Use of placebo in clinical trials of psychotropic medication. Can J Psychiatry. 2018 May;63(5):338–341. doi: 10.1177/0706743717752917. PMID: 29668328; PMCID: PMC5912304.

[7] Armstrong PW, Pieske B, Anstrom KJ, Ezekowitz J, Hernandez AF, Butler J, Lam CSP, Ponikowski P, Voors AA, Jia G, McNulty SE, Patel MJ, Roessig L, Koglin J, O'Connor CM; VICTORIA Study Group. Vericiguat in patients with heart failure and reduced ejection fraction. N Engl J Med. 2020 May 14;382(20):1883–1893. doi: 10.1056/NEJMoa1915928. Epub 2020 Mar 28. PMID: 32222134.

[8] Mast J. The $1B Merck-Bayer drug that divided cardiologists in March gets priority review. Endpoints News. July 16, 2020. https://endpts.com/the-1b-merck-bayer-drug-that-divided-cardiologists-in-march-gets-priority-review/. Accessed October 15, 2021.

[9] Whitley E, Ball J. Statistics review 4: Sample size calculations. Crit Care. 2002 Aug;6(4):335–341. doi: 10.1186/cc1521. Epub 2002 May 10. PMID: 12225610; PMCID: PMC137461.

[10] Cadeddu M, Farrokhyar F, Thoma A, Haines T, Garnett A, Goldsmith CH; Evidence-Based Surgery Working Group. Users' guide to the surgical literature: How to assess power and sample size. Laparoscopic vs. open appendectomy. Can J Surg. 2008 Dec;51(6):476–482. PMID: 19057738; PMCID: PMC2592579.

[11] Schoenfeld DA. Sample-size formula for the proportional-hazards regression model. Biometrics. 1983 Jun;39(2):499–503. PMID: 6354290.

[12] Machin D, Campbell MJ. *Statistical Tables for the Design of Clinical Trials.* 1st ed. Wiley; 1987.

[13] Plieth J. Lupuzor reminds UK investors that there's no easy money in biotech. Evaluate Vantage. April 17, 2018. https://www.evaluate.com/vantage/articles/news/lupuzor-reminds-uk-investors-theres-no-easy-money-biotech. Accessed October 15, 2021.

[14] Navarra SV, Guzmán RM, Gallacher AE, Hall S, Levy RA, Jimenez RE, Li EK, Thomas M, Kim HY, León MG, Tanasescu C, Nasonov E, Lan JL, Pineda L, Zhong ZJ, Freimuth W, Petri MA; BLISS-52 Study Group. Efficacy and safety of belimumab in patients with active systemic lupus erythematosus: A randomised, placebo-controlled, phase 3 trial. Lancet. 2011 Feb 26;377(9767):721–731. doi: 10.1016/S0140-6736(10)61354-2. Epub 2011 Feb 4. PMID: 21296403.

[15] Safety, tolerability, and efficacy of NBI-98854 for the treatment of pediatric subjects with Tourette syndrome. ClinicalTrials.gov identifier: NCT03325010. Updated June 28, 2021. Accessed October 15, 2021.

[16] Du YS, Li HF, Vance A, Zhong YQ, Jiao FY, Wang HM, Wang MJ, Su LY, Yu DL, Ma SW, Wu JB. Randomized double-blind multicentre placebo-controlled clinical trial of the clonidine adhesive patch for the treatment of tic disorders. Aust N Z J Psychiatry. 2008 Sep;42(9):807–813. doi: 10.1080/00048670802277222. PMID: 18696285.

[17] Neurocrine Biosciences announces topline data from Phase IIb T-Force GOLD study demonstrating valbenazine did not meet primary endpoint in pediatric patients with Tourette syndrome. Neurocrine Biosciences press release. December 12, 2018. https://neurocrine.gcs-web.com/news-releases/news-release-details/neurocrine-biosciences-announces-topline-data-phase-iib-t-force. Accessed October 15, 2021. Permalink: https://perma.cc/CND6-U7XR.

[18] Cainap C, Qin S, Huang WT, Chung IJ, Pan H, Cheng Y, Kudo M, Kang YK, Chen PJ, Toh HC, Gorbunova V, Eskens FA, Qian J, McKee MD, Ricker JL, Carlson DM, El-Nowiem S. Linifanib versus Sorafenib in patients with advanced hepatocellular carcinoma: Results of a randomized Phase III trial. J Clin Oncol. 2015 Jan 10;33(2):172–179. doi: 10.1200/JCO.2013.54.3298. Epub 2014 Dec 8. Erratum in: J Clin Oncol. 2017 Aug 1;35(22):2590. PMID: 25488963; PMCID: PMC4279237.

[19] Cheng AL, Kang YK, Chen Z, Tsao CJ, Qin S, Kim JS, Luo R, Feng J, Ye S, Yang TS, Xu J, Sun Y, Liang H, Liu J, Wang J, Tak WY, Pan H, Burock K, Zou J, Voliotis D, Guan Z. Efficacy and safety of sorafenib in patients in the Asia-Pacific region with advanced hepatocellular carcinoma: A Phase III randomised, double-blind, placebo-controlled trial. Lancet Oncol. 2009 Jan;10(1):25–34. doi: 10.1016/S1470-2045(08)70285-7. Epub 2008 Dec 16. PMID: 19095497.

[20] Toh HC, Chen PJ, Carr BI, Knox JJ, Gill S, Ansell P, McKeegan EM, Dowell B, Pedersen M, Qin Q, Qian J, Scappaticci FA, Ricker JL, Carlson DM, Yong WP. Phase 2 trial of linifanib (ABT-869) in patients with unresectable or metastatic hepatocellular carcinoma. Cancer. 2013 Jan 15;119(2):380–387. doi: 10.1002/cncr.27758. Epub 2012 Jul 25. PMID: 22833179.

[21] Llovet JM, Montal R, Villanueva A. Randomized trials and endpoints in advanced HCC: Role of PFS as a surrogate of survival. J Hepatol. 2019 Jun;70(6):1262–1277. doi: 10.1016/j.jhep.2019.01.028. Epub 2019 Mar 31. PMID: 30943423.

[22] Llovet JM, Ricci S, Mazzaferro V, Hilgard P, Gane E, Blanc JF, de Oliveira AC, Santoro A, Raoul JL, Forner A, Schwartz M, Porta C, Zeuzem S, Bolondi L, Greten TF, Galle PR, Seitz JF, Borbath I, Häussinger D, Giannaris T, Shan M, Moscovici M, Voliotis D, Bruix J; SHARP Investigators Study Group. Sorafenib in advanced hepatocellular carcinoma. N Engl J Med. 2008 Jul 24;359(4):378–390. doi: 10.1056/NEJMoa0708857. PMID: 18650514.

14.

STATISTICAL TESTS

EVEN FOR EXPERT BIOSTATISTICIANS, it is often difficult to perform an in-depth analysis of the methods used in a published report from a biopharma study. In most trials, there are several plausible and technically appropriate statistical options available, and without access to the raw data and a significant level of detail about the trial and analytic approach, it is typically not feasible to determine whether the investigators chose the best one and executed it appropriately.

That challenge notwithstanding, in this chapter we briefly cover a few key statistical concepts that merit attention from non-expert readers of clinical trials. We focus on issues related to three extremely common types of analyses: comparisons of proportions, comparisons of means or medians, and comparisons over a time course. Statistical considerations related to a fourth common situation, time-to-event analyses, are discussed in Chapter 11. Note that because of our focus on interventional trials, we do not cover issues related to meta-analyses or epidemiologic case-control studies.

For non-expert readers who are looking for more depth and breadth than we provide here, our main recommendation for further self-study is *Intuitive Biostatistics*, by Harvey Motulsky.[1] Other solid choices include *Statistical Thinking for Non-Statisticians in Drug Regulation*, by Richard Kay;[2] *Clinical Trials: A Practical Approach*, by Stuart Pocock;[3] and *Strategy and Statistics in Clinical Trials*, by Joseph Tal.[4]

Comparisons of proportions

The simplest randomized controlled trial design divides patients into a control arm and an experimental arm and assesses each patient's response to therapy as "yes" or "no" by some criterion. Some of these studies assay a particular positive or negative event, whereas others define response by whether a patient ended up above or below a set cutoff point on a specific clinical scale or laboratory test.

The common feature of these studies is that there are exactly two possible outcomes for each patient. This means that the results can be summarized in a simple table. The example in Table 14-1 is from TULIP-2, a Phase 3 study reported in 2020 of anifrolumab (AstraZeneca) versus placebo in systemic lupus erythematosus.[5] This 362-patient trial used the British Isles Lupus Assessment Group-based Composite Lupus Assessment to define each patient as either a "responder" or a "non-responder" after 52 weeks of therapy based on a set of defined criteria.

TABLE 14-1: Example of data from a comparison of proportions.

	Responder	**Non-responder**	**Total**
Placebo	57	125	**182**
Drug	86	94	**180**
Total	**143**	**219**	

Table note: Adapted from the TULIP-2 trial; see text for source information.

The classic statistical method in this scenario is either Fisher's exact test, which is valid for any sample size, or the chi-squared test, which is more convenient for large sample sizes but inappropriate if the value in any cell of the table is less than 5, although other statistical tools are also used depending on the specific details of the study. The key analytic question is whether the proportion of responders in the anifrolumab arm (86 of 180, or 47.8%) is statistically different from that in the placebo arm (57 of 182, or 31.3%). Applying Fisher's exact test to the TULIP-2 data yields a significant two-tailed *P* value of .0018.

Comparisons of proportions sometimes also report the **relative risk (RR)** or risk ratio, which is the quotient of the two risks. So in TULIP-2, the RR is 47.8% divided by 31.3%, or 1.53. In this case, because the event (response) is positive for patients, an RR value greater than 1 indicates a benefit from the drug compared with the control.

Trials will sometimes report an **odds ratio (OR)** instead of an RR. These two parameters do not measure the same thing, and although they are similar for low event rates, they diverge considerably for common events.[6] "Odds" are defined in terms most easily related to gambling: the chance of experiencing the event divided by the chance of *not* experiencing it. If you roll a fair six-sided die, the chance of rolling a six is 1/6, and the chance of not rolling a six is 5/6, making the odds 1/6 ÷ 5/6, or 0.20. So in TULIP-2, the odds of responding in the drug arm were 0.91 (86/180 ÷ 94/180) versus 0.46 for the control. Then, the odds ratio is the ratio of those two odds, that is, 0.91 ÷ 0.46 = 1.98, in contrast to the RR of 1.52. Between the two, RRs have the benefit of being more intuitive as the ratio of two probabilities, and thankfully, although ORs are frequently reported in epidemiologic studies, they are relatively uncommon in drug trials.

The interpretation of comparisons of proportions in a drug trial usually requires looking at the **absolute risk difference** in its appropriate clinical context. In TULIP-2, the absolute improvement was that 16.3% more patients achieved a favorable outcome with anifrolumab versus placebo. The clinical impact of this difference generally depends on outcomes with current clinical management and the safety and tolerability profile of the experimental therapy. Assessing it typically requires one to review the literature and talk to practicing physicians in the particular therapeutic area.

Finally, some papers report the **number needed to treat (NNT)**, which is the inverse of the absolute risk difference. TULIP-2 has an NNT of 1 ÷ 0.163 = 6.13, which means one would need to treat between six and seven patients with anifrolumab to get one response. Some academics argue that the NNT adds important context for practitioners, particularly when discussing treatment options with patients, but in most discussions of drug development and approval it does not add any significant insight or value.

Comparisons of proportions that use cutoffs of continuous endpoints

Many comparisons of proportions reflect a choice to set a fixed cutoff level on a continuous scale that separates responders from non-responders instead of measuring an absolute numerical change in the scale, as discussed in a later section. Statisticians frown upon this approach because it involves a loss of information and statistical power, and it can make a drug appear highly effective even if its actual effect is fairly small.[7] But in practice, this is a common approach, and often an appropriate one in drug development.

The most important factor to consider when a trial dichotomizes a continuous endpoint into responders and non-responders is whether the cutoff value is considered relevant to drug developers, regulators, and clinicians. For example, a hemoglobin A1c concentration of 6.5% is the accepted level that distinguishes diabetic from pre-diabetic patients, and it is at least theoretically plausible to imagine designing a study to calculate the fraction of patients who cross this threshold after therapy instead of or alongside a direct measurement of the drug's effect on absolute HbA1c concentrations. Similarly, in drug development for acute migraine treatment, the U.S. Food and Drug Administration (FDA) recommends assessing headache pain on a four-point scale and then analyzing the fraction of patients whose scores went to zero (no pain) at two hours after dosing.[8] Although this may seem somewhat arbitrary, it presumably arose out of expert discussions and has now become the standard in the field.

In other situations, however, the clinical justification for dichotomizing a scale into two categories is much weaker. For example, two ongoing Phase 3 studies of PledOx (calmangafodipir; PledPharma AB) for prevention of chemotherapy-induced peripheral neuropathy use an instrument that rates pain from zero to 16 using four questions on a four-point scale (FACT/GOG-NTX-4).[9,10] Instead of analyzing the scores numerically, however, the trials dichotomized the primary endpoint to measure the proportion of patients with "moderate or severe" symptoms, which they defined as scoring 3 or 4 on at least one of the questions. Notably, this definition does not appear elsewhere in the literature, and several other Phase 3 trials in this indication assessed the pain scale endpoint differently.[11]

One should be particularly cautious about interpreting results from studies with arbitrarily dichotomized endpoints if the statistical analysis plan was not pre-specified. This scenario raises the possibility that positive results were cherry-picked after testing a range of possible dichotomized and non-dichotomized analytic approaches, which would violate statistical rules for multiple hypothesis testing, discussed in Chapter 12 on *P* values. Positive findings from trials that may have defined the endpoint threshold after analyzing the data should be viewed as exploratory and hypothesis-generating at best.

Other considerations in comparisons of proportions

The dichotomization case above is a specific example of a general problem of how to define responders in a drug study. In every trial, it is important to understand what the standards are in the clinical area and how the choice of endpoint may have affected the results. For example, the TULIP-2 trial was run after an initial study of anifrolumab failed using a different definition based on the SLE Responder Index-4 (SLE-4) as its primary endpoint. In some therapeutic areas there may be debate about which definitions are most appropriate for clinical trials of new therapies, and guidance from clinical and regulatory experts is essential.

Comparisons of means or medians

A common situation in randomized controlled trials (RCTs) is when a single parameter is compared between drug-treated patients and those in the control arm. A main factor that determines which statistical tests are appropriate is whether the data assume the classic symmetric bell-shaped curve of a normal, or Gaussian, distribution.[12] So-called parametric tests like the t-test assume normality and have greater statistical power than non-parametric ones like the Mann-Whitney or Kruskal-Wallis tests, which do not make this assumption. In other words, if the data are normally distributed so one has the option of using either a parametric or a non-parametric test, the parametric test is more likely to detect a difference if one actually exists.

Even expert readers may struggle to determine whether the correct test was used in a specific situation. Investigators with access to the raw data can assess normality graphically or by using commonly accepted approaches like the Kolmogorov-Smirnov, Shapiro-Wilk, or Anderson-Darling tests,[13] but results of these analyses are infrequently reported publicly in journal articles and virtually never in press releases or investor presentations. The most practical approach for most readers is to use a general rule of thumb based on the sample size.[14] In general, data from fewer than 30 individuals per arm are rarely normally distributed and should almost always be analyzed using non-parametric methods. As the sample size increases above 30 per arm—and especially when it exceeds 100 per arm—normality is more likely, and parametric tests are probably appropriate. A Phase 2 RCT in autoimmune pulmonary alveolar proteinosis randomized

64 patients to receive either inhaled recombinant GM-CSF or placebo for 24 weeks.[15] The primary endpoint was the mean change in alveolar-arterial oxygen gradient from baseline to the end of the study, and the trial demonstrated a statistically significant improvement due to the experimental therapy (mean [SD] change of −4.50 [9.03] mm Hg vs. +0.17 [10.50] mm Hg; P=.02). The investigators appropriately used the non-parametric Mann-Whitney U test to perform the analysis.

In single-arm studies, it is common to assay a parameter in the single group of patients and then retest the same patients after exposure to an experimental therapy. Although this looks superficially similar to comparing means or medians between study arms, here each patient's ending value is highly dependent on his or her starting value. This situation necessitates the use of so-called paired analytic tests such as the paired t-test (for parametric data) or the Wilcoxon signed-rank test (for non-parametric data). A single-arm study published in 2020 tested the ability of the recombinant fusion protein pabinafusp alfa (Izcargo; JCR Pharmaceuticals) to reduce cerebrospinal fluid concentrations of heparin sulfate in 28 male patients with Hunter syndrome.[16] The authors used a paired t-test to determine that the difference between the pre- and post-treatment concentrations was 5,856 ± 2,614 ng/mL versus 2,124 ± 882.6 ng/mL, with P<.001. Note that the small sample size raises the possibility that the data are not normally distributed and suggests that a paired non-parametric test might have been more appropriate.

Comparisons over a time course

As noted, a common scenario when biotech trials compare means or medians between study arms occurs when patients have been treated for a period of time. A simple approach employed by many investigators is to define a single summary statistic for each patient, such as the absolute or relative difference between the beginning and ending values or the slope of the line.[17] This topic is also discussed in Chapter 10 on figures.

However, problems arise when a study that administers an experimental treatment over time compares the two arms at multiple intermediate points during the study and reports a P value for statistical significance at each. This is particularly common in early- and mid-phase trials, in which it might not yet be clear when the maximum effect is expected to occur. There are two problems with this approach. First, in many cases this type of analysis is performed after the study has already failed to achieve significance on its primary endpoint, which makes the statistical comparisons invalid. Second, this approach is susceptible to the problem of multiple hypothesis testing of subgroups, as discussed in Chapter 7 on analysis. Even if it were appropriate to make statistical comparisons at intermediate time points, the investigators may need to use specialized methods like multiplicity corrections based on mixed models for repeated measures to avoid spuriously declaring at least one statistically significant result.

A representative example is provided by a single-arm Phase 2 trial published in 2013 that assessed the ability of a combination of naltrexone and bupropion (Contrave; Orexigen Pharmaceuticals) to reduce depression symptoms in overweight and obese individuals with major depression.[18] The primary endpoint, which was positive, was a statistically significant difference in the MADRS depression score from baseline to week 12. The paper also reported six comparisons at intermediate time points, which were also declared statistically significant with $P<.001$. It does not appear from the methods that the investigators used any specific tools to account for multiple hypothesis testing, but given that the pre-specified primary endpoint was positive, the chance that the outcomes at the intermediate time points may not have all been statistically significant does not substantively change the interpretation of the trial.

A more worrisome situation arises when the primary outcome of a difference at some time point is negative, but a subsequent analysis of intermediate time points suggests that some of them were statistically significant. The STRIDE-1 Phase 3 study reported in 2020 of the NMDA receptor antagonist AXS-05 (Axsome Therapeutics) versus buproprion in patients with treatment-resistant depression failed to meet its primary endpoint, a statistically significant change in the MADRS depression score from baseline to week 6. But the company highlighted the apparently significant improvement at weeks 1 and 2, with *P* values of .020 and .035, respectively.[19] These intermediate assessments are at best useful for hypothesis generation only, and the absence of any evidence of statistical correction for multiple hypothesis testing suggests that the barely significant differences are unlikely to be meaningful even for this purpose.

[1] Motulsky H. *Intuitive Biostatistics: A Nonmathematical Guide to Statistical Thinking.* 4th ed. Oxford University Press; 2017.

[2] Kay R. *Statistical Thinking for Non-Statisticians in Drug Regulation.* 2nd ed. Wiley; 2014.

[3] Pocock SJ. *Clinical Trials: A Practical Approach.* John Wiley & Sons; 1983.

[4] Tai J. *Strategy and Statistics in Clinical Trials: A Non-Statisticians Guide to Thinking, Designing, and Executing.* 1st ed. Academic Press; 2011.

[5] Morand EF, Furie R, Tanaka Y, Bruce IN, Askanase AD, Richez C, Bae SC, Brohawn PZ, Pineda L, Berglind A, Tummala R; TULIP-2 Trial Investigators. Trial of anifrolumab in active systemic lupus erythematosus. N Engl J Med. 2020 Jan 16;382(3):211–221. doi: 10.1056/NEJMoa1912196. Epub 2019 Dec 18. PMID: 31851795.

[6] Knol MJ, Algra A, Groenwold RH. How to deal with measures of association: A short guide for the clinician. Cerebrovasc Dis. 2012;33(2):98–103. doi: 10.1159/000334180. Epub 2011 Dec 13. PMID: 22156574.

[7] Kirsch I, Moncrieff J. Clinical trials and the response rate illusion. Contemp Clin Trials. 2007 Jul;28(4):348–351. doi: 10.1016/j.cct.2006.10.012. Epub 2006 Dec 19. PMID: 17182286.

[8] Migraine: Developing drugs for acute treatment: Guidance for industry. U.S. Food and Drug Administration. February 2018.

[9] Preventive treatment of oxaliplatin induced peripheral neuropathy in adjuvant colorectal cancer (POLAR-A). ClinicalTrials.gov identifier: NCT04034355. Updated October 14, 2020. Accessed October 15, 2021.

[10] Preventive treatment of oxaliplatin induced peripheral neuropathy in metastatic colorectal cancer (POLAR-M) (POLAR-M). ClinicalTrials.gov identifier: NCT03654729. Updated October 14, 2020. Accessed October 15, 2021.

[11] Smith EM, Pang H, Cirrincione C, Fleishman S, Paskett ED, Ahles T, Bressler LR, Fadul CE, Knox C, Le-Lindqwister N, Gilman PB, Shapiro CL; Alliance for Clinical Trials in Oncology. Effect of duloxetine on pain, function, and quality of life among patients with chemotherapy-induced painful peripheral neuropathy: A randomized clinical trial. JAMA. 2013 Apr 3;309(13):1359–1367. doi: 10.1001/jama.2013.2813. PMID: 23549581; PMCID: PMC3912515.

[12] Altman DG, Bland JM. Statistics notes: The normal distribution. BMJ. 1995 Feb 4;310(6975):298. doi: 10.1136/bmj.310.6975.298. PMID: 7866172; PMCID: PMC2548695.

[13] Mishra P, Pandey CM, Singh U, Gupta A, Sahu C, Keshri A. Descriptive statistics and normality tests for statistical data. Ann Card Anaesth. 2019 Jan-Mar;22(1):67–72. doi: 10.4103/aca.ACA_157_18. PMID: 30648682; PMCID: PMC6350423.

[14] Ghasemi A, Zahediasl S. Normality tests for statistical analysis: A guide for non-statisticians. Int J Endocrinol Metab. 2012 Spring;10(2):486–489. doi: 10.5812/ijem.3505. Epub 2012 Apr 20. PMID: 23843808; PMCID: PMC3693611.

[15] Tazawa R, Ueda T, Abe M, Tatsumi K, Eda R, Kondoh S, Morimoto K, Tanaka T, Yamaguchi E, Takahashi A, Oda M, Ishii H, Izumi S, Sugiyama H, Nakagawa A, Tomii K, Suzuki M, Konno S, Ohkouchi S, Tode N, Handa T, Hirai T, Inoue Y, Arai T, Asakawa K, Sakagami T, Hashimoto A, Tanaka T, Takada T, Mikami A, Kitamura N, Nakata K. Inhaled GM-CSF for pulmonary alveolar proteinosis. N Engl J Med. 2019 Sep 5;381(10):923–932. doi: 10.1056/NEJMoa1816216. PMID: 31483963.

[16] Okuyama T, Eto Y, Sakai N, Nakamura K, Yamamoto T, Yamaoka M, Ikeda T, So S, Tanizawa K, Sonoda H, Sato Y. A Phase 2/3 trial of pabinafusp alfa, IDS fused with anti-human transferrin receptor antibody, targeting neurodegeneration in MPS-II. Mol Ther. 2021 Feb 3;29(2):671–679. doi: 10.1016/j.ymthe.2020.09.039. Epub 2020 Sep 30. PMID: 33038326; PMCID: PMC7854283.

[17] Matthews JN, Altman DG, Campbell MJ, Royston P. Analysis of serial measurements in medical research. BMJ. 1990 Jan 27;300(6719):230–235. doi: 10.1136/bmj.300.6719.230. PMID: 2106931; PMCID: PMC1662068.

[18] McElroy SL, Guerdjikova AI, Kim DD, Burns C, Harris-Collazo R, Landbloom R, Dunayevich E. Naltrexone/bupropion combination therapy in overweight or obese patients with major depressive disorder: Results of a pilot study. Prim Care Companion CNS Disord. 2013;15(3):PCC.12m01494. doi: 10.4088/PCC.12m01494. Epub 2013 Jun 20. PMID: 24171147; PMCID: PMC3795584.

[19] Axsome Therapeutics. STRIDE-1 Phase 3 trial of AXS-05 in TRD—topline results (investor presentation). March 30, 2020. https://axsometherapeuticsinc.gcs-web.com/static-files/ea125d9e-1b04-447f-80f3-f4cd7ad1f248. Accessed October 15, 2021. Permalink: https://perma.cc/QC7K-4BJQ.

15.

ADAPTIVE TRIALS

ADAPTIVE CLINICAL TRIALS are studies that rely on interim analyses of the data to refine the design or execution in mid-study, before the full trial is complete.[1] Most adaptive trials are based on the idea that under well-controlled circumstances, one can adjust the design of an experiment in response to collected data.[2] This is in contrast to more conventional approaches, in which one designs a trial, runs it to completion, and only at the end examines the data to test whether the findings supported or refuted the hypothesis.

As a simple illustration, a drug trial might be designed with a certain sample size to detect a certain magnitude of effect compared with the control. But if the results from the first few patients are much more positive or negative than expected, one might adjust one's prediction about the likely effect size and stop the trial after enrolling far fewer patients than originally planned.

When executed correctly, adaptive trials can significantly improve the efficiency of drug development.[3] Their main drawbacks are that they are more complicated to design and analyze, and they require additional operational capabilities to execute the study and ensure that interim looks at the data do not compromise its integrity. Adaptive trials require stringent information-handling protocols to ensure that investigators and patients remain blinded to the results from interim analyses, and any trial using adaptive approaches needs to transparently report its methods. The U.S. Food and Drug Administration (FDA) has issued draft guidance on how to design, execute, and analyze data from adaptive drug trials[4] that readers should review for additional context.

In this chapter, we discuss the main components of adaptive design that are seen in studies of novel therapeutics. We also cover more complex adaptive trials that use a master protocol to test combinations of multiple drugs or indications in the context of a single study.

Common components of adaptive trials

Several components of adaptive design have been put into practice with increasing frequency in studies of new drugs. Some that are most commonly encountered are described here:

- **Pre-planned stopping rules:** Interim analyses can include parameters for ending the study before all the patients have been analyzed if either efficacy is confirmed or it is futile to continue because the drug no longer has a chance of showing efficacy. This can allow a trial to reduce the time and number of patients needed to determine the benefit or lack thereof. This approach is typically used in Phase 3 studies intended for regulatory approval.

  Example: The PARADIGM-HF trial published in 2014 compared LCZ696 (Entresto; Novartis), a fixed-dose combination of a neprilysin inhibitor and an angiotensin receptor blocker, with the ACE inhibitor enalapril for the management of heart failure.[5] The study was halted early when the experimental drug demonstrated superior efficacy at the third pre-planned interim analysis.

- **Response-adaptive randomization:** This approach initially randomizes patients equally to one of several experimental arms, either different therapies or different doses of the same treatment. Later it preferentially assigns newly enrolled patients to study arms that appear to be yielding the most favorable outcomes. The effect of this method is to gain efficiency by minimizing the number of patients subjected to treatments that have shown preliminary evidence of lesser or no efficacy. This feature can be used in Phase 2 studies but would not be permitted in a trial intended for registration.

  Example: The ASTIN trial published in 2003 tested the ability of a novel neutrophil inhibitor (UK-279,276; Pfizer) to improve recovery from acute ischemic stroke.[6] The placebo-controlled trial included 15 dose levels of the drug, and efficacy was continuously reassessed to drive adaptive allocation to the best-performing doses. Testing so many different doses would have been impractical using standard trial designs. The study was negative, and Pfizer subsequently terminated its license for the drug.

- **Sample size re-estimation:** Some trials with interim analyses pre-specify an "intermediate zone" of efficacy at an interim time point that triggers an expansion of the study to take the smaller likely effect size into account. With a smaller effect size, more patients are needed to maintain statistical power, as discussed in more detail in Chapter 13. This approach allows investigators to choose an initial sample size based on an optimistic effect size but maintain the flexibility to test for a smaller but still clinically meaningful effect in the same trial. It is often combined with pre-planned stopping rules if the drug is convincingly shown to be either highly effective or grossly ineffective at the interim analysis. As with pre-planned stopping rules, this feature is typically seen in Phase 3 studies.

  A variation on this theme that is being explored is to incorporate sample size re-estimation into a seamless Phase 2/3 study (see below) as a so-called 2-in-1 adaptive Phase 2/3 trial.[7] In this scenario, the results of a Phase 2 study trigger either continuation into Phase 3, with or without adding more patients, or continuation as a Phase 2 trial. If the study continues into Phase 3, all patients from the Phase 2 portion are rolled over into Phase 3. The intention is to speed up development in comparison to the conventional approach after Phase 1 of running sequential, unlinked Phase 2 and Phase 3 trials while maintaining an appropriately high threshold for initiating a large Phase 3 program.

  Examples: Sunesis's Phase 3 VALOR trial tested the company's experimental drug vosaroxin versus placebo in acute myeloid leukemia.[8] An interim analysis in 2012 showed results in a pre-set "promising zone" that triggered an automatic, fixed upsizing of the study,[9] although the trial subsequently failed.[10] Separate from its impact on study execution, the design also formed the basis for a novel financing deal for the company, with funding dependent on the outcome of the interim analysis.[11]

INDUCE-3 was a Phase 2/3 trial that tested pembrolizumab (Keytruda; Merck) plus either an ICOS inhibitor (GSK3359609; GlaxoSmithKline) or placebo in head and neck cancer.[12] The Phase 2 portion failed to show improved progression-free survival (PFS) in 2021, and enrollment was halted.[13]

In another Phase 2/3 study, RELATIVITY-047, Bristol Myers Squibb tested the efficacy of its anti-PD-1 antibody nivolumab (Opdivo) plus its anti-LAG-3 antibody relatlimab in melanoma. The PFS portion of the study was deemed successful in 2021, and the trial continued into Phase 3 to assess overall survival (OS).[14]

- **Seamless design:** Many trials are designed to progress directly from one phase to the next instead of formally stopping the first and then beginning the next with a new set of patients. In the most common seamless Phase 1/2 or Phase 2/3 studies, an initial phase tests patients' responses to a range of doses. Then, one is selected to form the basis of a larger efficacy phase of the study, and the others are discontinued. This approach can be substantially more efficient than running two separate studies for dose finding and efficacy.

  Example: Merck's Phase 2/3 study published in 2015 of its 9-valent vaccine against human papilloma virus initially recruited patients into four arms. One received a 4-valent vaccine as an active control, and the others received different doses of the new agent.[15] After an interim analysis using surrogate markers of immune response, the middle dose of the 9-valent vaccine was chosen for the remainder of the study. The low- and high-dose arms were discontinued.

Master protocol trials: Baskets, umbrellas, and platforms

Basket, platform, and umbrella trials share in common the use of master protocols that allow one to more efficiently study multiple treatments or patient populations under the auspices of the same clinical study, without having to file formal amendments.[16,17,18] Beyond that, however, they are actually quite different from one another:

- **Basket:** The goal of a basket trial is to test a new therapy in multiple diseases at once. Many Phase 1 studies of new anti-cancer agents are essentially basket trials as they enroll patients with any advanced cancer, independent of type, to detect signals worthy of following up in subsequent studies. More recently, however, the term has mainly been applied to later-stage studies that include patients with the same molecular marker, like a particular gene mutation or amplification, regardless of the specific clinical classification of their disease. They are most common in oncology, where they are sometimes referred to as "marker-specific, histology-independent" studies because inclusion depends solely on the results of a molecular test, not the pathologic classification of the tumor. In this context, they are most often used when the molecular marker is relatively rare in each individual type of cancer, and it would not be practical to test the drug separately in the relevant subset of each tumor.

  The 2017 approval of Keytruda (pembrolizumab; Merck) in cancers with high microsatellite instability (MSI-H), independent of tumor type, was the first example of a basket trial leading to marketing authorization.[19] Its registrational data package included 90 patients with MSI-H colorectal cancer, and an additional 49 patients with various other MSI-H solid tumors.[20]

- **Umbrella:** Whereas a basket trial tests one drug in a mix of clinical indications, an umbrella trial enrolls patients with a single disease and assigns them to treatment arms with different experimental drugs. These studies can incorporate interim analyses to decide which arms should be continued or halted and can also adjust recruitment to favor promising arms with response-adaptive randomization.

  In cancer, umbrella trials typically assign patients to particular arms on the basis of specific biomarkers. The ongoing FOCUS4 study assigns patients with advanced colorectal cancer to different therapeutic arms depending on their molecular profiles.[21] The completed CheckMate 370 study in lung cancer, initially described in 2016, assigned patients to different combinations with nivolumab based on the cancer's histology and mutational status.[22] In both cases, each molecularly defined sub-trial includes a randomized control.

- **Platform:** Platform studies typically test a variety of potential therapies in a given indication, with the distinguishing feature that they allow for the addition of new arms as the trial progresses to test emerging experimental agents and hypotheses.[23] The ongoing BATTLE,[24] GBM AGILE,[25] and I-SPY2[26] studies are platform trials that explore potential therapies and predictive biomarkers of response in lung cancer, glioblastoma, and breast cancer, respectively. The HEALEY platform trial tests a suite of potential therapies for amyotrophic lateral sclerosis.[27] Like umbrella trials, these studies commonly incorporate interim analyses that allow for the termination of arms testing ineffective therapies.

  Most platform trials, including the ones cited, are executed by cooperative trial consortia, but there are uncommon examples of tests run by individual companies. Roche is sponsoring five MORPHEUS platform trials to explore multiple cancer immunotherapy combinations across various cancer indications and flexibly open and close treatment arms as data emerge and new therapeutic options become available.[28]

---

[1] Park JJ, Thorlund K, Mills EJ. Critical concepts in adaptive clinical trials. Clin Epidemiol. 2018 Mar 23;10:343–351. doi: 10.2147/CLEP.S156708. PMID: 29606891; PMCID: PMC5868584.

[2] Thorlund K, Haggstrom J, Park JJ, Mills EJ. Key design considerations for adaptive clinical trials: A primer for clinicians. BMJ. 2018 Mar 8;360:k698. doi: 10.1136/bmj.k698. PMID: 29519932; PMCID: PMC5842365.

[3] David FS, Bobulsky S, Schulz K, Patel N. Creating value with financially adaptive clinical trials. Nat Rev Drug Discov. 2015 Aug;14(8):523–524. doi: 10.1038/nrd4682. Epub 2015 Jul 24. PMID: 26205464.

[4] Adaptive designs for clinical trials of drugs and biologics: Guidance for industry. U.S. Food and Drug Administration. November 2019.

[5] McMurray JJ, Packer M, Desai AS, Gong J, Lefkowitz MP, Rizkala AR, Rouleau JL, Shi VC, Solomon SD, Swedberg K, Zile MR; PARADIGM-HF Investigators and Committees. Angiotensin-neprilysin inhibition versus enalapril in heart failure. N Engl J Med. 2014 Sep 11;371(11):993–1004. doi: 10.1056/NEJMoa1409077. Epub 2014 Aug 30. PMID: 25176015.

[6] Krams M, Lees KR, Hacke W, Grieve AP, Orgogozo JM, Ford GA; ASTIN Study Investigators. Acute stroke therapy by inhibition of neutrophils (ASTIN): An adaptive dose-response study of UK-279,276 in acute ischemic stroke. Stroke. 2003 Nov;34(11):2543–2548. doi: 10.1161/01.STR.0000092527.33910.89. Epub 2003 Oct 16. PMID: 14563972.

[7] Chen C, Anderson K, Mehrotra DV, Rubin EH, Tse A. A 2-in-1 adaptive Phase 2/3 design for expedited oncology drug development. Contemp Clin Trials. 2018 Jan;64:238–242. doi: 10.1016/j.cct.2017.09.006. Epub 2017 Sep 28. PMID: 28966137.

[8] Ravandi F, Ritchie EK, Sayar H, Lancet JE, Craig MD, Vey N, Strickland SA, Schiller GJ, Jabbour E, Erba HP, Pigneux A, Horst HA, Recher C, Klimek VM, Cortes J, Roboz GJ, Odenike O, Thomas X, Havelange V, Maertens J, Derigs HG, Heuser M, Damon L, Powell BL, Gaidano G, Carella AM, Wei A, Hogge D, Craig AR, Fox JA, Ward R, Smith JA, Acton G, Mehta C, Stuart RK, Kantarjian HM. Vosaroxin plus cytarabine versus placebo plus cytarabine in patients with first relapsed or refractory acute myeloid leukaemia (VALOR): A randomised, controlled, double-blind, multinational, Phase 3 study. Lancet Oncol. 2015 Sep;16(9):1025–1036. doi: 10.1016/S1470-2045(15)00201-6. Epub 2015 Jul 30. PMID: 26234174; PMCID: PMC4822512.

[9] Sunesis Pharmaceuticals to implement one-time sample size increase to Phase 3 VALOR trial in AML. Sunesis Pharmaceuticals press release. https://www.globenewswire.com/news-release/2012/09/11/490067/10004723/en/Sunesis-Pharmaceuticals-to-Implement-One-Time-Sample-Size-Increase-to-Phase-3-VALOR-Trial-in-AML.html. Accessed October 15, 2021. Permalink: https://perma.cc/M3JU-2R2W.

[10] Sunesis announces results from pivotal Phase 3 VALOR trial of vosaroxin and cytarabone in patients with first relapsed or refractory acute myeloid leukemia. Sunesis Pharmaceuticals press release. October 6, 2014. https://www.globenewswire.com/en/news-release/2014/10/06/670800/14761/en/Sunesis-Announces-Results-From-Pivotal-Phase-3-VALOR-Trial-of-Vosaroxin-and-Cytarabine-in-Patients-With-First-Relapsed-or-Refractory-Acute-Myeloid-Leukemia.html. Accessed October 15, 2021. Permalink: https://perma.cc/3ZLN-QDJH.

[11] Sunesis and Royalty Pharma announce $25 million vosaroxin agreement. Royalty Pharma press release. March 29, 2012. https://www.royaltypharma.com/news-releases/news-release-details/sunesis-and-royalty-pharma-announce-25-million-vosaroxin-royalty. Accessed October 15, 2021. Permalink: https://perma.cc/4DEF-J3X8.

[12] Hansen AR, Stanton TS, Hong MH, Cohen EEW, Mehanna HM, Chisamore MJ, Turner D, Yadavilli S, Bell K, Baccan C, Leone R, Chen H, Zhou H, Ellis CE, Ballas MS, Hoos A, Rischin D. INDUCE-3: A randomized, double-blind study of GSK3359609 (GSK609), an inducible T-cell co-stimulatory (ICOS) agonist antibody, plus pembrolizumab (PE) versus placebo (PL) plus PE for first-line treatment of PD-L1-positive recurrent/metastatic head and neck squamous cell carcinoma (R/M HNSCC). J Clin Oncol. 2020;38(suppl):TPS6591. doi: 10.1200/JCO.2020.38.15_suppl.TPS6591.

[13] Taylor NP. GSK stops Keytruda combo trials after ICOS drug falls short. FierceBiotech. April 15, 2021. https://www.fiercebiotech.com/biotech/gsk-stops-keytruda-combo-trials-after-icos-drug-falls-short. Accessed October 15, 2021.

[14] Storrs C. RELATIVITY-047 trial interim analysis: Combination of anti-LAG-3 antibody and nivolumab improves PFS in advanced melanoma. ASCO Daily News. June 6, 2021. https://dailynews.ascopubs.org/do/10.1200/ADN.21.200597/full/?cid=DM7797&bid=82513548. Accessed October 15, 2021. Permalink: https://perma.cc/3FSB-LBBQ.

[15] Joura EA, Giuliano AR, Iversen OE, Bouchard C, Mao C, Mehlsen J, Moreira ED Jr, Ngan Y, Petersen LK, Lazcano-Ponce E, Pitisuttithum P, Restrepo JA, Stuart G, Woelber L, Yang YC, Cuzick J, Garland SM, Huh W, Kjaer SK, Bautista OM, Chan IS, Chen J, Gesser R, Moeller E, Ritter M, Vuocolo S, Luxembourg A; Broad Spectrum HPV Vaccine Study. A 9-valent HPV vaccine against infection and intraepithelial neoplasia in women. N Engl J Med. 2015 Feb 19;372(8):711–723. doi: 10.1056/NEJMoa1405044. PMID: 25693011.

[16] Woodcock J, LaVange LM. Master protocols to study multiple therapies, multiple diseases, or both. N Engl J Med. 2017 Jul 6;377(1):62–70. doi: 10.1056/NEJMra1510062. PMID: 28679092.

[17] Park JJH, Siden E, Zoratti MJ, Dron L, Harari O, Singer J, Lester RT, Thorlund K, Mills EJ. Systematic review of basket trials, umbrella trials, and platform trials: A landscape analysis of master protocols. Trials. 2019 Sep 18;20(1):572. doi: 10.1186/s13063-019-3664-1. PMID: 31533793; PMCID: PMC6751792.

[18] West HJ. Novel precision medicine trial designs: Umbrellas and baskets. JAMA Oncol. 2017 Mar 1;3(3):423. doi: 10.1001/jamaoncol.2016.5299. PMID: 27930754.

[19] Cooper S, Bouvy JC, Baker L, Maignen F, Jonsson P, Clark P, Palmer S, Boysen M, Crabb N. How should we assess the clinical and cost effectiveness of histology independent cancer drugs? BMJ. 2020 Jan 2;368:l6435. doi: 10.1136/bmj.l6435. PMID: 31896539.

[20] FDA approves Merck's Keytruda (pembrolizumab) for adult and pediatric patients with unresectable or metastatic, microsatellite instability-high (MSI-H) or mismatch repair deficient (dMMR) solid tumors. Merck press release. May 25, 2017. https://www.merck.com/news/fda-approves-mercks-keytruda-pembrolizumab-for-adult-and-pediatric-patients-with-unresectable-or-metastatic-microsatellite-instability-high-msi-h-or-mismatch-repair-deficient-dmmr/. Accessed October 15, 2021. Permalink: https://perma.cc/848U-LZSU.

[21] FOCUS4 trial home page. MRC Clinical Trials Unit at University College London. http://www.focus4trial.org/. Updated June 27, 2019. Accessed October 15, 2021. Permalink: https://perma.cc/6BKA-MPQ7.

[22] Blumenschein G, Chandler J, Garon EB, Waterhouse D, Goldman JW, Gunuganti VK, Boccia R, Spigel D, Glaspy J, Berry DA, Korytowsky B, Zhu J, Lin WH, Bennett K, Reynolds C. PS01.59: CheckMate 370: A master protocol of Phase 1/2 studies of nivolumab as maintenance or first-LIne +/- standard-of-care therapies in advanced NSCLC. J Thoracic Oncol. 2016 Nov 1;11(11 suppl):S307. doi: 10.1016/j.jtho.2016.09.094.

[23] Park JJH, Harari O, Dron L, Lester RT, Thorlund K, Mills EJ. An overview of platform trials with a checklist for clinical readers. J Clin Epidemiol. 2020 Sep;125:1–8. doi: 10.1016/j.jclinepi.2020.04.025. Epub 2020 May 13. PMID: 32416336.

[24] Kim ES, Herbst RS, Wistuba II, Lee JJ, Blumenschein GR Jr, Tsao A, Stewart DJ, Hicks ME, Erasmus J Jr, Gupta S, Alden CM, Liu S, Tang X, Khuri FR, Tran HT, Johnson BE, Heymach JV, Mao L, Fossella F, Kies MS, Papadimitrakopoulou V, Davis SE, Lippman SM, Hong WK. The BATTLE trial: Personalizing therapy for lung cancer. Cancer Discov. 2011 Jun;1(1):44–53. doi: 10.1158/2159-8274.CD-10-0010. Epub 2011 Jun 1. PMID: 22586319; PMCID: PMC4211116.

[25] Alexander BM, Ba S, Berger MS, Berry DA, Cavenee WK, Chang SM, Cloughesy TF, Jiang T, Khasraw M, Li W, Mittman R, Poste GH, Wen PY, Yung WKA, Barker AD; GBM AGILE Network. Adaptive global innovative learning environment for glioblastoma: GBM AGILE. Clin Cancer Res. 2018 Feb 15;24(4):737–743. doi: 10.1158/1078-0432.CCR-17-0764. Epub 2017 Aug 16. PMID: 28814435.

[26] The I-SPY2 trial. Quantum Leap Healthcare Collaborative. https://www.ispytrials.org/i-spy-platform/i-spy2. Accessed October 15, 2021. Permalink: https://perma.cc/G3VT-88X3.

[27] Healy ALS platform trial. Massachusetts General Hospital. https://www.massgeneral.org/neurology/als/research/platform-trial. Accessed October 15, 2021. Permalink: https://perma.cc/S46Q-AXLC.

[28] Chau I, Haag GM, Rahma OE, Macarulla TM, McCune SL, Yardley DA, Solomon BJ, Johnson M, Vidal GA, Schmid P, Argiles G, Dimick K, Mahrus S, Abdullah H, He X, Sayyed P, Barak H, Bleul C, Cha E, Drakaki A. 1239TiP—MORPHEUS: A Phase Ib/II umbrella study platform evaluating the safety and efficacy of multiple cancer immunotherapy (CIT)-based combinations in different tumour types. Ann Oncol. 2018 Oct;29(suppl 8): viii439–viii440. doi: 10.1093/annonc/mdy288.110.

MISCELLANEA

Legal notes

All information in this book is provided for informational purposes only. Nothing in it should be construed as investment advice. Any opinions expressed or references to specific companies or products are not, and should not be taken as, recommendations or guarantees of any specific outcome. Do your own diligence and seek advice from your own financial or investment adviser.

Pharmagellan advises many pharmaceutical and biotech companies, medical device companies, and investors. Although none of these companies had any role in the content of this book, you should conservatively assume that any company mentioned is a past, current, or prospective client of the firm.

Looking ahead

We expect to publish updated versions of this book in the future. If you have suggestions for corrections, improvements, expansions, or additional examples, please let us know at info@pharmagellan.com. We'll reward you with our heartfelt thanks as well as a personal acknowledgment in the next edition if we incorporate your feedback.

ACKNOWLEDGMENTS

Several experts helped shepherd this book toward publication. Tracy Cutchlow provided strategic oversight of the entire project, and her enthusiastic support was indispensable during the most difficult writing periods. Alex Dmitrienko gave critical advice on how to accurately convey complex statistical concepts to a non-expert audience. Editor Bob Simison was invaluable in helping refine the structure and prose, notwithstanding a friendly disagreement over em dashes. The book's functional and stylish design is the skilled handiwork of Denise Clifton.

Many friends, colleagues, experts, and supporters generously gave their time and intellect to review the final complete draft or provided highly valuable input for specific sections. Special thanks to Mark Casey, Valay Desai, Donna Francher, Neil Lineberry, Brad Loncar, Andy Matthews, David Sable, Bryan Takasaki, Emily Walsh, Sam Wang, and Stan Ward. Their contributions were critical to the quality of the book, although none of these individuals bears any responsibility for the final product.

ABOUT THE AUTHOR

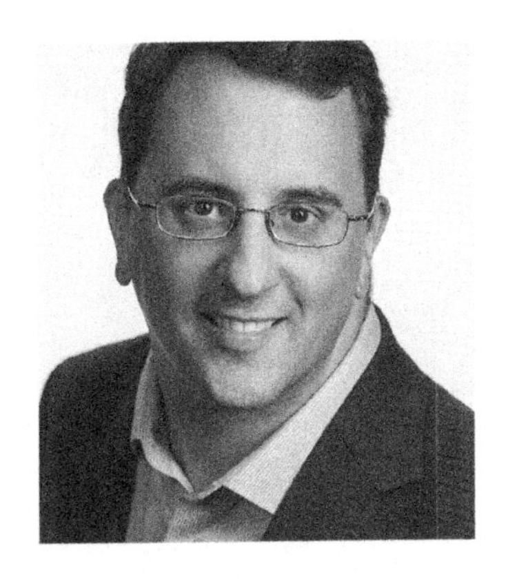

FRANK S. DAVID, MD, PHD, is the founder and managing director of Pharmagellan, a biotech advisory firm that focuses on maximizing the strategic and financial value of R&D. He has advised C-suite, commercial, R&D, business development, and investor clients across all major therapeutic areas and life sciences sectors. He previously co-led the Transactional Consulting practice at Leerink Partners (now SVB Leerink) and served as director of strategy in AstraZeneca's Oncology Innovative Medicines Unit. Besides his consulting activities, Frank is a member of the Harvard-MIT Center for Regulatory Science and an innovation strategist at the Brigham Research Institute of Mass General Brigham.

Frank's research and analyses on biopharma innovation, strategy, and policy have appeared in *Nature Reviews Drug Discovery*, *Health Affairs Blog*, *BMJ Open*, *JAMA Network Open*, and other venues. He is also the lead author of *The Pharmagellan Guide to Biotech Forecasting and Valuation.*

A board-certified pathologist, Frank began his career as a physician-scientist at Harvard Medical School and Brigham and Women's Hospital. He received his BS in molecular biophysics and biochemistry at Yale University and his MD and PhD degrees at Columbia University's College of Physicians and Surgeons, and completed his clinical training in anatomic pathology at Brigham and Women's Hospital.

For more information about Frank and Pharmagellan, please visit www.pharmagellan.com.

Made in the USA
Las Vegas, NV
28 February 2024